Eating Expectantly

A Practical and Tasty Approach to Prenatal Nutrition

by

Bridget Swinney M.S., R.D.

with

Tracey Anderson R.N., B.S., F.A.C.C.E.

 **Meadowbrook Press**
Distributed by Simon & Schuster
New York

Library of Congress Cataloging-in-Publication Data
Swinney, Bridget, 1960–
     Eating expectantly : a practical and tasty approach to prenatal nutrition / by Bridget Swinney,
     with Tracey Anderson.
          p. cm.
     Includes bibliographical references and index.
     ISBN 0-671-57048-X (Simon & Schuster). – ISBN 0-88166-257-7 (Meadowbrook Press)
     1. Pregnancy–Nutritional aspects. I. Anderson, Tracey, 1957–. II. Title.
     RG559.S949   1996
     618.2'4–dc20   96-21804
                                                                      CIP

ISBN # 0-88166-257-7
Simon & Schuster Ordering # 0-671-57048-X

Coordination Editor, Copyeditor: Liya Lev Oertel
Production Manager, Text Design: Amy Unger
Production Coordinator: Danielle Dickey
Cover Design: Linda Norton
Cover Art: Vicki Wehrman
Proofreader: Victoria Hall

Text © 1996 by Bridget Swinney, M.S., R.D.
The cover illustration © by Vicki Wehrman.

Published by Meadowbrook Press, 18318 Minnetonka Boulevard, Deephaven, MN 55391.

BOOK TRADE DISTRIBUTION by Simon & Schuster, a division of Simon and Schuster, Inc.,
1230 Avenue of the Americas, New York, NY 10020.

The contents of this book have been reviewed and checked for accuracy and appropriateness by professionals in the field of nutrition. However, the authors, editors, reviewers, and publisher disclaim all
responsibility arising from any adverse effects or results that occur or might occur as a result of the inap-
propriate application of any of the information contained in this book. If you have a question or concern
about any of the information in this book, consult your health care professional.

99 98 97 96   10 9 8 7 6 5 4 3 2 1

Printed in the United States of America.

Dedication

This book is dedicated to the memory of two people:
to my mother, Marjorie Morgan Swinney,
and to my friend and mentor, Robert Chambers.
It is also dedicated to the three special men
in my life, Frank, Nicolas, and Robert.

Acknowlededgments

I would like to mention the people who contributed to the making of this book.

Tracey Anderson, a registered nurse and a childbirth educator, who wrote the "Trimester Challenges" and "How Baby Is Growing" sections. Tracey lives in Colorado with her husband and two young daughters. In addition to having fun being a full-time mom, she can be found teaching a scripture-based Lamaze series that she developed. Tracey also enjoys teaching childbirth education classes to teens and low-income moms at the Life Support Center and speaking on parenting issues to Moms of Preschoolers and to other Mom support groups.

Michael Hambidge, M.D., Sc.D., who wrote the foreword for this book, is a professor of pediatrics at the University of Colorado Health Sciences Center in Denver. He is also the director of the Center for Human Nutrition at UCHSC. Dr. Hambidge served on the Subcommittee on Dietary Intake and Nutrient Supplements of the National Academy of Sciences that produced the report *Nutrition during Pregnancy*. Dr. Hambidge now serves on the Food and Nutrition Board of the National Research Council.

Thank you to the many people who reviewed chapters or the full manuscript of this book. Your input and expertise is greatly appreciated.

Roseanne Ainscough, R.D., C.D.E., Becky Bass, M.S., R.D., Barb Berntsen, Mike Bolger, Ph.D., Food and Drug Administration, Ruth Bowling, R.D., Jacquie Craig, M.S., R.D., C.D.E., Betty Crase, La Leche League International, Pat DeKam, L.V.N., Liz Diemand, M.S., R.D., Kathy Fraser, Maggie Garfield, R.N., C.C.E., Michael Hambidge, M.D., Kathy Glaaser, M.S., R.D., Anita Hall, R.N., Lori Hannah, R.D., Janis Harsila, R.D., Sue Havala, R.D., Betty Hopkins, Pat Kendall, Ph.D., R.D., Linda Kohlman, R.N., C.D.E., Shirley Lippincott, R.D., Ginny Murphy, R.D., Mary Peet, M.A., R.D., Marilyn Prost, R.N., M.S.N., Gordon Silver, M.D., FACOG, Julie Smith, R.D., Leslie Weddell, Gazette Telegraph food editor, and DeeAnn Whitmire, M.S., R.D.

In addition, thank you to the individuals and organizations that assisted directly or indirectly: Alan and Denise Fields, authors of *Baby Bargains*, the Vegetarian Resource Group, Michelle Kling with the March of Dimes, Connie Evers, Kate Ruddon with the American College of Obstetricians and Gynecologists, Virlie Walker with the Food and Drug Administration, Kathy Glaaser, Wendy Gregor, Diane Dimperio, Miriam Erick, Michelle Williams, Candi McNany, Wayne Valey, the staff of the Diabetes Education and Support Center, and to my other friends and colleagues who were supportive during this project. Also, thanks to my family: Gene, Kay, Colleen, Gary, Judy, and, especially Frank, Nicolas, and Robert for their endless patience.

Thanks to those who helped test recipes: Kathy Fraser, Melissa Wiles, Laura Albaum, Peggy Braley, Shawna Walker, and Peggy Connor; to my recipe tasters: Scott and Sean Fraser, Barb Berntsen, Sue Richardson, Kathy Irwin, Robert, Frank, and Nicolas; and to those who graciously allowed me to publish their recipes: Janet Boyd, Deborah Compton, Andy Hawk, Linda Hood, Cindy McKee, Margo Morrow, Brenda Ponichtera, The Colorado Dietetic Association, Norma Robinson, Debbie Russell, Ceacy Thatcher, and the Vegetarian Resource Group.

Also thanks to the American College of Obstetricians and Gynecologists, the Food and Drug Administration, the Center for Science in the Public Interest, and the Vegetarian Resource Group for allowing me to reprint their documents.

A special thanks to Bruce Lansky, who saw the same vision for *Eating Expectantly* that I did, to Liya Lev Oertel for her wonderful and understanding editorial direction, and to Amy Unger for the crisp typesetting.

Contents

Section I

Nutrition Needs, Challenges, and Eating Tips

Section II

Shopping, Cooking, and Eating Out

Foreword

Eating Expectantly has been written at a most favorable moment in our perception of the value of optimal maternal nutrition during pregnancy for both mother and baby. The report of the Food and Nutrition Board of the National Academy of Sciences, entitled "Nutrition during Pregnancy" (1990), has had a special role in focusing our attention on nutrition during pregnancy and has provided a thorough, up-to-date review of the major issues.

This report comes exactly twenty years after the Food and Nutrition Board's 1970 report on "Maternal Nutrition and the Course of Pregnancy." The convening of an expert committee, including leaders in the field of nutrition and obstetrics, to write this recent report reflects the substantial advances in our knowledge during the intervening years and the need to apply recent findings to prenatal care.

Of the many conclusions reached by this expert committee, two are especially noteworthy. The first of these is the recommendation for greater maternal weight gain than has been recommended previously. This is in recognition of the association between maternal weight gain during the second and third trimesters and the growth of the baby prior to birth. The specific recommendation is for a minimum weight gain of twenty-five pounds unless the mother is overweight prior to pregnancy. For mothers who are underweight prior to pregnancy, even greater weight gain is recommended.

The second recommendation of particular note is that routine micronutrient supplements be limited to a daily iron supplement of thirty milligrams. While other specific micronutrient supplements are advised in a number of special circumstances, a routine prenatal vitamin/mineral supplement is not recommended. Rather, the emphasis is on optimal diet as the source of micronutrients.

The reasons for this emphasis on the foods we eat reach far beyond the simple fact that we don't need to take supplements if we consume an adequate, nutritionally well-balanced diet. One important reason is the very real risk that we will consciously or subconsciously pay less attention to an optimal diet if we take our daily multivitamin/mineral pill. Shortcomings of the latter approach include the risk of nutrient/nutrient interactions and imbalances, an area about which we continue to learn more. "New" micronutrients that are important for human health continue to be "discovered." Not surprisingly, regular consumption of fruits and vegetables results in health benefits that are far greater than those of vitamin supplements.

One of the most important reasons for selecting an optimal diet rather than a substitute pill is the fact that prenatal vitamins are not prescribed until the first prenatal visit to an obstetrician. This visit usually does not occur prior to conception or prior to the critical early development of the baby during the first four to six weeks of pregnancy. We now know, for example, that an adequate intake of folate, one of the B vitamins, in the pre-conceptional period will greatly reduce the risk of spina bifida and other neural tube defects. To be protective, however, adequate folate must be taken prior to conception and in those first few weeks of pregnancy. The bottom-line message is that the emphasis on optimal diet is of the greatest importance to all women of childbearing age at all times–not only when pregnant–has been confirmed.

I commend Bridget Swinney for her timely and informative guide. You should get your copy now and not wait until you are pregnant.
Michael Hambidge, M.D., Sc.D., Professor of Pediatrics, Director of the Center for Human Nutrition, University of Colorado Health Sciences Center.

Introduction
Why You Need this Book!

When a woman became pregnant years go, she didn't change her life that much. The health of the baby was thought to depend mostly on chance and the placenta was thought to protect the fetus from all dangerous substances. Things are different today. We have an abundance of knowledge about pregnancy and nutrition, and the amount of research on the subject grows daily. Now we know that the placenta only acts as a "screen" and many toxic substances can still get through to the baby. So mom is the true "gatekeeper."

You will probably find pregnancy to be much more "high tech" than it was as recently as ten years ago. But even with all the diagnostic tests and fancy equipment now available, good nutrition is still the most important factor in giving your baby a healthy start in life.

Eating Expectantly puts nutrition and health during pregnancy into perspective for the nineties. It gives you answers to questions you may want to ask, but are not quite sure whom to ask. This book is based on a realistic and practical approach to eating, instead of relying on theoretical advice that doesn't work in the "real world."

And, *Eating Expectantly* not only gives you guidance on what to eat, it carries through with over one hundred delicious recipes developed specifically for the stages of pregnancy. In addition, it has over one hundred and fifty menus to meet different needs; you'll find Don't Feel Like Cooking Menus, Meals in Minutes, I Could Cook All Day Menus, Healthiest Fast-Food Menus, and Company's Coming! Menus.

If you are vegetarian or trying to eat meatless meals more often, you'll find the vegetarian chapter helpful. If you experience one of the unexpected conditions of pregnancy, such as gestational diabetes, high blood pressure, or bed rest, *Eating Expectantly* will guide you through by explaining the facts and providing tips for eating and food preparation.

If you're not pregnant yet, you will benefit even more from this book. You'll know how your diet should be and you'll know what to expect during pregnancy. I suggest that you read the whole book, skipping the chapter on high-risk pregnancies (unless you already have a chronic disease such as diabetes). Then, start using the menus and recipes now! This will get you used to eating right and the healthy eating will be easy to keep up when you're pregnant. Just keep in mind that you won't need to increase your calories until you are pregnant.

Eating Expectantly answers the following questions—and more:

- What can I do before I get pregnant to help ensure I have a healthy baby?
- Will pesticides and preservatives in foods affect my baby?
- What if I can't drink milk—do I really need a lot of calcium?
- I'm vegetarian. How can I meet my nutrient needs?
- Help! I was just diagnosed with gestational diabetes; what do I do?
- Should I take a vitamin supplement?
- How much weight should I gain?
- How is my current diet?
- Do I need to go on a low-salt diet if I start to have high blood pressure?
- How can I eat right when I'm on bed rest?
- I don't feel like cooking. Help!
- What are the best fast-food and restaurant choices for me while I'm pregnant?
- Should I exercise?

This book uses knowledge and experience gathered from hundreds of pregnant women and mothers, including myself. I've also collected answers from scientific experts; those who do nutrition research and work with pregnant and breast-feeding women daily.

If you have any questions or concerns about what to eat, how much to eat, or how to practice good nutrition–before, during, or after your preg-nancy–this book is a must! I hope you enjoy reading it as much as I enjoyed writing it. More importantly, I hope that by reading and following the advice in *Eating Expectantly,* you can give your baby and yourself the gift of good nutrition and good health!

Section I

Nutrition Needs, Challenges, and Eating Tips

Contemplating Pregnancy

Why Prepregnancy Planning Is Best

Thinking about having a baby? If you are thinking about starting or adding to your family and are seeking information about pregnancy, you're making a smart move! In addition to reading about pregnancy on your own, you may also want to visit with your health care provider when you decide you'd like to become pregnant. Prepregnancy counseling is recommended for several reasons:

1. You have time to change the lifestyle habits that may affect your pregnancy: smoking, drinking, caffeine intake, and eating habits.

2. You have time to start eating a well-balanced diet, build up nutrient stores, start exercising regularly, and lose or gain weight, if needed.

3. You can learn about fetal development and understand the importance of changing your habits before the first weeks of pregnancy. During the first weeks after conception much of the critical development takes place, and during this time the effects of poor diet or lifestyle habits can damage the fetus the most. Most of the brain cell division occurs when most women don't know they're pregnant.

4. If you have any chronic medical conditions, such as high blood pressure, diabetes, or kidney disease, getting them under control before you become pregnant is vital to having the healthiest baby possible!

5. If you have had an unsuccessful pregnancy, or have delivered a baby with birth defects, you can find out how to improve the outcome of your next pregnancy and the health of your next baby.

6. If this is your first pregnancy but you have a history of genetic defects in your family, or you have a genetic condition that you could

pass on to your children, you will have time to receive genetic counseling.

Who Should Have Genetic Counseling?

According to the March of Dimes, anyone who has unanswered questions about diseases in the family or who is concerned about being at increased risk of having a child with a birth defect or inherited disorder should consider genetic counseling. It is also suitable for:

Couples who:

- already have a child with mental retardation, an inherited disorder, or a birth defect.
- have or are concerned that they might have an inherited disorder or birth defect.
- have an infant who has a genetic disease diagnosed by routine newborn screening.
- are concerned that their job, lifestyle, or medical history may pose a risk to pregnancy, including exposure to radiation, medications, chemicals, infections, or drugs.

- would like testing or more information about genetic defects that occur frequently in their ethnic group (such as Tay-Sach, thalassemia, and sickle-cell anemia).
- are first cousins or other close blood relatives.

Women who:

- will be thirty-four years or older at the time of pregnancy.
- have had two or more miscarriages or babies who died in infancy.
- based on tests such as ultrasound or alphafetoprotein, have been told that their pregnancy may be at increased risk for complications or birth defects.

If you would like more information on genetic counseling and other helpful information for pregnancy, contact your local chapter of the March of Dimes Birth Defects Foundation.

The Importance of Good Nutrition before Pregnancy

The following examples illustrate the importance of good nutrition and early prenatal care for a healthy pregnancy:

- A landmark study done in several countries found that a B vitamin called folacin (also called folate and folic acid) could prevent up to 72 percent of such neural tube defects as spina bifida.[1] The U.S. Public Health Service now recommends that all women of childbearing age who are capable of becoming pregnant should consume 400 micrograms of folic acid per day.[2] To reduce your risk for birth defects, you should consider a multivitamin containing folic acid.[3] Women who have had a child with a neural tube defect are much more likely to have another child with the same problem; those women should talk to their health care provider about a larger supplement of folic acid. (See page 27 for the key nutrients of pregnancy, including folacin.)
- According to certain studies, your child's health as an adult could be affected by your eating habits during pregnancy. Recent research shows that babies who are born small for gestational age and are small during the first year have a higher risk later in life for insulin resistance (which could lead to diabetes), elevated

triglycerides, and lower HDL cholesterol levels, as well as a higher risk for heart disease.[4]

• Another study showed that women's lower weight gain between fifteen and thirty-five weeks gestation was related to higher blood pressure when their child was ten to twelve years old. A strong association also exists between the mothers' thin triceps skinfold (indicating impaired nutritional status) and increased blood pressure in their child when the child is ten to twelve years old.[5]

• Women with preexisting diabetes are several times more likely to have a baby with birth defects than the nondiabetic women. This fact may be related to glucose control before conception and in the very early weeks of pregnancy.[6] However, this increased risk can be reduced significantly with good control of blood sugars and early prenatal counseling.

• Recent research shows that iron and folic acid intake is related to increased infant body weight and length—another reason to make sure your diet is adequate during pregnancy.[7]

• Anyone who is unknowingly pregnant might drink alcohol or take medication that could harm the fetus. Excessive alcohol intake can cause birth defects and long-lasting problems such as mental and physical retardation, hyperactivity, and smaller birth weights. Because researchers aren't sure what small amounts of alcohol could do to the fetus, the safest recommendation is to avoid alcohol during pregnancy and the prepregnancy period.

• According to researcher Michael Crawford, of the Institute of Brain Chemistry and Human Nutrition in London, "The individual responsibility for the development of the brain rests with the mother. Some 70 percent of the total number of brain cells to last an individual's lifetime have divided before birth." He also proposes that developmental disorders common to low-birth-weight infants (such as mental retardation, cerebral palsy, and blindness) are the result of poor maternal nutrition before and during the first trimester.[8]

• Brain growth continues until the age of two. The continued importance of essential fats in the infant's diet gives a critical role to breast milk as the best source of nutrition; presently, formula is not fortified with the same types of essential fats found in breast milk.

The main trend for eating today is definitely "low fat". However, the type of fat necessary for brain development comes from vegetable fat, so make sure you have at least several teaspoons per day of vegetable oil such as canola oil. Other sources of vegetable fat include nuts, seeds, wheat germ, olives, and avocado. Also remember that fat can be an important calorie source during pregnancy if you are not able to eat enough calories from other types of foods.

• Evidence shows that smoking during pregnancy is not only related to lower birth rate, but may also affect neurological development.[9] Also, smoking by either parent during pregnancy is related to a higher risk of childhood cancer for the child.[10]

• In general, women may not get enough of some vitamins and minerals when they aren't pregnant. The Total Diet Study found that women aged twenty-five to thirty ate less than 75 percent of the RDA for calcium, magnesium, and iron, and only 80 percent of the RDA for zinc.[11] A 1987

The Prepregnancy Quiz

The following quiz will help you and your partner know if your diet and lifestyle habits are ready for pregnancy. Circle "yes" or "no"; then follow the directions for scoring on the next page.

1. I eat at least three servings of fruit and three servings of vegetables on most days. **Yes** **No**

2. I eat a vitamin C-rich food daily (examples include citrus fruit or juice, berries, papaya, mango, pineapple, melon, broccoli, cauliflower, tomato, and vegetable juice). **Yes** **No**

3. I eat a wide variety of foods from all food groups, including many types of protein foods. **Yes** **No**

4. I do some form of aerobic exercise at least twice each week. **Yes** **No**

5. I don't smoke and avoid secondhand smoke. **Yes** **No**

6. I consume one or fewer caffeinated beverages a day. **Yes** **No**

7. I avoid taking drugs of any kind: prescription, over-the-counter, herbal preparations, or "street drugs." **Yes** **No**

8. I am currently at or close to my desirable body weight. **Yes** **No**

9. I avoid exposure to radiation, pesticides, herbicides, solvents, PCBs, and other chemicals. **Yes** **No**

10. I limit my consumption of shark, swordfish, or lake whitefish to once a month or less. **Yes** **No**

11. I usually eat three balanced meals a day and watch my saturated fat intake. **Yes** **No**

12. I eat three servings of calcium-rich foods daily (examples include milk, yogurt, cheese, high-calcium vegetables, tofu made with calcium, and juice fortified with calcium). **Yes** **No**

13. I take a multivitamin/mineral supplement containing 400 micrograms of folic acid daily. **Yes** **No**

14. I avoid taking any single vitamin supplements (such as Vitamin A or C) without my physician's approval. **Yes** **No**

15. I avoid drinking alcohol. **Yes** **No**

16. I avoid eating raw milk, eggs, shellfish, or foods that are made with these (examples include caesar salad dressing, mousse with uncooked egg, sushi). **Yes** **No**

17. I eat three servings of whole-grain breads, cereals, or other whole-grain products on most days. **Yes** **No**

The Prepregnancy Quiz

18. I live a moderately paced lifestyle, get eight hours of sleep most nights, and feel generally happy. **Yes** **No**

19. I have not followed any severe diets or had an eating disorder in the last three months. **Yes** **No**

20. I am a vegetarian who eats no animal products, though I do take a vitamin B_{12} and calcium supplement, if warranted and discussed with my physician. **Yes** **No**

21. I have made a visit to my physician and discussed a future pregnancy. **Yes** **No**

How did you do?

Count the number of "Yes" answers and see how you scored below.

17-21: Congratulations! Your body is ready for pregnancy!

13-16: You're doing pretty well; you have just a few things to work on to have the healthiest pregnancy possible.

9-12: Start working; you may need a few months to make the changes necessary to have the healthiest pregnancy possible.

9 or less: Oops! Your lifestyle may need an overhaul! Talk to your health care provider before beginning a pregnancy.

report showed that one out of four women between the ages of twenty-five and thirty-four skipped breakfast regularly. Skipping a meal can significantly cut down on needed nutrients.[12] One out of five women has no iron reserves. Many women eat only half the recommended amount of calcium.[13] Thus, women may be starting their pregnancy with a depleted supply of many nutrients that play vital roles in the development of the fetus.

• The death rate seems to be higher for babies of overweight women than for babies of women at their ideal weight, primarily due to an increase in premature deliveries.[14] Also, two studies have recently shown that obese women are two to four times more likely to have a baby with a neural tube defect than women who are not significantly overweight.[15,16] The solution? If you are overweight, and especially if you are 20 percent or more over your ideal

weight, lose weight before you conceive. (See the resources section for weight control resources.)

A few words of advice: make sure that you don't become pregnant while you are on a weight loss diet–your intake of certain vitamins may not be enough for the important stages of early development. Taking a vitamin/mineral supplement during the weight loss period is advisable. (See page 33.)

Eating at least the number of servings of each food listed in the Before-Baby Diet will help you become a healthy "future mom." As soon as you find out you're pregnant, you can switch over to the Eating Expectantly Diet on page 44. The two diets are not very different, so the transition will be easy. (See Chapter Eleven, Stocking the Pregnant Kitchen, if you're wondering how to begin to eat healthy.)

▼

A Few Words about Infertility

Infertility, defined as not conceiving after one year of unprotected intercourse, affects more than five million women and their partners. Some of these numbers may be a result of delaying pregnancy. Generally, the older we are, the longer we need to conceive. Seeking assistance for infertility can be an emotionally charged venture, to say the least.

Nutrition can and does play a role in fertility. If you are seeking help for infertility, please make sure you are not underweight. If you are underweight when you become pregnant, your chances of having a low-birth-weight infant are much higher. Some fertility treatments greatly increase your chances of having twins or more and this

further increases your chance of having low-birth-weight infants.

Here is an overview of some of the effects body weight, nutrition, and activity levels have on fertility.

Body Weight

The body appears to be very protective of the unborn baby. Conceiving is more difficult if you are underweight or overweight. According to one estimate, up to 12 percent of infertility associated with ovulatory dysfunction is a result of being excessively underweight or excessively overweight.[17]

In the natural order of things, this makes sense because under- and overweight women have a higher risk of having a low-birth-weight or preterm baby. Body fat seems to be the synchronizing factor (or the conductor, if you will) for the harmonious hormonal symphony that must take place for a pregnancy to occur and be carried to term.

In fact, the first period of teens who are very lean athletes is often delayed for years until their body fat increases. In those cases, the body creates a delay that will not allow pregnancy to occur until the amount of body fat necessary to sustain a pregnancy is present.

Reductions in body fat in men also affect their sperm produc-

tion, which could be a cause of infertility.

Having too much body fat can also affect fertility. Part of the body's estrogen is made in the body fat of the breasts and abdomen. Excess body fat can affect the amount and types of circulating hormones that affect fertility.[18]

Nutrition

Caffeine

The results of studies about the effects of caffeine on fertility are conflicting. However, a link does exist between caffeine intake and increased risk of miscarriage.[19] If you are having trouble conceiving, staying away from caffeine is a good idea. (See page 38 for caffeine content of foods.)

Vegetarian Diet

A meatless eating plan can be very healthy. (See Chapter Six for more information.) However, one study showed that a low-calorie vegetarian weight loss diet caused seven out of nine women in the study to stop ovulating. The same study related an abrupt switch to a vegetarian diet to lack of ovulation.[20] If you are vegetarian and are having trouble conceiving, take a very close look at your diet to make sure you are not lacking any nutrients. Compare your diet to the recommended diet in Chapter Six. You may also want to take a multivitamin supplement.

Eating Disorders

Amenorrhea (lack of menstrual periods) is a symptom of anorexia nervosa. Amenorrhea and oligomenorrhea (decreased menses) often occur in women with anorexia nervosa and are also seen in about 50 percent of women with bulimia. Reproductive hormones are also reduced in women who maintain a lower than normal body weight.[21] An increase in body weight and a balanced food intake will help restore normal reproductive functions.

If you have an eating disorder, you should try to resolve the underlying causes of the disorder for a permanent recovery. The eating habits and health problems associated with some eating disorders can put your baby at risk for birth defects, low birth weight or prematurity. So, it is best to normalize your eating habits and make sure you are not below your ideal body weight prior to pregnancy.[22] Comprehensive programs that involve a psychologist, physician, and dietitian are most helpful.

Depleted Iron Stores

Women whose depleted iron stores were supplemented with iron and vitamin C had increased chances of conception;[23]

another good reason to make sure your diet is good quality and has ample amounts of iron from food or a supplement.

Alcohol

If you are trying to conceive, you should stay away from alcohol. Research shows that, besides being dangerous to the fetus, excessive alcohol intake can also have an effect on fertility in women and men. Alcohol is a male reproductive tract toxin, and the degree of impairment varies with the amount of alcohol ingested and the duration of drinking.[24]

Vitamin C

Two different studies demonstrated that vitamin C supplements of 200 milligrams improved fertility in men, in both heavy smokers as well as in nonsmokers.[25,26] Vitamin C may also

The Before-Baby Diet	
Food	Daily Servings
Grains/Starches	6 or more
Fruits	3 or more
Vegetables	3 or more
Be sure to include at least 1 vitamin C- and 1 vitamin A-rich fruit or vegetable daily.	
Protein or equivalent	4–6 ounces
Dairy or calcium-rich foods	3 or more

protect against DNA damage to sperm—all the more reason to make sure your partner also follows the Before-Baby Diet! He may especially want to increase intake of vitamin C foods or take a supplement.

Zinc

Zinc is important in the male and female reproductive systems. A zinc deficiency in men is related to decreased sperm count, decreased sperm motility, and decreased serum testosterone (a sex hormone) levels.[27] All of these factors could have a large impact on fertility. (See page 31 for food sources of zinc.)

Selenium

Inadequate and excess selenium are both related to male fertility. To make sure both partners' intake of selenium is adequate, eat plenty of seafood and whole grains.

Too Many Carrots

Women who ate no red meat and who supplemented their diet of mostly vegetables and salads with up to a pound of carrots a day had stopped ovulating. After reducing carrot intake, most women improved menstrual function, which points to the conclusion that their infertility problem could be completely diet related.[28] Although this information is speculative, it does draw attention to the important concept of moderation!

Activity Level

Women involved in sports on a competitive level sometimes reduce their body fat level so low that they stop menstruating. Strenuous exercise and decreased levels of body weight and body fat are related to reproductive problems, including infertility. Regular exercise is important for good health. However, if you take exercise to the extreme and are having trouble conceiving, you may have to slow down!

▼

Keys for Planning a Healthy Pregnancy

Several months before you become pregnant, both you and your partner should follow the advice below. Although men are often left out of the prepregnancy planning stage, they must also take good care of themselves since sperm is also affected by diet and the environment.

▶ **Don't drink alcohol or take drugs.**

That includes aspirin! If you take a prescription medication, ask your doctor if it is safe to take during pregnancy. If your medicine is not safe, your doctor can possibly substitute a medication that is. Find out from your health care provider which over-the-counter medications are safe during pregnancy, especially during the first trimester.

▶ **Make a prepregnancy visit to your health care provider.**

At this time you can discuss your current health as well as your immunity to diseases such as chicken pox and rubella. These diseases are fairly harmless most of the time, but if you contract them during pregnancy, they could cause serious problems to the fetus. You may want to get immunized.

▶ **Both you and your partner should follow the Before-Baby Diet.**

Since one cycle of sperm production takes ten weeks, you should both follow the diet for three months prior to pregnancy.[29] When couples discuss pregnancy, they often ignore the father's diet. However, current research now shows that the father's diet can affect his sperm and, ultimately, the fetus. A joint project at U.C. Berkeley and USDA's Western Human Nutrition Research Center have linked low dietary intakes of vitamin C to increased genetic damage in sperm, which presumably translates into a higher risk of birth defects and genetic disease.[30] (See page 31 for good food sources of vitamin C.)

Study leader Dr. Bruce Ames says, "All we know now is that if your dietary intake of vitamin C gets below a certain level—about 60 milligrams per day, which is the Recommended Daily Allowance—you get into trouble. This strongly indicates that vitamin C protects against DNA damage."

▶ **Keep your environment safe.**

For both partners, this means avoiding exposure to pesticides and herbicides, radiation (X-rays), fumes from paint, extermination chemicals, and glue. Avoid exposure to lead, which can cause premature birth, brain damage, learning disabilities, and kidney and liver damage. Up to forty million people have too much lead in their drinking water.[31] (See page 36 for the important details.)

If you smoke, try to quit or reduce your amount. Avoid or limit exposure to secondhand smoke.

▶ **Avoid or limit caffeine.**

The pendulum seems to swing back and forth on caffeine and its effects on fertility and other reproductive issues. Low birth weight and birth defects don't seem to be related to caffeine consumption. On the other hand, caffeine intake may be linked to infertility and miscarriage. Common sense says to avoid caffeine or limit to one serving a day.

▶ **Take a multivitamin supplement containing 400 micrograms of folic acid and no more than 100 percent of the RDA of other nutrients...**

...recommends the March of Dimes. The main reason is to prevent neural tube defects such as spina bifida. Some evidence shows that vitamin supplementation may also prevent other birth defects, such as heart and limb defects and oral cleft problems. On the other hand, avoid taking supplements of individual vitamins, especially vitamin A; as mentioned earlier, extreme doses of certain vitamins may have unwanted results.

▶ **Reduce stress or learn how to cope with it effectively.**

Extreme stress is thought to affect fertility. However, stress is hard to measure since all of us perceive it differently. Exercise is a good stress reliever.

▶ **Avoid exposure to high temperatures.**

For example, sperm production is reduced in men who weld inside storage tanks, who drive a truck and literally sit on a "hot seat" for hours, and even in those who regularly sit in a hot tub. Tight briefs or pants can also reduce sperm production. However, most experts believe that to have a real effect on fertility, a man's exposure to high temperatures would have to be continuous over a long period of time.[32]

Also, women who take long hot baths or sit in the hot tub or sauna can actually damage the embryo's nervous system during the first thirty days after conception.

▶ **Analyze your workplace for reproductive hazards.**

Many occupations use chemicals or energy that are dangerous to future children. Much controversy surrounded a lawsuit that addressed removing women from jobs involving exposure to lead because of the reproductive hazard. However, your baby or your ability to become pregnant could be affected by what you and your partner are exposed to at the workplace (and other places too). One study showed that the wives of men exposed to ethylene oxide, rubber chemicals, solvents used in refineries, and solvents used in the manufacturing of rubber products had increased risk of miscarriage.[33] Other known hazards include radiation, exposure to lead, solvents, paints, anesthetic gases, glues, exposure to copper, arsenic and cadmium, solder fumes, polyvinyl chloride, aerosol sprays, and dyes.[34]

If you are exposed to any of the above or any other chemicals of which you are unsure, ask your supervisor about the Material Safety Data Sheets. For more information, contact the National Institute for Occupational Safety and Health (in the phone book under Government Agencies), which can refer you to government agencies about specific health concerns. Or contact the Women's Occupational Health Resource Center, Columbia University School of Public Health, 21 Audubon Avenue, New York, NY 10032.

For a copy of *Art Material Safety Alert,* send a postcard to CSPC, Washington, D.C. 20207.

▶ **Prevent toxoplasmosis.**

Babies exposed to the toxoplasmosis parasite (toxoplasma gondii) before birth may be born with mental retardation and blindness. Toxoplasmosis is ex-

Best Sources of Folate

The RDA for folate is 400 micrograms during pregnancy; 280 micrograms for breastfeeding.

Food	Serving Sizes	Folate in micrograms*
Chicken liver	3.5 ounces	763
Veal liver	3.5 ounces	752
Chicken giblets	3.5 ounces	372
Lentils	1 cup	358
Cowpeas	1 cup	356
Sunflower seeds	1 cup	317
Pinto beans	1 cup	294
Baked beans, homemade	1 cup	256
Navy beans	1 cup	255
Asparagus	1 cup	242
Spinach, frozen, drained	1 cup	220
Beef liver	3.5 ounces	217
Refried beans	1 cup	211
Turnip greens	1 cup	171
Pork liver	3.5 ounces	163
Black bean soup	1 cup	158
Hummus	1 cup	146
Split peas	1 cup	127
Mixed nuts	1 cup	118
Creamed corn	1 cup	115
Orange juice	1 cup	109
Trail mix	1 cup	107
Broccoli, frozen	1 cup	104
Peas, frozen	1 cup	94
Tempeh	1 cup	86
Boysenberries	1 cup	84
Taco Bell Bean Tostada	1	75
Taco Bell Bean Burrito	1	73
Iceberg lettuce	¼ head	73
Beets	1 cup	73
Arby's Ham and Cheese Sandwich	1	71
Artichoke	1	61
Wakame (seaweed)	1 ounce	55
Papaya	1 cup	53
Kombu (seaweed)	1 ounce	51
Vegetable juice	1 cup	51
Blackberries	1 cup	49
Melon balls	1 cup	44

*Numbers are rounded to nearest whole number; numbers are for cooked foods, as applicable.

Source: Nutritionist III Nutrition Software.

creted in cat feces and is also found in raw meats. So avoid changing the cat litter box, keep cats away from eating and food preparation areas, and wear gloves while gardening. Toxoplasmosis can also be transmitted through uncooked or undercooked meat and unwashed fruits and vegetables.[35] So, don't feed your cats raw meat, and cook meats, especially lamb and pork, to a temperature of 160 degrees throughout.

Focus on Folate

Folate, also called folic acid or folacin, is a B vitamin that is very important during pregnancy; it is needed for cell division and for blood cells. Folacin is water soluble and can be destroyed in cooking. Thus, when you cook your vegetables, cook in as little water as possible for as short a time as possible.

People who may need more folacin in their diet are those who have been on such medications as anticonvulsants and some birth control pills. The U.S. Public Health Service now recommends that all women of childbearing age who are capable of becoming pregnant should consume 400 micrograms of folic acid per day.[36] If you have had a child with a neural tube defect, you will need to take much higher doses—check with your health care provider.

? Questions You May Have

Q: I drink about four or more cups of coffee every day. Any advice on cutting down?

A: Caffeine is a stimulant, and as most people know, it is habit forming. In addition, caffeine is a diuretic: it causes your body to lose fluid, and during pregnancy your need for fluid increases. Substances found in coffee and tea also interfere with the absorption of iron. All of the above are good reasons for reducing coffee, caffeinated soda, and tea intake. Cut down gradually to avoid such side effects as headaches. You may want to substitute other, lower caffeine, drinks such as "half the caffeine" coffee, decaffeinated tea or coffee, or hot cocoa.

Q: Help! I'm a junk food junkie! I eat fast food every day and actually crave it. How can I improve my diet?

A: Fast food can fit into a balanced diet if done right. However, if you eat fast food often

(and depending on your choices), you are likely to have decreased intakes of vitamin A, vitamin B_6, vitamin C, and calcium, which are all important nutrients during pregnancy.[37] The other problem is that most restaurant meals are higher in fat and calories than those eaten at home.

Try switching to healthier choices, such as bean burritos, grilled chicken sandwiches, or salads with low-fat meats. Add a salad bar or side salad with lots of fruits and vegetables, drink low-fat or skim milk with your meal, and bring along a fruit for dessert. Be sure to eat more fruits, vegetables, and whole grains at other meals to reach your totals. (See page 206 for more information and suggested menus from fast-food restaurants.)

Q: I've been taking birth control pills for five years. Is there anything special I should do before I become pregnant?

A: Physicians usually recommend that you have at least two periods "off the pill" to make sure your hormone levels are back to normal. However, the American College of Obstetricians and Gynecologists no longer has a recommendation regarding this. They state, "Using birth control pills before you become pregnant does not cause birth defects,

no matter how close to conception you stop using them."[38] However, your periods may be irregular at first, which makes it difficult to determine your fertile times, or to calculate your due date when you become pregnant. If you had painful or heavy periods before you started taking the pill, you may experience those types of menstrual cycles again.

Nutritionally, you should make sure your diet is better than average, since any medication taken over a long period of time can affect your nutritional status. Oral contraceptives can increase your need for B vitamins, including folacin. If you've had a poor diet over the past six months, you might consider a vitamin/mineral supplement.

Q: I am diabetic and always thought trying to have a baby would be dangerous, but I hear things are different now.

A: You're right! The important thing is for your diabetes to be under control before you get pregnant because high blood sugar could cause birth defects in the first few weeks of pregnancy. Also, during pregnancy your insulin needs will change often and you will need close monitoring. Visit your primary physician and talk about your plan. Your physician will probably refer you to an obstetrician who specializes in taking care of diabetic moms. You may also want to see an eye doctor. (See page 98 for more advice for diabetic moms-to-be.)

Q: I'm thirty-eight and my biological clock just went off. Anything I can do before pregnancy to ensure the health of my baby?

A: Make a visit to your health care provider to get a checkup and a "bill of good health." Older women who are in good health and have early and regular prenatal care can have perfectly healthy babies. Preparing for your pregnancy and getting into some good lifestyle habits can start your baby out on the right foot! However, older moms do have some increased risks of a few problems during pregnancy, mostly because as we get older, some conditions are more common, such as diabetes and high blood pressure. (See page 124 for more information.)

Q: Before I realized I was pregnant, I drank too much at a party; what shall I do?

A: Your situation is not uncommon since many pregnancies are a "surprise." The best thing to do is to stay calm; don't panic. Start right now following all the above advice and try not to think about what you've done in the past. Do discuss your concerns with your health care provider, who will help you put them in perspective.

CHAPTER TWO

The Knowledgeable Pregnancy

What Every Woman Needs to Know

So you're pregnant—or planning to be. Congratulations! You are about to begin the most exhilarating, exhausting, challenging, and special time of your life. No doubt you will find yourself daydreaming in the months to come…what will my baby look like?…how will I be as a first-time (or second- or third-time) mom?…what will he or she grow up to be—will he discover the cure to cancer, or will she be the first woman president? But your thoughts will inevitably drift back to one important question…will my baby be healthy?

Fortunately, the answer to that question mostly depends on you. Although genetics and pure chance can affect your baby's health, taking good care of yourself can give your baby the best odds of being born healthy.

If you are just considering pregnancy, you are one step ahead of the game and have time to get your body and personal habits into great shape. (See Chapter One, Contemplating Pregnancy.) Pre-conception counseling seems to be the new buzz word among hopeful moms-to-be, and with good reason. Your health care provider can give you advice on eating, exercise, alcohol, and so on. If you are diabetic, or have another medical condition, this type of counseling is an especially good idea.

As a pregnant or soon-to-be-pregnant woman, you have a unique opportunity to make your health the best it can be. The good habits you start now can be with you and your family for life—it's up to you! In fact, exciting research shows that your diet and nutritional status before and during pregnancy and your baby's birth weight can have an effect on your baby's risk of such chronic diseases as diabetes, high blood pressure, and cardiovascular disease. Apparently, a poor diet before and during pregnancy leads to lower birth weight and so "programs" your baby to have health problems as an adult. (See Chapter One for more specifics.)

Good nutrition is not something you should worry about only during pregnancy. I've seen many a fifty-year-old who needed to change his or her eating habits to lose weight, reduce blood sugar, or lower cholesterol. However, to "teach an old dog new tricks" truly is tough. So if your children learn good eating habits from the start, they will never have to worry about changing them!

Ten Steps to a Healthy Diet

Because so much conflicting advice is available on nutrition today, I've put together ten easy eating tips to follow, now and after your pregnancy.

1. *Variety for good balance.* We've all known those people who eat a tuna sandwich and apple for lunch, day in, day out. What's missing is variety. Variety is not only the spice of life, it also helps provides the right balance of nutrients, vitamins, and minerals you need. Not that a tuna sandwich is a bad lunch. But just think about all the other foods and nutrients you are missing! The concept of variety and balance is especially important during pregnancy, to ensure you don't get too much of certain vit-

amins or additives and that you get the right mix of all vitamins and minerals that are important for your baby's growth and development.

2. *Moderation is the key* to an enjoyable life and also the key to good health. In a recent survey of fourth- to eighth-graders, 85 percent of the students said that you should avoid all high-fat foods and 77 percent thought that you should never eat foods that have a lot of sugar.[1] Wrong! There is not one food that you should never eat, regardless of its fat or sugar content! Just eat it in small amounts. (The exception would be diabetics who must strictly control their blood sugar. The occasional sweet is probably okay, but you should discuss this with your health care provider or diabetes educator first.)

3. *Follow the food pyramid guide.* The food pyramid is a wonderful pictorial example of how our diet should be built. Start with a base of whole grains and cereals, and build on with fruits, vegetables, protein, milk, and, finally, tiny amounts of sugar and fat. If your grocery cart doesn't reflect the food pyramid, you should reconsider your shopping list! Below is the food pyramid modified for pregnancy.

4. *Bone up on calcium.* Calcium has never been more important in the diet. In fact, a recent National Institutes of Health panel recently recommended calcium intakes above the RDA for all age and sex groups. During pregnancy, supplemental calcium has been shown to lower blood pressure and reduce the

The Eating Expectantly
Food Pyramid

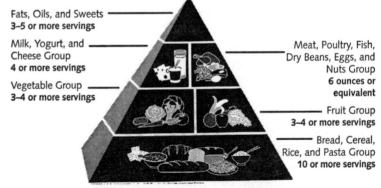

Fats, Oils, and Sweets
3–5 or more servings

Milk, Yogurt, and
Cheese Group
4 or more servings

Vegetable Group
3–4 or more servings

Meat, Poultry, Fish,
Dry Beans, Eggs, and
Nuts Group
**6 ounces or
equivalent**

Fruit Group
3–4 or more servings

Bread, Cereal,
Rice, and Pasta Group
10 or more servings

Source: Modified for pregnancy based on the Food Pyramid Guide from the U.S. Department of Agriculture/U.S. Department of Health and Human Services.

risk of preeclampsia (a form of hypertension occurring in pregnancy).[2] But even after pregnancy, you should try to have two or three servings of calcium-rich food a day (more if breastfeeding). Research on calcium is promising–higher calcium intake is linked to lower blood pressure and is also related to a lower risk of colon cancer.[3,4]

Of course, calcium is well known for building bones to their maximum strength and keeping them that way, thus helping to prevent osteoporosis. You start losing bone mass in your thirties–so be sure to have adequate calcium, either in your diet or by supplement, throughout your lifetime.

5. *Don't skimp on iron.* Getting enough iron in your diet may be a real challenge: while we need more iron than men, we generally eat much fewer calories. Add to that sometimes nutritionally unbalanced diets and too many meals eaten on the run, and the result is often iron deficiency anemia. Anemia during pregnancy carries a large price–a three-times-higher risk of delivering a low-birth-weight baby and double the chance of having a premature infant. (See page 60 to find out more about this important mineral.)

6. *Go for the whole grains–*three are key. Women often shy away from such foods as bread, pasta, and corn because they're thought of as fattening. Because of their "nutritional punch," such foods should be the foundation of every meal. They provide energy, fiber, vitamins, and minerals. Recent research links eating more fiber from whole grains with reduced risk of fatal colon cancer, breast cancer, and endometrial cancer.

Whole grains contain trace minerals that have important implications for chronic disease prevention, but are in short supply in the American diet. Examples of those minerals are chromium, selenium, zinc, copper, manganese, and magnesium. Examples of whole grains are whole-grain (such as whole-wheat) breads and cereals, brown rice, and whole-grain pastas.[5]

7. *Don't forget the exercise.* We've become a nation of couch potatoes, and as the saying goes, couch potatoes have tater tots! But that is changing as people realize the many benefits of exercise: stress reduction, improved endurance, lowered resting heart rate, blood pressure control, cardiovascular efficiency, improved self-esteem and body image, better sleep habits, and lowered risk of heart attack, stroke, diabetes and even some types of cancer.

During pregnancy, staying limber can help those aches and pains, can help reduce fatigue, and also gets you ready for the "Mother's Marathon"–labor and delivery! However, you should tone down exercise during pregnancy. (See Chapter Ten, Fitting Fitness In, for more information.)

8. *Get your fill of fluids.* Our body is comprised of about 60 percent water, so drinking plenty of it makes sense. Thirst is the first sign of dehydration, though it lags behind actual need. Thus, by the time you feel thirsty, you are already behind in your fluid intake! Eight to ten glasses a day are recommended during pregnancy. With your increased blood supply, amniotic fluid, and extra tissue to support, the more fluids you have, the better. You can have fluid in the form of juices and decaffeinated teas and sodas, but try to have most of it as clear, clean water!

9. *Focus on fiber.* Most of us don't get enough fiber; the National Cancer Institute recommends twenty to thirty-five grams.[6] During pregnancy, you'll find yourself trying to eat more high-fiber foods to combat constipation. Adequate fiber in the diet may reduce risk of colon cancer, breast cancer, and, during pregnancy, can prevent constipation and hemorrhoids. (See page 47 for more fiber facts.)

10. *Spare the extras.* As mentioned before, no food should be totally off limits. However, you can also go overboard in fat, sugar, and even artificial sweeteners if you let your taste buds rule. You should eat such extras as candy, "junk food," and ice cream as a treat after you have eaten all the "must" foods. With all the extra nutrients you need during pregnancy, you can't afford to eat many "empty calorie" foods.

Suggested Weight Gain	
Prepregnancy Weight	**Suggested Weight Gain**
Underweight (10% below ideal body weight)	28–40 pounds
Normal Weight (Average weight for height)	25–35 pounds
Overweight (20% or more over ideal body weight)	15–25 pounds

Teens and African American women should strive for gains at the upper end of the range. Women under 5'3" should gain an amount of weight at the lower end of the range.

Source: *Nutrition during Pregnancy: Part I, Weight Gain: Part II, Nutrient Supplements,* Subcommittee on Nutritional Status and Weight Gain during Pregnancy, National Academy of Sciences.

▼

Everything You Ever Wanted to Know about Weight Gain During Pregnancy

Putting on pounds is probably every woman's nightmare, but during pregnancy, the amount of weight you gain and how you gain it may be the distinguishing factor between a healthy, term baby and one that is born small and premature.

In one study, women with a low rate of weight gain were more than twice as likely to have a preterm delivery than those with an average weight gain.[7] Happily watching yourself gain weight may be tough, but try to get used to it.

Where the Weight Goes

You have probably seen life-sized pictures of a fetus, no bigger than a spoon and weighing no more than an ounce. So why have you gained five pounds?! Since the average birth weight is about seven pounds and the average weight gain is thirty, pregnancy weight gain is obvi-

Where the Weight Goes	
Tissue	**Pounds**
Breast	1–2 lbs.
Placenta	1½ lbs.
Enlarged Uterus	2 lbs.
Increased Blood and Fluids	8½ lbs.
Baby	7½ lbs
Fat stores	4–14 lbs.
Total gained	**25–35 lbs.**

ously more than just baby; your blood supply increases, your breasts and uterus enlarge, there are miscellaneous extra fluids, plus, you guessed it–FAT! The fat provides additional calories for breastfeeding. During pregnancy, your body also builds additional muscle to carry the extra weight. The chart below left shows where your weight goes.

Historically, weight gain recommendations have gone from one extreme to another. Once, health practitioners thought that toxemia of pregnancy (now called preeclampsia) and high blood pressure could be prevented if the mom-to-be gained as little as possible. Now we know that good nutrition and increased weight gain are the keys to having healthier babies.

According to U.C. Berkeley nutritional epidemiologist Barbara Abrams, coauthor of a large study that looked at weight gain in pregnant women, "Our study shows that maternal weight gain is an important factor in pregnancy outcome, especially the baby's birth weight. Since low birth weight is the major cause of infant mortality and mental and physical disability, it can be dangerous to restrict a pregnant woman's weight gains."[8]

Twenty-five to thirty-five pounds is the recommended weight gain for the "average woman," but many don't fit into the average mold. The amount of weight you should gain depends on your weight before you were pregnant, and on whether you are having twins or more. (See page 117 on information for multiple births.) Refer to the chart on page 22 to see how much you should gain.

What's "Ideal Weight"?

Ideal weight has different definitions. Some health professionals use insurance weight charts, some use the "rule of five," and others use the recent Suggested Weights for Adults from the U.S. Department of Agriculture and U.S. Department of Health and Human Services. You could also define ideal body weight as the weight at which you feel best.

"Rule of five"(for women): Start with 100 pounds for five feet tall. Add five pounds for every inch over five feet you are. There is always a plus or minus 10 percent factor to account for bone and body build, etc.

Monitoring Your Own Weight Gain

Keep in mind that what's important isn't just the *amount* of weight you gain, but *how* you gain it, or the *pattern* of weight gain. The weight gain should be gradual and should somewhat follow the curves on the Weight Gain Chart (next page). You should gain approximately two to four pounds during the first trimester, and close to a pound a week during the second and especially the third trimester,

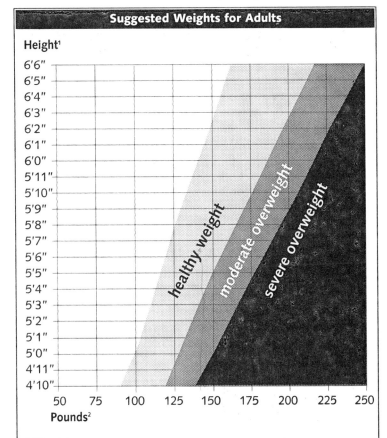

Suggested Weights for Adults

Height (without shoes): 6'6", 6'5", 6'4", 6'3", 6'2", 6'1", 6'0", 5'11", 5'10", 5'9", 5'8", 5'7", 5'6", 5'5", 5'4", 5'3", 5'2", 5'1", 5'0", 4'11", 4'10"

Pounds: 50, 75, 100, 125, 150, 175, 200, 225, 250

Regions: healthy weight, moderate overweight, severe overweight

[1] Without shoes

[2] Without clothes. The higher weight in the ranges generally apply to men, who tend to have more muscle and bone.

Note: This chart refers to *prepregnancy* weights.

Source: *Report of the Dietary Guidelines Advisory Committee on the Dietary Guidelines for Americans,* 1995, pages 23–24.

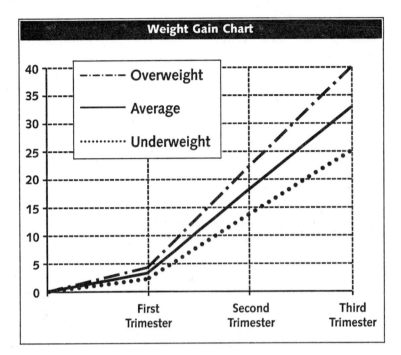

Weight Gain Chart

40
35
30
25
20
15
10
5
0

------- Overweight
——— Average
.... Underweight

First
Trimester

Second
Trimester

Third
Trimester

Scales are often different, and all the above factors also come into play, so compare only weights from the same scale.

Gaining Too Fast or Too Much

Most women fear gaining too much, because they think the weight will be difficult to take off. Also, gaining too much weight can cause excessive infant size and increased risk of a C-section. However, regardless of how much you gain, pregnancy is never the time to try to lose weight. If you have reached your goal of a thirty-pound weight gain by week thirty-five, don't think that you should not gain any more for the remaining five weeks!

Here are several explanations for gaining too much weight or gaining too fast:

- Overeating or simply eating too many high-fat, high-calorie foods (are you trying to truly "eat for two")? (See the quiz on the next page to evaluate the "extras" in your diet.)
- Multiple fetuses. If you don't feel that your weight gain is related to eating, consult your health care provider about the possibility that you are carrying more than one baby.

when the baby grows the most. If your goal is more or less than average, adapt those numbers accordingly.

In general, if you are eating all the right foods, with just a few splurges, your weight gain will follow the right pattern for you. Remember that women have fluctuating weights, which vary even more during pregnancy. A few tips for weighing are listed below.

▶ **Weigh yourself at the same time of day and under the same conditions.**

For example, always weigh yourself first thing in the morning,

after you use the restroom, naked, or wearing the same nightgown.

▶ **Weigh yourself weekly, not daily!**

Weighing daily could drive a person nuts! Since your weight depends on what you have had to eat and drink, how much sodium you've consumed, and even your bowel habits, you could show a three-pound "weight gain" on Monday, and a four-pound "weight loss" on Wednesday.

▶ **Compare only weights from the same scale.**

If your health care provider's scale shows a four-pound weight gain compared to your home scale, don't go into a panic!

- Inaccurate weighing or weighing after eating or drinking. (Weighing after drinking a quart of water, for example, will add two pounds to your weight!)
- Preeclampsia/high blood pressure. If you gain three or more pounds a week in the second or third trimester of pregnancy, and you also experience swelling of feet and/or hands, severe headaches, or problems with vision, contact your health care provider immediately! Those could be the first signs of preeclampsia, a potentially serious problem.

(See page 116 for more information.)

How to Avoid Gaining Too Much Weight

Now that the recommended weight gain is higher than it was a few years ago, you will definitely "look" pregnant! However, two things control your weight gain, and how it looks on you—your diet and your activity level. The distribution of the gained weight varies among women. You will hear myths about your weight gain. Some people will tell you that if you're having a boy, the weight will be all in

your stomach. And if your weight gain is spread out all over, many will predict a girl! The truth is, your genes control where the weight goes.

If you start a low-impact exercise program of which your health care provider approves (such as swimming or walking) or continue an established exercise program, you will be well toned and so will look and feel better. Being in good overall physical shape will make you feel good about your expanding waistline. Having more lean muscle tissue will also help you lose weight after you have your baby.

An experienced mother of two says: "I lost all my weight within a few months of having Brian. I swam regularly right up to delivery. However, with Emily, I was very sick with bronchitis the last six weeks of pregnancy and spent a lot of time in bed. Overall, I was much less active when I was pregnant with Emily and it took me much longer to take the weight off after Emily was born."

Of course, your diet may need critical analysis. If you follow the Eating Expectantly Diet, you shouldn't have any problem with excess weight gain. The quiz below may shed some light on your eating habits.

Not Gaining Enough

There are as many reasons for not being able to gain enough

Will You Gain Too Much Weight? Quiz

1. Do you eat sweets four times a week or more?
2. Do you snack on chips, nuts, nachos, French fries, etc., four times a week or more?
3. Do you use a lot of margarine, salad dressing, sour cream, and cheese?
4. When you cook, do you pour more than one teaspoon of oil, per serving, into the pan?
5. Do you regularly eat the skin on the chicken, fat on your steak, etc.?
6. Do you eat "typical" fast food or fried food more than once a week?
7. Do you often eat when bored, depressed, angry, or happy but not hungry?
8. Do you usually eat while doing something else, such as reading, watching television, etc.?
9. Do you eat snacks such as regular ice cream and regular cheese?

If you answered "yes" to three or more of the above questions, you have a good chance of gaining too much weight (or too much fat) during your pregnancy. Keeping an eye on fat intake will help you now, and later, when you are trying to lose your "baby fat."

weight as there are for gaining too much. Though not gaining enough weight may seem a blessing to some, the lack of weight can cause major problems for your baby. Women who don't gain enough are more likely to deliver their babies before they are due, and their babies are likely to be smaller. Newborn death is more related to prematurity and low birth weight than to any other cause.[9] So if you are having problems gaining enough weight, be sure to find the reason below and do something about it.

- Fast metabolism. Women who were underweight before pregnancy may simply burn calories more quickly. You may need to closely analyze your diet for ways to increase calories—and may need individual help from a registered dietitian.
- You can't eat much because of nausea, heartburn, stress, or other problems. First, you need to get to the root of the problem. Nausea usually goes away after the first trimester. The other problems may have simple solutions. Psychosocial stress has been known to decrease weight gain and you may need help from a counselor or social worker. Ask your health care provider for assistance.

- You go a mile a minute. Some moms-to-be have a very active lifestyle and don't slow down for pregnancy. This could result in burning too many calories, or not taking the time to eat enough. Either scenario leaves fewer calories left for baby to grow on. If your lifestyle is interfering with your weight gain, you may need to look at slowing down your activities, reducing exercise, and/or increasing calories.
- Psychological factors. If you have ever had a weight problem or a history of eating disorders, you might find gaining weight psychologically difficult. Your overall psychosocial well-being may also have an effect on your weight status. Depression, anxiety, low self-esteem, and lack of social support may all affect your weight gain.[10] You may need your health care provider or a psychotherapist to help you.
- You smoke. Smoking is associated with reduced weight gain as well as placenta previa (an abnormal placement of the placenta that may cause complications during delivery).[11] Do your best to quit or cut down.

What You Can Do If You Are Not Gaining Enough Weight

▶ **Make sure your diet is similar to the Eating Expectantly Diet on page 44.**

▶ **Slow down!**

▶ **Increase the amount of food you eat. If you are having trouble eating more, increase fat intake–the easiest way to increase calories without increasing the bulk.**

The best foods to add are those rich in unsaturated fats, such as vegetable oils, salad dressings, wheat germ, nuts, seeds, avocado, margarine, and peanut butter.

▶ **Don't forget the snacks.**

If you're eating just three meals a day, chances are you're not eating enough. Most women need a few snacks every day to fit in all the nutrients and calories they need for pregnancy. (See page 218 for snack ideas for high-energy moms.)

▶ **Increase what I call "Healthy Splurges"– foods that have some nutritive value, but have extra calories too, such**

as milkshakes, frozen yogurt, breads made with fruits or vegetables (like banana bread or zucchini bread), sweet potato or pumpkin pie, pudding, and egg custard.

To add calories, you may also want to add a food supplement such as Carnation Instant Breakfast to your milk.

▼

All about Fat

Watching the types and amounts of fat you eat is important—for the short and long term—for several reasons:

- Ounce per ounce, fat has more than twice as many calories as carbohydrate or protein.
- Some types of fat are absolutely essential for humans because the body cannot make them. EPA and DHA, two omega-3 oils found in fish are important for the building of fetal brain (which is 60 percent lipid) and eye tissue. Alpha-linoleic acid found in poly-unsaturated vegetable oils, can be converted to EPA and DHA in the body, but not very efficiently. Best

sources of alpha-linoleic are canola oil and soybean oil.

Another essential fat that can't be made in your body is linoleic acid (omega-6). All vegetable oils contain linoleic acid, but safflower oil is richest. Most people's diets contain too much of omega-6 and not enough omega-3. Omega-6 and omega-3 oils form biologically active compounds that affect body functions such as blood pressure, blood clotting, and immune response, so the right balance could make a profound difference to overall health. To get enough of these essential fats in your diet, try to have a balance of oils rich in omega-6 and omega-3. Eating fish (especially fatty fish) a few times per week can help ensure adequate omega-3 intake. (See page 188 for "The Facts on Fish.")

- Fat calories are stored easier than calories from other sources. Meaning, the more fat you eat, the more fat you wear.
- A high-fat intake is implicated in heart disease and certain types of cancer, especially breast, prostate, and colon cancer.[12]
- A high-fat diet, or eating fried foods, can aggravate the nausea of early preg-

nancy and heartburn later in pregnancy.

- Types of fat called trans-fatty acids are made when liquid oils are hydrogenated for storage or cooking purposes—for example, oil that is made into shortening or stick margarine. These types of fat appear worse than saturated fat in terms of heart disease and may have widespread implications for other diseases. Recent research also shows that trans-fatty acids get into the fetal blood stream in relation to the mother's consumption; trans-fat could restrict birth weight.[13] Trans-fatty acids are mostly found in margarines, shortening and products made from these, such as bakery goods, commercially fried foods, and snack foods. You may want to avoid margarine or use as little as possible and keep processed, high-fat foods to a minimum. Look at the label of several margarines and choose a "tub" product that has liquid oil as the first ingredient. Currently, the amount of trans-fatty acids is not listed on the food label.

To put your own fat intake in perspective, fat should be about 30 percent of your calories. If you are having difficulty gaining weight, you may need to increase your intake of fat, but try to get the extra fat from vegetable sources (such as avocado, nuts, peanut butter, vegetable oils, etc.).

Most health organizations recommend that we eat 30 percent or less of our calories from fat. A specific guideline for pregnancy hasn't been established, but somewhere around 30 percent fat is a prudent recommendation. Sonja Connor, M.S., R.D., research associate professor at the department of medicine at Oregon Health Science Center, says that a case can be made for watching fat intake during pregnancy, though she cautions intake below 20 percent, saying, "You may have trouble gaining weight and not laying down the fat you need to support lactation."

"The average pregnant woman needs 2,200 to 2,400 calories and 30 percent of those calories would work out to be about 70 to 90 grams of fat. This may sound like a lot. Are you savvy about fat? Look at the following diet and guess how much fat it contains.

How Much Fat?

Breakfast
Cereal with 1 cup 2% milk
2 slices toast with 2 teaspoons
    margarine
Fresh fruit

Snack
1 ounce cheese
10 wheat crackers

Lunch
Deluxe cheeseburger
Fries
Side salad with 2 tablespoons
    dressing

Snack
2 tablespoons peanut butter
    on melba toast
1½ cups 2% milk

Dinner
6 ounces fish sautéed in
    safflower oil
Baked potato with 2 table-
    spoons sour cream and
    2 teaspoons margarine
Fresh, steamed spinach
Tomatoes and cucumbers
    with 2 tablespoons
    vinaigrette dressing

Snack
Ice cream
Chocolate chip cookie

Believe it or not, the above menu has 160 grams of fat, or double the amount recommended. Let's change a few things and see how the fat adds up in our modified menu:

Breakfast
Cereal with 1 cup skim milk
2 slices of toast with 1 tea-
    spoon margarine and
    2 teaspoons fruit spread
Banana

Snack
1 ounce low-fat cheese
8 wheat crackers

Lunch
Grilled chicken sandwich
Side salad with pasta salad
    and light vinaigrette
    dressing
Peaches and pineapple
1 cup 2% milk

Snack
2 tablespoons peanut butter
½ bagel
Vegetable juice

Dinner
6 ounces fish baked with
    a crumb topping of
    Parmesan cheese and
    1 teaspoon margarine
Boiled new potatoes with
    2 teaspoons margarine
Fresh, steamed spinach
Melon balls
Skim milk

Snack
Frozen yogurt
Graham crackers

We've cut the fat in half with just a few changes! The menu now has under eighty grams of fat, a much better number. You can check the vitamin and mineral aspect of your diet by taking the nutrition quiz on page 61, or send in the Nutrition Analysis form at the back of the book.

Changing Your Mindset for Pregnancy

Up to now you've been the perfect model of health. You don't eat eggs, you work out five times a week, and you haven't eaten red meat in years. Now you're craving a steak, don't feel like exercising (or doing much of anything, for that matter), and eggs seem to go down really well. What's a woman to do? First, let's set a few things straight.

True, the average American diet contains too much protein, but eating lean red meat in moderation is fine. You just need to choose lean cuts, such as top round, eye of round, and flank steak. Red meat is rich in iron, and small amounts can help your body absorb iron from nonmeat sources. It is also a good source of zinc, an important nutrient during pregnancy.

Eggs are a great source of protein and eating them in moderation is not a problem for most people. Even the American Heart Association allows three to four egg yolks a week in their Eating Plan for Healthy Americans.[14] Speaking from experience, sometimes eggs are easier to "get down." So don't feel guilty about eating extra eggs–

just watch the accompaniments (bacon, sausage, biscuits, hash browns, cheese, etc.).

Your body is going through a tremendous amount of change (no kidding!), and not feeling quite as energetic as you used to is normal. You also may not feel comfortable about the size or look of your "body with baby," which may make you uncomfortable getting into an exercise outfit or bathing suit. Try to keep up some exercise, even if just walking around the neighborhood. Exercise will help keep muscle tone and will make you feel good–mentally and physically. (See Chapter Ten for more on exercise.)

Lastly, remember that pregnancy doesn't last forever, even though sometimes it feels as though it might!

The Essential Guide to Vitamins and Minerals

The body needs many different nutrients every day. Every vitamin and mineral plays an important, if minor, role in the making of a healthy baby.

The Energy-Releasing Nutrients

You have probably heard people say "vitamins give me more energy." Actually vitamins have no calories; but you must have them to be able to use the energy in your food.

Thiamin (Vitamin B₁)

RDA for pregnancy: 1.5 milligrams; for breastfeeding: 1.6 milligrams.

Functions: Releases energy from carbohydrate–the higher your carbohydrate intake, the higher your need for B_1. Used in appetite and nervous system function.

Sources: Brewer's yeast, enriched cereals and breads, pork, sunflower seeds, oatmeal, wheat germ, dried beans, and peas.

Note: Thiamin is unstable in heat and light. Vegetables high in thiamin and other water-soluble vitamins should be cooked minimally, with as little water as possible.

Riboflavin (Vitamin B₂)

RDA for pregnancy: 1.7 milligrams; for breastfeeding, first six months: 1.8 milligrams; for second six months: 1.7 milligrams.

Functions: Helps release energy from all foods–the more energy you use, the more riboflavin you need. Maintains normal vision and skin health.

Sources: Liver, fortified cereals, milk, yogurt, and cheese.

Niacin (Vitamin B₃)

RDA for pregnancy: 1.7 milligrams; for breastfeeding: 2.0 milligrams.

Functions: Helps release energy from food–the more energy you use, the more niacin you need. Supports health of skin, nervous system, and digestive system.

Sources: Fortified cereals, poultry, fish, meat, legumes, and nuts.

Pantothenic Acid

The estimated safe and adequate daily dietary intake is four to seven milligrams.

Functions: Helps release energy from food. Involved in antibody production.

Sources: Widespread in many foods. Beef and chicken liver, salmon, trout, and avocado are good sources.

Biotin

The estimated safe and adequate daily dietary intake is 30 to 100 micrograms.

Functions: Helps release energy from food. Assists in fat synthesis and carbohydrate storage.

Sources: Widespread in many foods. Beef and chicken liver, oatmeal, hazelnuts, and peanuts are good sources.

The Building Nutrients

These nutrients are responsible for helping to build bone, muscle tissue, hormones, and other tissues.

Calcium

RDA for pregnancy and breastfeeding: 1,200 milligrams. The National Institutes of Health Consensus Conference on Optimal Calcium Intake recommends an intake of 1,200 to 1,500 milligrams of calcium daily for pregnant and nursing women.[15]

Functions: Principal material of bones and teeth; vital in muscle contraction, nerve functioning, blood clotting, blood pressure and immune defense. Research shows a possible relationship between adequate calcium in the diet and reduced risk of hypertension and colon cancer.[16] Adequate calcium over the life-span protects against osteoporosis.

Sources: Milk and milk products, small fish with bones, blackstrap molasses, tofu that has calcium added during processing, broccoli, greens, legumes, some seaweed, and sea vegetables.

Vitamin B₁₂ (Cobalamin)

RDA for pregnancy: 2.2 micrograms; for breastfeeding: 2.6 micrograms.

Functions: Helps in new red blood cell production; helps maintain health of nerve cells.

Sources: Liver, muscle meats, fish, eggs, milk and milk products, and fortified foods.

Note: Only foods of animal origin and certain fortified foods contain Vitamin B₁₂. Check the label of foods to see whether B₁₂ is added. (See page 79 for more information.)

Phosphorus

RDA for pregnancy and breastfeeding: 1,200 milligrams.

Calcium and phosphorus make up three-fourths of the total weight of minerals found in the body. Unlike calcium, a deficiency of phosphorus is rare.

Functions: Used in building bones and teeth; needed in every cell membrane, in genetic material, as part of energy production, and in the body's buffering system.

Sources: Primary sources of phosphorus in the American diet are animal protein and carbonated sodas.

Note: Excess phosphorus may draw calcium out of the body.

Magnesium

RDA for pregnancy: 320 milligrams; for breastfeeding, first six months: 355 milligrams; for second six months: 340 milligrams.

Functions: Used in bone mineralization, protein building, enzyme action, muscle contraction, transmission of nerve impulses, and maintenance of teeth. Also helps in the regulation of blood sugar and insulin. Low intakes of magnesium have recently been implicated in increased risk of heart disease.

Sources: Nuts, legumes, whole grains, dark green vegetables, and seafood.

Vitamin A

RDA for pregnancy: 800 retinol equivalents; for breastfeeding, first six months: 1,300 retinol equivalents; for second six months: 1,200 retinol equivalents. One retinol equivalent is equal to one microgram of vitamin A or six micrograms of beta-carotene. The body converts beta-carotene into vitamin A.

Functions: Helps in cell growth and development and in formation of bones and teeth. Needed for healthy skin, mucous membranes, cornea of the eye, and reproductive health. Very promising research is going on regarding beta-carotene, cancer, and heart disease.

Sources: Liver, fortified milk, cheese, eggs. Fish liver oils are also good sources. However, because toxins tend to accumulate in the fat of fish, fish oils are not recommended during pregnancy.

Warning: Excess Vitamin A is very toxic to the fetus, so if you are taking an individual supplement of Vitamin A, or a high-potency multivitamin containing several times the RDA for the vitamin, STOP IMMEDIATELY and consult your health care provider. Recent research shows that women who took a supplement of just four times the RDA for vitamin A were nearly five times more likely to have a baby with a birth defect.[17] Also, if you are trying to conceive or are already pregnant, you should not be taking any medication containing Vitamin A, such as Retin-A.

Beta-Carotene

The body converts beta-carotene to Vitamin A as needed, so there is no worry in having too much beta-carotene in the diet. However, people who have consumed large amounts of carrots or carrot juice have had their skin turn orange! The skin returns to normal after the person resumes a moderate diet.

Sources: Spinach and dark leafy greens, broccoli, deep-orange fruits such as apricots, peaches, cantaloupe, and orange vegetables such as squash, carrots, sweet potatoes, and pumpkin.

Vitamin K

RDA for pregnancy and breastfeeding: 65 micrograms.

Vitamin K is made in the digestive tract, though infants are given a dose at birth before their own production starts.

Functions: Needed in the synthesis of blood-clotting proteins.

Sources: Seaweed (dulce and rockweed), green tea, soybean oil, turnip greens, and lettuce.

Vitamin D

RDA for pregnancy and breastfeeding: 10 micrograms or 400 International Units (IU).

Functions: Used in bone mineralization through control of calcium and phosphorus in the body.

Sources: Sunshine, fortified milk, fortified cereals, egg yolks, fish liver oil, and liver.

Note: The best source of vitamin D is sunlight! Your skin produces its own vitamin D when exposed to sufficient sunlight. Women who develop deficiencies generally avoid dairy products, have very dark skin, or do not regularly expose their skin to the sun (because of being covered in clothes or sunscreen). Women who live in northern latitudes such as Alberta, Canada or Boston, Massachussetts, are also potentially at risk for vitamin D deficiency because those areas don't get sufficient sunshine in the winter.[18] If any of the above risk factors apply to you, you will want to make sure to eat more foods fortified with vitamin D, spend more time in the sun, or ask your health care provider about taking a supplement. (Use caution in supplementing vitamin D on your own—it is toxic in large doses.)

Another good reason to make sure your body makes enough vitamin D from sunshine—recent studies show that sunlight deprivation and the associated reduced circulating vitamin D may lead to increased risk for breast, colon, and prostate cancer.[19]

Vitamin B₆ (Pyridoxine)

RDA for pregnancy: 2.2 milligrams; for breastfeeding: 2.1 milligrams.

Functions: Used in amino acid and fatty acid metabolism; helps to make red blood cells. Vitamin B_6 is needed in amounts proportional to the amount of protein in the diet.

Sources: Green and leafy vegetables, meats, fish, poultry, shellfish, legumes, fruits, and whole grains.

Note: Women—pregnant and not—don't seem to have enough vitamin B_6 in their diet. Some women who take birth control pills may have a slightly increased need for the vitamin. Deficiency of the vitamin can cause anemia, irritability, and abnormal brain wave pattern.

B₆ and Morning Sickness: Research regarding the use of vitamin B_6 for morning sickness is conflicting. Large amounts of B_6 can be neurotoxic, so please discuss B_6 supplements with your health care provider before self-prescribing.

Folate (Folacin, Folic Acid)

RDA for pregnancy: 400 micrograms; for breastfeeding, first six months: 280 micrograms; for second six months: 260 micrograms.

Functions: Needed for all new cell production and use of amino acids. Also needed for some enzymes.

Sources: Spinach, leafy green vegetables, liver, black-eyed peas, lentils, red kidney beans, broccoli, Brussels sprouts, beets, okra, green peas, asparagus, legumes, orange and grapefruit juice, and fortified cereals.

Note: The need for folacin during pregnancy more than doubles, due to vast increases in the number of new cells being made. Folate can be easily destroyed in cooking. Certain medications, such as oral contraceptives, anticonvulsants, aspirin, chemotherapy drugs, and antacids, can affect your folate status. Alcohol and smoking can also increase the need for folate.[20] If you take any of the above medications, smoke, or drink regularly, or if you did just prior to pregnancy,

your need for folate is probably greater than average. You will need to choose your diet more carefully and may want to discuss additional folacin supplementation with your health care provider.

Folacin and Birth Defects: A landmark study done in several countries showed that folacin supplementation at around the time of conception could prevent about 70 percent of recurrent neural tube defects. It is thought that folic acid supplementation can also prevent first-time occurrences. The U.S. Public Health Service now recommends that all women of childbearing age who are capable of becoming pregnant should consume 400 micrograms of folic acid per day.[21]

Iron

RDA for pregnancy: 30 milligrams; for breastfeeding: 15 milligrams.

Functions: Plays a very important role in pregnancy: part of the blood protein hemoglobin, which carries oxygen in the body; part of muscle protein. Necessary for the use of energy in the body.

Sources: Clams, fortified cereals, chicken liver, tofu, beef liver, lentils, eggs, chicken, legumes, and dried fruit.

Note: Iron deficiency anemia is still a public health problem in the U. S. Pregnant women with iron deficiency anemia are more likely to have a premature birth or low-birth-weight baby. In the 1985 Continuing Surveys of Food Intakes of Individuals (CSFII) only 4 percent of women met or exceeded the RDA for iron.[22]

Zinc

RDA for pregnancy: 15 milligrams; for breastfeeding, first six months: 19 milligrams; for second six months: 16 milligrams.

Functions: Promotes normal growth of tissues and bones; needed for the normal development of a fetus; involved in making genetic material, in immune reactions, in taste and smell perception, and in wound healing. Zinc is also required for sperm production.

Sources: Shellfish (oysters), meat, poultry, whole grains, dried beans, and nuts.

Note: Zinc deficiency during pregnancy can cause low birth weight, increased pregnancy complications, and premature births. A zinc deficiency during fetal brain development could cause fetal brain injury.[23]

Vitamin C (Ascorbic Acid)

RDA for pregnancy: 70 milligrams; for breastfeeding, first six months: 95 milligrams; for second six months: 90 milligrams.

Functions: Needed for thyroid hormone, collagen synthesis, and the production of amino acids. Strengthens resistance to infection, helps in the absorption of iron, and acts as an antioxidant to protect cell membranes.

Sources: Papaya, citrus fruits, melons, peppers, berries, green leafy vegetables, tomatoes, broccoli, cauliflower, and cabbage.

The Support Nutrients

These nutrients help all the other nutrients with their functions.

Vitamin E (Tocopherol)

RDA for pregnancy: 10 milligrams; for breastfeeding, first six months: 12 milligrams; for second six months: 11 milligrams (all based on alpha-tocopherol equivalents).

Functions: Strong antioxidant, meaning it breaks down oxidants, or free radicals, which can be destructive to cell membranes. Vitamin E works together with other antioxidants, vitamin C, and beta-carotene. Promising research is being done with vitamin E and cancer, heart disease, and cataracts. If you followed a low-fat diet or took cholesterol-lowering drugs before your pregnancy, your body may be partially depleted of vitamin E.

Sources: Wheat germ and wheat germ oil, sunflower oil, safflower oil, almond oil and almonds, hazelnuts, and mayonnaise and salad dressings made with the above oils.

Sodium

There is no RDA for sodium; estimated minimum requirement for pregnancy is 570 milligrams; for breastfeeding, 635 milligrams.

Functions: Maintains normal fluid balance. Needed for nerve impulse transmission.

Note: Historically, pregnant women lowered their salt and sodium intake during pregnancy to reduce water retention, and sometimes to prevent toxemia or preeclampsia. Now, moderation rather than restriction is the key for pregnant women.

Potassium

There is no RDA for potassium; estimated minimum requirement for pregnancy is 2,000 milligrams; for breastfeeding, 2,500 milligrams.

Functions: Maintains fluid balance and helps maintain normal blood pressure. Helps with nerve impulses and muscle contractions.

Sources: Bananas, oranges and orange juice, watermelon, cantaloupe, vegetables, meats, milk, grains, and legumes.

Note: A high intake of potassium has been linked to a reduced incidence of high blood pressure in certain populations.[24] In the 1985 Continuing Survey of Food Intakes of Individuals, women's intakes of potassium were well below the Estimated Safe and Adequate Daily Dietary Intake.[25]

Other Trace Elements

Zinc and iron are considered trace elements, but they are so important during pregnancy, they were included in the section above. Other trace elements include copper, iodine, selenium, fluoride, manganese, chromium, and molybdenum. According to the Subcommittee on Dietary Intake and Nutrient Supplements, routine supplementation of trace elements during pregnancy does not seem to be necessary, with the exception of iron.

Copper

The estimated safe and adequate daily dietary intake for adults is 1.5 to 3 milligrams.

Functions: Helps in red blood cell production; is found in nerve coverings and connective tissue. Also assists in energy production and in respiration. Copper deficiency during pregnancy is unknown.

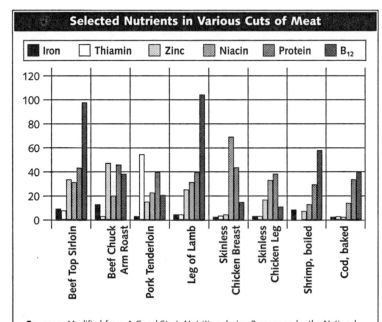

Selected Nutrients in Various Cuts of Meat

Legend: Iron, Thiamin, Zinc, Niacin, Protein, B₁₂

Categories (x-axis): Beef Top Sirloin, Beef Chuck Arm Roast, Pork Tenderloin, Leg of Lamb, Skinless Chicken Breast, Skinless Chicken Leg, Shrimp, boiled, Cod, baked

Sources: Modified from *A Good Start; Nutrition during Pregnancy*, by the National Livestock and Meat Board, and *Food Values of Portions Commonly Used*, 15th edition, by Jean Pennington.

Sources: Whole grains, shellfish, liver, kidney, raisins, nuts, peas, and beans.

Iodine

The RDA for pregnancy is 175 micrograms; for breastfeeding: 200 micrograms.

Functions: An essential component of the thyroid hormone thyroxine, which is responsible for regulating the metabolic rate (the amount of energy the body needs at rest). Iodine deficiency during pregnancy can cause disorders in the fetus, including stillbirth, birth defects, and neurological impairment. However, there is no evidence of iodine deficiency in the U.S.

Sources: Seafood, iodized salt, and food grown in ocean areas that contain iodine-rich soil.

Selenium

The RDA for pregnancy: 65 micrograms; for breastfeeding: 75 micrograms.

Functions: As an antioxidant, selenium works to protect body compounds from oxidation. Promising research links selenium and other antioxidants with reduced cancer risk.

Sources: Seafood, meats, and grains.

Fluoride

The estimated safe and adequate daily dietary intake for adults is

1.5 to 4 milligrams.

Functions: Bonds calcium and phosphorus in bones and teeth; prevents cavities in teeth.

Sources: Water that naturally contains fluoride or water that has fluoride added. (If you are not sure whether your water contains flouride, you might want to have it tested.)

Manganese

The estimated safe and adequate daily dietary intake for adults is 2 to 5 milligrams.

Functions: Part of enzymes that are active in many cell processes and a component of an important antioxidant.

Sources: Whole grains, beans, peas, and nuts.

Chromium

The estimated safe and adequate daily dietary intake for adults is 50 to 200 micrograms.

Functions: Associated with insulin; needed for the release of energy from glucose. Inability to use glucose results in diabetes-like deficiency symptoms. There is some concern that increased refinement of foods such as whole grains could lead to decreased intake of this trace mineral.

Sources: Whole grains, meat, mushrooms, asparagus, and brewers' yeast.

Molybdenum

The estimated safe and adequate daily dietary intake for adults is 75 to 250 micrograms.

Functions: A component of enzymes used in many body processes.

Sources: Legumes, cereals, and organ meats.

Of Special Concern

Studies of pregnant women's diets have shown that intakes of folate, iron, calcium, zinc, magnesium, and vitamins B_6, D, and E, were below the RDAs. Check the preceding pages to see if you have sources of these nutrients in your diet.

Selected Nutrients in Various Cuts of Meat

All animal proteins are not equal; they provide varying amounts of zinc, iron, and vitamins B_6 and B_{12}. The table on page 32 shows why you should eat a variety of meats.

▼

To Supplement or Not to Supplement?

The need for vitamin/mineral supplements has been contro-versial for years, and their use during pregnancy also has two sides.

Prenatal vitamins have generally been prescribed across the board for most pregnant women. However, a National Academy of Sciences subcommittee recommends in its report, *Nutrition during Pregnancy*, that prenatal vitamin supplements should be prescribed on an individual basis, based on the woman's current nutritional status.[26]

The reason for the concern over supplementation is that certain nutrients in large doses can be toxic to the fetus, including iron, zinc, selenium, and vitamins A, B_6, C, and D. Moreover, an increase in the amount of one nutrient may negatively affect how other nutrients are absorbed and used.[27]

Because of the evidence about folic acid and neural tube defects, several organizations have come out in favor of either folic acid supplementation or a multivitamin supplement containing folic acid–before conception. A new federal regulation now mandates that any grain products calling themselves fortified must also be fortified with folic acid. The rule doesn't go into effect until January 1, 1998, and even when grains are fortified, you must still eat other foods containing folic acid to meet the recommended intake. For example, the March of Dimes Foundation recommends that all women capable of becoming pregnant take a multivitamin supplement that contains 400 micrograms of folic acid.

To prevent birth defects, the insurance of having the proper mix of nutrients in your body before conception makes sense. Since up to 60 percent of pregnancies in the U.S. may be unplanned, all women of childbearing age who could become pregnant should take a supplement.

If You Take Supplements

Most women don't make their first visit to the doctor until the tenth or twelfth week of pregnancy, after much of the organ development has taken place. Here are some words of advice about taking vitamin supplements:

▶ **DO NOT TAKE INDIVIDUAL SUPPLEMENTS, except for calcium or vitamin C.**

Large amounts of certain vitamins can be toxic to the fetus and cause birth defects, or can create imbalances, with certain nutrients competing with other nutrients for absorption. Recent research shows that women who took more than 10,000 IU of vitamin A–just four times the

RDA–had five times the risk of birth defects as compared to women who consumed 5,000 IU or less.[28]

▶ **Before you are pregnant, take a multivitamin/ mineral supplement that contains 400 micrograms of folic acid and no more than 100 percent of the RDAs.**

You can find this information on the label. When you confirm your pregnancy, your health care provider will probably suggest you take a prenatal vitamin. Remember that a vitamin/mineral supplement is no substitute for a healthy diet!

▶ **Remember that vitamin supplements are not the only sources of substantial amounts of vitamins.**

Fortified cereals such as Total also provide 100 percent of the RDA for many nutrients. If you were to take a multivitamin in addition to several servings of fortified food, you could potentially get too many vitamins, and the excess could build up to a toxic level.

▶ **If your health care provider suggests a supplement that is making you nauseated, consider taking the**

supplement with a light snack before you go to bed.

> "The bottom-line message: the emphasis on optimal diet is of the greatest importance to all women of the childbearing age at all times–not only when pregnancy has been confirmed."
>
> – *Michael Hambidge, M.D., Sc.D., Director of the Center for Human Nutrition, University of Colorado Health Sciences Center.*

Calcium Supplements

Calcium is vital during pregnancy for the health of your baby and, especially, for your future bone health. Preliminary research also shows some correlation between increased calcium in the diet and reduced incidence of high blood pressure during pregnancy.[29,30,31]

Yet so many women, both pregnant and not, don't have enough calcium in their diet. Women often start thinking about osteoporosis around the time of menopause, but they should actually consider their bone health all their lives; bone continues to grow until age twenty-five and gradually starts losing mass after age thirty-five. (See page 58 for information on how to sneak calcium into your diet.)

Recent research shows another good reason to have enough calcium in your diet: as your bones lose calcium to make up for the calcium missing from your diet, lead stored in your bones is also released. You are exposed to small amounts of lead over a lifetime, from drinking water and other sources, and it is stored in your bone. During times when the bones lose calcium (during pregnancy, lactation, and after menopause, in women), lead is released into the bloodstream.

Adequate dietary calcium is essential in preventing, or keeping to a minimum, the turnover of bone. For women who had a substantial lead exposure earlier in life (such as living in a house with lead pipes or eating leaded paint chips as a child), adequate calcium is even more important to prevent possible lead poisoning of yourself and your child.[32]

The National Institutes of Health recommend 1,200 to 1,500 milligrams of calcium a day for pregnant and breastfeeding women. They suggest you try to get your calcium from your food first. If you can't, then take a supplement.

If you are currently taking a calcium or iron supplement, you should consider a few things about the way you take them:

Type of calcium

Calcium is best absorbed from calcium citrate and calcium carbonate. Calcium carbonate is the most concentrated and economical form of calcium. Many women take Tums because it contains calcium carbonate. If you take too much calcium carbonate at one time, it can cause "rebound hyperacidity"–excess stomach acid. If this becomes a problem, consider taking the calcium supplement in several doses during the day, since it is absorbed better that way. Avoid oyster shell calcium and dolomite due to possible lead and heavy metal contamination.

What you take with it

Calcium is best absorbed when taken with food; iron is best absorbed on an empty stomach. However, if you take an iron supplement along with calcium citrate or calcium phosphate (types of supplements) on an empty stomach, the amount of iron you absorb may be decreased.[33]

The solution

If you take both iron and calcium, take them at different times. Take your iron supplement on an empty stomach (or with a light snack when you are not having a dairy product). Take your calcium supplement with a light snack. Registered pharma-

cist Nellie Whaley suggests that if you take calcium and iron, take the calcium at least two hours after, or one hour before, you take the iron.

Some women find that iron or prenatal vitamin supplements make them nauseated. Taking them right before bedtime or with a snack usually helps. Whenever you decide to take your supplements, make sure to make it a ritual; calcium or iron left in the bottle won't bring you any benefit!

▼

Keeping Your Baby's Environment Safe

You knew they were coming, "the don'ts." A physician who specializes in high-risk pregnancies once told me, "You have only one chance to give your baby what it needs. Why not do everything you can to help your baby along–it's only nine months." To give advice is easy, but following it may not be as easy. If you are having problems with your habits, talk to your health care provider.

Smoking

The first trimester, and before pregnancy if possible, is a good time to kick some bad habits and pick up some good ones. Kiss your cigarettes good-bye, because babies of smokers weigh an average of half a pound less that those of nonsmokers. Research shows that to quit smoking is the single most important thing you can do to improve the growth and long-term health of your baby.

Other adverse affects of smoking while pregnant include higher risk of preterm delivery, early infant death and possible long-term growth problems, problems with intellectual performance and behavioral development. Babies of mothers who smoked during pregnancy were found to have a greater risk of obstructive sleep apnea (infants stop breathing while sleeping).[34] Smoking while you are pregnant may also affect your baby's neurological development.[35] Smoking by either parent during pregnancy is related to a higher risk of childhood cancer for the child.[36] And after your baby is born, he or she will also suffer the ill effects of secondhand smoke.[37,38,39]

Smokers may need extra nutrients, such as vitamins B_{12} and C, amino acids, folate, and zinc, and thus taking a multivita-min/mineral supplement may be necessary.[40]

Quitting smoking has many benefits—but it may be easier said than done. For help, call the Cancer Information Service at 1-800-4CANCER.

Lead Exposure

Although lead may not be something that you consume consciously, you may receive a regular dose of lead from your drinking water. According to the Environmental Protection Agency (EPA), as many as forty million people may have too much lead in their drinking water. Pregnant women and children run the highest risk of problems from lead exposure because of increased absorption. Lead exposure can cause increased rates of miscarriage and stillbirths and may lead to such long-term effects as learning disability, brain damage, hyperactivity, high blood pressure, and kidney disease.[41] You may have exposure to too much lead if:

- Your home was built between 1978 and 1988. Lead solder was used in home plumbing during those years. In older homes with lead solder, minerals usually coat the pipes and keep the lead from leaching out.
- Your home was built before 1930. These homes often used lead pipes instead of copper ones. Also, water companies installed lead pipes underground to bring water to homes built during the first part of the century.
- You have "soft" or acidic water. Soft or acidic water can strip away the coating or the solder on the inside of water pipes. If no lead was used either in your pipes or in the service pipes carrying water to your home, you are safe, even if you have soft water.

To be safe, you should have your water tested for lead; this costs from fifteen to twenty-five dollars (avoid do-it-yourself tests—they are often inaccurate). Beware of scam artists who provide free lead testing and then sell you a treatment system you don't really need. The EPA action level for lead is fifteen parts per billion. You should take action to decrease the lead in your water if it has fifteen parts per billion of lead in "first draw" (or five parts per billion after you have let the water run for a minute or more).[42]

A reverse-osmosis or distillation system can remove the lead, but can be expensive and may waste resources. (Some systems can also remove many other potentially harmful substances in your water: Watkins has a system that is also supposed to remove the dangerous cryptosperideum bacteria.) Less-expensive treatments are available, such as filter systems and even a drip carafe (Brita Water Filter System, for example); make sure that the equipment is certified by the Water Quality Association or the National Sanitation Foundation (NSF).

Note: To decrease the lead in your water until you can do further testing or treatment, run the cold water for several minutes before using. (Instead of wasting the water, consider saving it to water plants, wash windows, etc.). If you usually use hot water to make coffee, tea, or for cooking, use cold water instead. For the first time, new faucets are available that don't leach unsafe levels of lead—make sure the faucet you buy is certified by the NSF.

Other possible sources of lead exposure include leaded crystal decanters, ceramic pottery with lead-containing glaze (especially imported), and lead-based paint that is chipping or being removed. (Paint applied before 1978 contains lead.)

Stripping lead paint from your home should only be done by a professional who is certified or licensed in lead safety. If not removed properly, the fine lead particles can circulate in the air and home environment and

cause even more problems.

Hot, acidic drinks such as coffee can cause lead to leach from lead-glazed mugs. Don't drink fruit juice or store acidic foods in leaded crystal because lead can be leached into the food or drink. If you eat canned imported foods regularly, be aware that their cans may contain lead solder.[43]

For More Information:
National Lead Information Center:
1-800-LEAD FYI

Water Quality Association:
4151 Naperville Road
Lisle, IL 60532
(Both can inform you which types of water filters handle lead removal.)

National Sanitation Foundation:
P.O. Box 1468
Ann Arbor, MI 48106
(This organization sets the standards for water treatment systems.)

Environmental Protection Agency (EPA) Safe Drinking Water Hotline:
1-800-426-4791 (202-382-5533 in Washington, D.C.)
(The EPA can give you a list of state-certified testing labs and can answer questions about the water supply.)

Frandon Enterprises:
1-800-359-9000
(Makes two inexpensive lead-testing kits; one for water and one for ceramic ware, crystal, and even children's toys.)

If you think your job is exposing you to dangerous amounts of lead, contact the nearest office of the Occupational Safety and Health Administration (OSHA–listed in the phone book under U.S. Department of Labor), or call OSHA's Office of Information and Consumer Affairs at 202-523-8151.

Illness during Pregnancy

Though no one plans to get sick or to be exposed to illness during pregnancy, knowing the facts can help.

Fever: If you have a fever during pregnancy, contact your health care provider immediately. Temperatures over 102.5 degrees may increase the risk of certain birth defects.

Rubella: Between 1988–1990, the number of rubella cases doubled. Rubella during pregnancy can cause stillbirth and birth defects. However, if you happened to receive a rubella vaccine before or during the first three months of pregnancy, chances are your baby will not have any of the problems associated with the disease. The March of Dimes recommends that women be tested for immunity to rubella before pregnancy.[44]

Caffeine Content of Your Favorite Beverages and Foods

Drink/Food	Caffeine, in milligrams
Soft Drinks (12 ounces)	
Mountain Dew	54
Mellow Yellow	52
Coke Classic, Cherry Coke, Diet Coke	46
Tab	46
Pepsi Cola	38
Diet Pepsi Light	36
Sprite, 7-Up, Slice, regular or diet	0
Any decaffeinated sodas	0
Coffee	
6 ounces, brewed	103
Instant (1 teaspoon, rounded)	57
Instant, decaffeinated (1 teaspoon, rounded)	2
Coffee Drinks (2 teaspoons, rounded)	
Orange cappuccino	75
Café Amaretto	60
Café Vienna	60
Café Francais	50
Suisse Mocha	40
Dutch Chocolate Mint	30
Viennese Chocolate Café	25
Tea	
6 ounces, brewed 3 minutes	36
Instant tea (1 teaspoon)	31
Herb teas	0
Cocoa Drinks	
Chocolate flavor mix in milk (2–3 heaping teaspoons)	8
Chocolate syrup in milk (2 tablespooons)	6
Hot cocoa (1-ounce packet)	5
Miscellaneous	
1 ounce milk chocolate (Cadbury)	15
¼ cup chocolate chips	12
½ cup Jell-O chocolate pudding	5
Jell-O chocolate pudding pop with chocolate coating	3

Sources: *Food Values of Portions Commonly Used*, 15th edition, by Jean Pennington, and General Foods.

Toxoplasmosis: The parasite that causes toxoplasmosis is passed in cat feces and can also be transmitted in uncooked and undercooked meats and in unwashed fruits and vegetables. (See page 13 for more details.)

Warning: Alcohol Can Cause Birth Defects

"Think before you drink" is a slogan that the March of Dimes has used to remind women of the risk of drinking alcohol when pregnant. Fetal Alcohol Syndrome (FAS) and a variation, Fetal Alcohol Effect (FAE), result in children who are scarred by the drinking habits of their mothers during pregnancy. According to certain estimates, FAE affects as many as 3 percent of all infants, making it the leading known cause of mental retardation and of learning and behavioral problems.[45] Some milder cases of FAE cause irritability, impulsiveness, and learning disabilities and aren't diagnosed for years; many kids affected by FAE end up dropping out of school.

Alcohol is now recognized as a potent teratogen (a substance capable of causing birth defects) that can cause growth retardation (both in the womb and after birth) and facial abnormalities. Chronic alcohol abuse has been defined as more than two drinks per day. One drink per day has been shown to decrease birth weight.[46] Since alcohol freely crosses the placenta, the fetus's blood alcohol level is equal to the mother's. So one drink in a day might not be risky, but a single drinking binge on a critical day of development could damage the fetus.

According to the Public Health Service, as many as 86 percent of women drink once during pregnancy; women with a higher level of education appear to drink more. Some women may be genetically susceptible to having a child with FAS. One study reported that black women are seven times more likely to have a child with the syndrome than white women with the same drinking habits.[47]

The good news is that if you are a drinker, whenever you stop, you increase your chances of having a healthy baby. Women who stopped drinking before their seventh month of pregnancy had healthy babies with no symptoms of FAS.[48]

What about an occasional drink? Research concerning low levels of alcohol consumption is limited and inconsistent. "Because there is no level of drinking that is known to be safe, it is best to completely avoid alcohol during pregnancy," says March of Dimes Medical Director, Richard B. Johnston, M.D. If you have other concerns about alcohol, discuss them with your health care provider.

Caffeine

You may be one of those people who "aren't worth a darn" before their first cup of coffee! The bulk of the research about caffeine and pregnancy shows that moderate consumption (one cup of coffee a day, for example) is probably safe, yet there is some conflicting research. In some studies, caffeine has been linked to miscarriage, growth retardation, and infertility.[49,50,51]

The Food and Drug Administration continues to advise pregnant women to consume caffeine in moderation. Caffeine stimulates the central nervous system, is addictive, acts as a diuretic, and interferes with mineral absorption. The best advice—instead of relying on caffeine, get more sleep and take a brisk afternoon walk for a pick-up! Or if you must have some caffeine, switch to lower-caffeine products and have as little as possible.

About Herbal Preparations and Teas

Many people turn to herb teas to cut their caffeine intake. However, you should stay away from teas containing coltsfoot, sassafras, calamus, or comfrey, all of which are carcinogenic.[52] Many herbal preparations, whether sold as teas or quasi-medications, can act as drugs because they contain natural active chemicals that can be harmful to the fetus. Dr. Varro Tyler, Professor of Pharmacognosy at Purdue University and author of *The Honest Herbal,* advises, "It is best to avoid herbal supplements during pregnancy unless you have expert knowledge about herbs or you are under the care of a physician who is. Because they aren't approved as drugs, herbs don't undergo long-term toxicity testing."

Remember that many of the drugs we use today first came from herbs, flowers, and trees. Exceptions are teas accepted as harmless, such as peppermint, chamomile, and ginger. You should be safe if you stay with name brand herbal and decaffeinated teas.

Drugs—Prescription, Over-the-Counter, and Others

All drugs, legal and illegal, have the potential to seriously harm your baby—even something as seemingly harmless as aspirin. So let your health care provider know if you are regularly taking any kind of drug. Also, ask what is safe to take for a cold, flu, or bad headache. Avoiding all medications is best when pregnant, especially during the first trimester. However, if you must take something, have your health care provider approve it first.

Just because you are pregnant doesn't mean you are immune to headaches, colds, flu, and other problems for which you might ordinarily take medication. You may be on vacation and suddenly have a bad case of hay fever. For these times, have a list of over-the-counter medications that your health care provider has approved.

Cocaine

It has been estimated that over half the people addicted to crack cocaine are women.[53] Three studies done in urban areas showed that between 10 and 17 percent of women registered for prenatal care showed evidence of cocaine use.[54]

Cocaine addiction is, of course, harmful to the mother, but it can also have lifelong effects on a baby. Cocaine may take up to six days to leave the fetal blood supply. This increased exposure to the drug can result in premature separation of the placenta, growth retardation of the fetus, decreased birth weight, length, and head circumference, and premature delivery. Cocaine may also cause miscarriages, birth defects, and increased neurological and behavioral problems that may last a lifetime.[55]

If you are addicted to cocaine or any other drug, seek help through your local health department or drug treatment center. (If you'd like to read further about drugs and pregnancy, I recommend an excellent handbook entitled *Drugs, Vitamins, and Minerals in Pregnancy* by Ann Karen Henry, Pharm. D., and Jil Feldhausen, M.S., R.D., Fisher Books, 1989.)

▼

Traveling during Pregnancy

Chances are that during the nine months of pregnancy, you will travel somewhere. Traveling while pregnant may offer yet another challenge, or it may be "business as usual." Traveling can affect your exercise schedule and the types and amounts of food that you eat.

In the Plane

▶ **Find out whether a meal will be served.**

If you'd like a bit more control over your food on the flight, call the airline at least twenty-four hours before your flight to request a special meal. Some options are low-fat, vegetarian, diabetic, and seafood.

▶ **If you have a layover between flights, use the time to exercise.**

Walk to your gate instead of using moving sidewalks or a bus.

▶ **Bring your own supply of snacks.**

Unless you are flying cross-country or overseas nonstop, you probably won't have a complete meal. And even the airline "meals" can be skimpy. You will need snacks! Bring along fresh or dried fruit, whole-grain or graham crackers, string cheese, granola bars, nuts, and other nonperishable snacks.

▶ **Request an aisle seat so you can get up to walk and stretch or go to the restroom.**

"Bulkhead" seats in the first row offer more leg room.

▶ **If your flight is a long one, such as cross-country or overseas, drink plenty of fluids before and during your flight.**

Flying can dehydrate you. During long flights, avoid carbonated beverages—they can increase gas.

▶ **Get up and walk around several times during the flight.**

Or you may want to go to the back of the plane and just stand or stretch for a while. While sitting down you can do isometric exercises, which can improve circulation.

▶ **Avoid taking heavy carry-on luggage unless someone else can carry it for you.**

The weight can increase back pain.

In the Car

▶ **Bring along a small cooler in which you can keep yogurt, cheese, veggies, milk, fruit, and other snacks.**

You can even bring the makings of a sandwich, which can save you money on restaurant food. If you forget a cooler, you can always stop at a grocery along the way and pick up fresh or dried fruit and ready-to-eat raw vegetables.

▶ **Instead of eating regular-sized meals when you stop, order appetizers, or eat just half a portion.**

Sitting in the car for extended periods of time may induce "boredom eating," although you won't need as many calories while just sitting. Try to limit snacking to when you are actually hungry.

▶ **Drink plenty of fluids.**

If you are traveling to a higher altitude, your fluid needs will increase. Lack of activity can slow down your digestion and increase constipation. "Pit stops" will allow you to get out and stretch, which can prevent back pain and increase circulation.

▶ **Plan "adventure stops."**

Try to include enough time in your itinerary to make extended stops to see something of interest. Use the stops as your exercise time to walk and stretch.

At Your Destination

▶ **If you are staying at a hotel, try to get a room with a mini-fridge or kitchenette.**

You can keep your own snack foods as well as high-fiber cereals for breakfast or snacks.

▶ **Try to make wise food choices when eating out.**

When people eat most meals out, diets tend to be lower in fiber, calcium, vitamin C, and folacin, and higher in fat and sodium.[56] (See page 201 for advice on eating out.)

▶ **If you are staying with friends or relatives,**

take with you a few of the foods you usually eat, such as high-fiber cereal, milk, and extra fresh or dried fruit.

This way your diet won't be lacking and you won't be embarrassed about asking your host to buy special foods for you.

▶ **Make sure you pack nonperishable snacks in your bag for those hectic tourist schedules.**

Good snacks are cheese or peanut butter crackers, boxes of raisins, wheat crackers, fiber bars, apples or bananas, and individual bags of pretzels. Don't forget to drink! Juice boxes pack well.

▶ **If you are traveling to a foreign country, talk to your physician before making your reservations.**

Vaccinations may normally be required that you can't take while pregnant. Or you may need to eat especially carefully to avoid bacterial poisoning or "turista." You may want to take some nonperishable foods with you to snack on if familiar foods aren't available where you are going, or if food safety may be an issue. A friend of mine who went to an Asian country lived on peanuts and beer because those were the only foods she felt were safe. Thankfully, she wasn't pregnant.

The Positives of Pregnancy

Although most people are familiar with only the negatives of pregnancy, pregnancy also has many positive aspects. For example, some women feel at their best when they're pregnant. And some women with chronic medical problems go into remission or have decreased symptoms. By concentrating on the good things that occur during these nine months, life will be a lot more pleasant. Here are just a few of the good things about being pregnant. Try to think of them often!

- Thick shiny hair.
- That warm, healthy glow of pregnancy.
- People open the door for you.
- Finally, a larger bra size!
- Weight gain without guilt!
- You don't have to tuck in your blouses.
- You have an excuse now for being tired.
- You feel great all over.
- You feel good about taking care of yourself.
- You have a great reason for starting a walking program and for eating right.
- You are the designated driver for the next nine months.
- Your husband brings you breakfast (or lunch or dinner) in bed.
- You're too tired to clean house–a good excuse to hire a cleaning service!
- Finally, a long vacation to look forward to (maternity leave).
- Your other kids learn how to help around the house.
- The love for your yet-to-be-born baby abounds.
- You don't have to worry about forgetting your birth control pill.
- You can wear "one-size-fits-all" clothes.
- You will become a member of "Universal Motherhood" clan.
- You are part of a miracle.
- You have a special new friend living close by.
- This is an experience you have only once or several times in your life, so enjoy it!

CHAPTER THREE

The First Trimester

This chapter answers such questions as:

• *How much weight should I gain?*
• *I've read that I should eat one hundred grams of protein; how much is that?*
• *How much protein is in an egg?*
• *How else can I get protein in my diet if I don't feel like eating meat?*
• *What can I do about morning sickness?*
• *How can I avoid constipation?*

Morning Sickness– Myths and Miseries

Before you can even think about eating, you may need to think about surviving the day. A touch of the "queasies" may give you the first clue that you are pregnant. Here are some facts and fallacies:

• You are not alone. Morning sickness is the greatest reported problem of pregnancy, occurring in 50 to 90 percent of pregnancies. About 1.5 percent of women with morning sickness have such severe symptoms that they must be hospitalized.
• Contrary to the name, morning sickness can happen any time of the day or night, and often does.
• According to Miriam Erick, M.S., R.D., author of *No More Morning Sickness, A Survival Guide for Pregnant Women*, the biggest myths about morning sickness are:
  –"By the first trimester it will go away."
  (Average duration: 17.5 weeks.)
  –"It's all in your head." *(It's not.)*
  –"It's only in the morning." *(For some, it's all day.)*

No one really knows what causes morning sickness–the current ten theories range from raging hormones to fetal/placental enzymes to hormonal-heightened sense of smell! Regardless of what causes it, you need to know what you can do about it! Here are some tips summarized from *No More Morning Sickness*.[1]

▶ **Trust your own intuition.**

Ask yourself–what would make you feel better? Something sweet, salty, sour, crunchy, soft, bland, wet, etc.? No matter how bizarre or atypical the food you conjure up sounds–it might just do the trick.

Believe it or not, potato chips are often that food. According to Miriam, "I'm not sure why–it could be the nutrient profile, the taste, the smell, or the mouth-feel."

Watermelon is another food that often sounds good–and it provides essential fluids. You may find "eating" your fluids more appealing than drinking them–that is, eating solid foods that have a high water content, such as melon, grapes, popsicles, etc.

▶ It's not in your head, it's in your nose.

Odors may be the trigger that is causing your nausea. When you feel queasy, take inventory of your surroundings. Smells are everywhere, as pregnant women with enhanced senses of smell know. Body odors, cooking odors, mold, mildew, air fresh-eners, burnt coffee, cologne, detergent, and so on. Getting away from odors is virtually impossible, which can be a prob-lem if odors make you turn "green". Miriam recommends tracking your environment, in-cluding keeping a "score" of how you feel, level of smells, amount of motion, noise, preferred taste and texture of food eaten, and the time. Hopefully, this will open your eyes to some environ-mental situations that you can change.

▶ Set out to change your environment as much as possible.

Often you won't be able to con-trol the smells around you–cigarette smoke from the car in front of you or the smell of Greek food coming from next door. But do try to control your environ-ment (to the point of moving out of your environment temporari-ly) as much as possible.

▶ Drink enough fluids.

"Fluids are the most necessary nutrients and the hardest to get in," says Miriam. Most women need ten cups of fluid a day. Dehydration from any cause (even severe morning sickness) is potentially fatal, which is why women with severe morning sickness are often hospitalized for intravenous rehydration.

▶ When life gives you lemons, make lemonade!

Miriam has had good luck with using lemon–as a way to mask other smells and to help keep food down. "No one really knows why lemon works. Smells really do communicate–bad ones can make people nauseous and good smells can really increase people's sense of well-being," advises Miriam.

▶ Rest assured that morning sickness does not indicate something is wrong with your baby.

On the contrary, women who have morning sickness have lower risk of miscarriage and, unless they lose a significant amount of weight as a result of morning sickness, their risk of having a baby that is low birth weight or has birth defects is not higher than average.

▼

The Eating Expectantly Diet

10 or more servings of starches/grains

1 serving is 1 slice of any type bread, 1 flour tortilla, ½ cup pasta, ⅓ cup rice or legumes, 6 crackers, or ½ cup of potato.

3 to 4 or more servings of fruit

1 serving is 1 medium piece of fresh fruit, ½ banana, ½ cup canned fruit in its own juice, 1 cup melon or berries, or 2 plums or nectarines.

3 to 4 or more servings of vegetables

1 serving is ½ cup of any cooked nonstarchy vegetable or 1 cup of lettuce.

Note: Be sure to include at least one fruit or vegetable that is a good source of vitamin A and one serving that is high in vitamin C.

6 or more ounces of protein or equivalent

1 protein equivalent is 1 ounce of lean meat, 1 ounce reduced-fat cheese, ¼ cup cottage cheese, ½ cup of tofu, 2 tablespoons peanut butter, ½ cup cooked dried beans, or 1 egg.

Note: Increase your protein intake one ounce for each serving of milk that you don't drink.

4 or more servings of dairy products

1 serving is 1 cup of any type milk or yogurt, preferably skim or low fat.

3 to 5 or more servings of fat

1 serving is 1 teaspoon margarine or butter or 2 teaspoons reduced-fat margarine, 1 teaspoon mayonnaise or 2 teaspoons reduced-fat mayonnaise, 1 slice bacon, ½ ounce cream cheese, 1 tablespoon sour cream, ⅛ avocado, 10 peanuts, or 5 olives.

And here is an example of a "real" meal plan:

Breakfast

Raisin bran cereal with strawberries
Whole-wheat bagel with light cream cheese
Milk

Snack

Vegetable juice
Whole-grain crackers
Low-fat string cheese

Lunch

Lean roast beef sandwich on wheat bread
Raw carrots and broccoli with dip
Melon balls
Sugar cookies
Milk

Snack

Popcorn

Dinner

Grilled salmon steak
Grilled corn on the cob
Spinach salad with tomato and mushrooms
Whole-grain roll
Fresh orange
Milk

Snack

Peanut butter and graham crackers
Yogurt with dried fruit

▼

Weight Gain/ Energy Needs

Are you one of those people who received a "special license to eat" because you are pregnant? Well your license was just revoked because "eating for two" is a bit of a misnomer. You do need larger amounts of many nutrients during pregnancy, but you don't need to eat twice the food and calories, especially in the first trimester.

The Subcommittee on Nutritional Status and Weight Gain During Pregnancy of the National Academy of Sciences recommends that you gain about a pound (or less) per month during the first trimester. That translates into 135 extra calories (or less) per day.[2] Uh oh, there go the visions of dancing chocolate sundaes in your head! Later in this chapter we'll talk about how to make your diet a winner without gaining too much weight!

▼

Protein Needs

Protein is essential during pregnancy because your body uses it to build each new cell for your baby. It is also needed for the placenta—the lifeline that brings nourishment from you to your baby. Protein helps make new blood cells and muscle tissue that supports your baby. To top it all off, protein is used to make all the hormones that are playing havoc in your body right now!

In the first trimester, your protein needs don't increase very much—only about 1⅙ grams extra each day, or the equivalent of ⅙ of an ounce of meat. The RDA

Protein Content of Food Groups		
Food	Serving sizes	Protein per serving, in grams
Dairy products	1 cup milk/ 1 ounce cheese	6–8
Legumes	½ cup	7–11
Meat, poultry, fish	1 ounce	6–8
Vegetables	½ cup	2–3
Fruits/juices	1 medium/½ cup	0–1
Bread/cereal	1 slice/1 ounce	2–4
Fat, oil	any amount	0

for protein throughout pregnancy is 10 grams higher than nonpregnant needs, or 60 grams per day.[3] The additional protein you need is equal to 1½ ounces of animal protein, 1¼ cups of legumes, 1½ eggs, or 1¼ ounces of cheese.

Several factors influence your body's protein needs. Most importantly, for your body to use the protein you eat for building tissues and cells, you must eat enough calories (energy). This is because your body's first priority is supplying energy. Thus, if you eat enough protein, but not enough calories, your body will use the protein for energy instead of for building tissues and other protein-dependent functions. For example, let's say you eat ten ounces of fish and chicken every day. You don't have much of an appetite so this fills you up and you don't eat much else, making your calorie intake from fats and carbohy-

drates inadequate. Because your body must use the protein for energy, your body will be deficient in the protein it needs for other important purposes.

Also, you won't have enough glucose (blood sugar) to supply your brain with energy, so your body will start breaking down fat into fragments called ketones. The presence of ketones is a sign that your body can't complete the metabolic process. If made in large amounts (usually only in diabetics) ketones can be harmful to your body. Avoid the production of ketones by having enough calories and carbohydrates in your diet.

However, consuming a certain *quantity* of protein is not the only goal. The *quality* of protein also affects your body's use of it. Protein needs are calculated by determining the need for high biological value, or high-quality, protein. High-quality protein

can be turned into body tissues. Examples are eggs, meat, chicken, milk, or fish. For all the bad press the egg has gotten over the years, it is well respected in this area. The egg's protein is of the highest quality and is often used as a standard to which other proteins are compared.

If you do not eat animal products, your body will need greater quantities of lower-quality plant proteins to meet protein needs. Vegetarians don't despair! You can meet your protein needs without eating meat, though you must look carefully at your intake of certain nutrients. (See page 81 for more information on vegetarian sources of protein.)

As a rule, Americans eat about twice as much protein as they really need. Pregnant women are no different, eating an average of 75 to 110 grams per day—well above the 60 grams per day recommended by the Food and Nutrition Board. However, some health care providers and birthing programs recommend up to 100 grams of protein, especially for high-risk pregnancies. A diet that contains approximately 100 grams of protein would, for example, contain 4 servings of dairy product, 6 ounces of animal protein (or the equivalent), 3 vegetables, 2 fruits, and 8 servings of starch or bread.

If you are similar to most of us, you won't have a problem meeting protein needs. In fact, the National Academy of Sciences advises pregnant women not to use specially formulated high-protein supplements, protein powders, or high-protein beverages because some evidence suggests possible harm from using these supplementary protein products.[4]

Why You May Need to "Work" to Meet Your Protein Needs

You might not be able to meet your protein needs if you:

- don't drink milk or eat dairy products and also don't eat many other protein sources.
- have nausea or vomiting that prevents you from eating much of anything.
- just don't have the desire to eat meat.

If you eat or drink the recommended four servings of dairy products each day, you will be meeting half your protein needs. If you don't, you'll need to increase protein from other sources.

If you just don't feel like eating meat, you are not alone. Most women have some food aversion; some stomachs turn at the thought of eating what used to be their favorite food.

If your favorite high-protein foods turn your stomach off, you can eat more dairy products,

which are also good sources of protein, or you can turn to other sources. Many of the women I've talked to could tolerate eggs and cheese well, even if they couldn't eat meat. You may also easily tolerate many vegetarian sources of protein. (See page 56 for a list of vegetarian sources of protein.) Experiment with what works for you.

If you can't eat much of anything due to first-trimester morning sickness, eat what you can. (See Chapter Thirteen for first-trimester recipes.)

If the condition persists to the point that you are losing weight, alert your health care provider, who may want to treat your nausea more aggressively, or may refer you to a registered dietitian for individual counseling.

Other Nutrient Needs

All vitamins and minerals have specific and essential roles during pregnancy, so be sure to have adequate amounts of all in your diet. Water is one of the most important nutrients in the first trimester—especially if you are suffering from morning sickness. Dehydration can be very serious! Folate is not only important in neural development, but

is also critical for cell production and division, which occur at leaps and bounds during the first trimester. Manganese is needed for developing the organs for hearing. Vitamin A is needed for developing tissues. A low intake of zinc early in pregnancy is related to a threefold increase in the risk of very preterm delivery.[5] Phosphorus, calcium, and vitamin D work together to produce a strong skeleton.

Focus on Fiber

After "low-fat," "high-fiber" may be the catch word of the nineties. Fiber is one of those things most people don't have enough of, even though every day new studies cite its benefits.

The old saying "An apple a day keeps the doctor away" may well relate to an apple's fiber content. Here's why:

- Adequate fiber is linked with reduced risk of colon, rectal, endometrial, and breast cancer.[6]
- Soluble fiber has been shown to reduce cholesterol, thus reducing risk of heart disease. Trace minerals and antioxidants in whole grains may also be beneficial in cutting heart disease risk.

• Soluble fiber also helps control blood glucose, which is particularly beneficial to people with diabetes.[7]
• Fiber fills you up, not out!
• Fiber keeps your bowels moving, which can help prevent constipation and hemorrhoids.

Eating Your Oats and Bran

Before we get into the specifics of fiber, following are a few simple ways to make sure you get enough fiber every day:

▶ **Follow the National Cancer Institute's slogan "Five a Day for Better Health."**

You'll be on your way to having adequate dietary fiber if you eat five fruits and vegetables daily.

▶ **Choose whole-wheat bread, crackers, and pasta.**

The American Dietetic Association supports the recommendation of three servings of whole-grain products daily.[8] Look at the label—"whole grain" or "whole-wheat flour" should be the first ingredient.

▶ **Eat brown rice, bulgur, or quinoa instead of white rice.**

▶ **Start your day with a high-fiber cereal.**

Choose cereals containing at least five grams of fiber per serving.

▶ **When baking, replace part of the white flour with wheat bran, whole-wheat flour, or oatmeal.**

▶ **Snack on other high-fiber foods such as bran muffins, dried fruit, fresh fruit, vegetables, and whole-grain crackers.**

Note: If your diet is normally low in fiber, make sure to increase the fiber in your diet gradually. Adding a lot of fiber to your meals all at once can result in bloating and gas. Also, remember to drink plenty of fluids while eating high-fiber foods, or the extra fiber might make matters worse.

If you follow the advice above, you will be sure to get the twenty to thirty-five grams of fiber currently recommended by the National Cancer Institute.[9] But if you want to be really aware of the specific amounts of fiber found in foods, look at the chart on page 49.

Snack Tip:

The fig may be the best-kept nutrition secret! Not only do figs have the highest amount of dietary fiber of any common fruit, nut, or vegetable, they are also higher in potassium than bananas and are considered a good calcium source! Pack this sweet and healthy treat as a between-meal snack.

Stuffed Figs

Make a large slice in fresh or dried fig. Fill with low-fat or fat-free cream cheese, or puree cottage cheese in the blender until it's the consistency of cream cheese. You can flavor the cheese with cinnamon or nutmeg for more flavor.

First-Trimester Challenges

Nausea or Morning Sickness

Following are some traditional tips for beating morning sickness. (See page 43 for more tips.)

Fiber Content of Foods

Fruits

Food	Serving sizes	Dietary fiber, in grams*
Figs	5	12
Prunes	5	8
Blackberries, canned (solid and liquid)	½ cup	7
Raspberries, fresh	½ cup	5
Dates	5	4
Pear, fresh with skin	1	4
Nectarine, fresh	1	3
Orange, fresh	1	3
Raisins	¼ cup	2
Pineapple, fresh	2 slices	2
Strawberries	½ cup	2

Most other fruits contain 1–3 grams of fiber per serving.

Vegetables

Food	Serving sizes	Dietary fiber, in grams*
Spinach, cooked, drained	½ cup	6
Corn, canned	½ cup	5
Broccoli, cooked, chopped	½ cup	4
Sweet potato, baked in skin	1 medium	3–5
Rhubarb, cooked	½ cup	3
Tomato, fresh	1 medium	2
Carrots, cooked	½ cup	2

Cereals, Grains, and Legumes

Food	Serving sizes	Dietary fiber, in grams*
Baked beans, canned	½ cup	6–8
Wheat bran, unprocessed	¼ cup	7
Refried pinto beans, canned	½ cup	5
Barley, light pearled	½ cup	4
Black beans	½ cup	4
Aunt Jemima whole-grain wheat frozen waffle	1 waffle	3
Corn tortilla	2	3
Bran muffin	1	2–5
Whole-wheat bread	1 slice	1–2
Rye crisp	¼ of large square	2
Brown rice, cooked, instant	½ cup	2
Popcorn	3½ cups	1
White rice, cooked	½ cup	1

*Numbers rounded off to the nearest whole number.

Sources: *Nutrients in Foods*, by Leveille, Zabik, and Morgan, 1983, *The Complete Book of Food Counts*, by Corrine Netzer, 1991, and manufacturer's labels.

What you can do:

▶ **Get up slowly when you awake in the morning.**

▶ **Have a snack before breakfast.**

A dry "prebreakfast" snack sometimes helps prevent nausea. You can leave food beside your bed at night, or let the father-to-be get involved and serve you "what sounds good" in bed. (This is a good habit to get into!) Many women feel better if they eat before they ever lift their head off the pillow!

▶ **Avoid getting very hungry.**

Eat small frequent meals with snacks in between, especially snacks that contain protein, to keep your stomach from being completely empty. You may need to eat as often as every hour to keep nausea at bay. (See page 217 for creative snack ideas.)

▶ **Have your partner do the cooking and use that time to go for a walk or take a catnap.**

This will help you avoid cooking odors and can give you time to do other important things. To cut down on cooking smells, you might want to consider getting "take-out" food from a restaurant that offers healthy choices. You might also want to eat on the patio or take a dinner "pic-nic" to the park to stay clear of indoor cooking fumes.

Note: If your nausea or vomiting becomes severe, notify your health care provider. Never take any medications without approval.

▶ **Drink fluids between, not with, meals.**

To avoid dehydration, you must not forget to drink, especially if you are vomiting. A way to improve your fluid intake is to make fluid more appealing; disguise it as Jell-O, broth, popsicles or frozen juice bars, slushy drinks, and fluid-packed fruits such as watermelon, frozen grapes, and frozen melon balls.

▶ **Avoid greasy, fried, highly seasoned foods, and any foods with an unpleasant or strong smell.**

Some women find cold, somewhat bland foods more appealing at this time.

Frequent Urination

In those first few months, you might feel as though you're making a path in the carpet to the bathroom! The increased frequency of your trips may give you the first hint that you're pregnant. Your baby, within the uterus, sits right above your blad-der. As your uterus engorges with blood and as the baby grows, the pressure on your bladder increases, while the space for storing urine decreases.

What you can do:

▶ **DON'T decrease your total fluid intake!**

However, if you're getting up several times during the night to use the restroom, you might want to slightly decrease your intake of fluids in the evening.

▶ **Sleep on your side.**

Lying on one side may help relieve pressure on the bladder.

▶ **Start doing Kegel exercises now and continue during and after your pregnancy.**

These exercises tone up the muscles that "hold in" urine. Have you ever sneezed or coughed and felt as though you nearly emptied your bladder? This can happen more frequently during the third trimester and again later in life. The weakened bladder control may be due to poor muscle tone in the area, along with added pressure from baby. Keeping these muscles toned during pregnancy can really help you get back in shape and heal more quickly after you have the baby. Ask your health care provider or childbirth educator for more information.

Note: If urination is painful, contact your health care provider.

Fatigue

You may feel as though you could sleep for the rest of your pregnancy. During the first trimester, when your hormones are playing tag and you're "it," fatigue is common.

What you can do:

▶ **Accept your need for rest and slow down your lifestyle.**

▶ **Eat regular, balanced meals that are high in the essential nutrients.**

If you're not eating enough calories or not getting enough essential nutrients, your diet could be partly to blame for the fatigue. (See page 27 for more information on essential vitamins and minerals.) During the first trimester, your health care provider will probably check the amount of iron in your blood. Iron-deficiency anemia can cause fatigue and is fairly common in pregnancy due to the greatly increased need for the mineral. Consuming adequate amounts of dietary iron before and during pregnancy can prevent anemia. (See pages 61–62 for good sources of iron.)

▶ **Exercise regularly.**

Even though you may not feel you have the energy to exercise, afterward you'll be glad you did. (See Chapter Ten, Fitting Fitness In.)

Cravings and Aversions

We've all seen and heard those stories about the husband who runs to the 7-Eleven in the middle of the night to get his wife a pint of Häagen-Dazs chocolate fudge ice cream. Now you may be experiencing something similar. No one is sure what causes cravings. Sometimes, a craving signals a dietary need. (Well, we don't have an RDA for chocolate fudge ice cream, yet!) For example, some women crave a nonfood item such as clay, starch, dirt, or ice. This particular type of craving, called pica, usually stems from an iron deficiency. Other cravings may just be due to—you guessed it—those crazy, mixed-up hormones of yours.

Cravings for sweets can be explained by drops in the blood sugar level, which can easily happen if you don't eat often enough. In that case, your body needs any carbohydrate food and you may, for example, turn the need into a "craving" for your favorite high-carbohydrate food such as ice cream or refried beans.

On the other hand, cravings can often be good. I'm generally not a grapefruit eater, but when pregnant with my second child, I asked for grapefruit frequently. I also often wanted a "stick-to-your-rib" food, such as a bean burrito or hamburger. This may have been just a need for more calories or protein.

Aversions to certain foods are just as common as cravings, so don't be surprised if your favorite food now turns your taste buds off. Sometimes an aversion acts as a protective factor to something that would be harmful to the baby, such as cigarettes or alcohol. Animal flesh is often not appealing during pregnancy. Eggs, cheese, milk, and beans are often more easy to tolerate. (See Chapter Six for more vegetarian eating tips.)

Whatever your particular fancy, rest assured it will probably change within your pregnancy and will be different with your next pregnancy!

What you can do:

▶ **To keep cravings in check, make sure to eat regular meals and snacks, including breakfast.**

▶ **If you *must* have something, then have it!**

If the craved-for food is less than nutritious, try to eat a small amount. Or try to steer your craving toward a healthier alternative—such as a whole-wheat raisin bagel instead of a donut.

Breast Changes

Often, breast enlargement and sensitivity are another of the first noticeable changes in pregnancy. In this first trimester, the fat layer of your breast is thickening and the number of milk glands is increasing. The veins close to the surface become larger due to the increase in blood flow within your body. Your nipples and areolas (the dark areas around your nipples) will enlarge and probably get darker.

What you can do:

▶ **Find a good supportive bra, preferably one with flexible straps.**

If you plan to breast-feed, you may find that a nursing bra suits your needs now and later.

▶ **If you are large-busted, you might want to sleep in a lightweight bra.**

Teeth and Gum Changes

Hormones and increased blood flow affect many areas of your

body, including your gums. They can soften and become more prone to developing gum infections.

What you can do:

▶ **Eat a balanced diet that contains plenty of vitamin C.**

Good nutrition is the first defense against gum disease.

▶ **Don't neglect teeth and gums during pregnancy.**

Continue regular flossing, brushing, and professional cleaning. Have a dental checkup during your pregnancy. However, be sure your dentist knows that you are pregnant before your visit.

Note: If you are planning a pregnancy, visit your dentist first for a checkup and for any dental work that might be needed.

▼

How Baby Is Growing

In the first three months, good nutrition is vital for your baby's development. Babies born to poorly nourished mothers are more susceptible to infections in early life and to birth defects. Many miraculous events are taking place within your body in just twelve weeks.

At the End of One Week

For the first seven days after the sperm fertilizes the egg, the group of cells (called a "zygote") is traveling down the fallopian tube toward the uterus. Although the zygote is no larger than the tiniest speck of sand, it carries all the genetic material (DNA) necessary for development. The zygote implants in the uterine wall seven to eight days after fertilization; then it is known as an "embryo."

During the first week, the cells are rapidly dividing into what will become organs, skin, hair, bones, and muscle. Even though the DNA and cells "know" the sex of the baby, genital formation does not take place yet, so we refer to the baby as "it."

The mass of cells that includes the embryo and that which will become the placenta is only about the size of a blueberry.

At the End of Four Weeks (One Month)

By this time, you may be confirming your pregnancy and may be experiencing some of the telltale signs. The embryo is no bigger than a grain of rice, and its heart is beating by the twenty-fifth day. The digestive system, backbone, and spinal cord are all beginning to form. Tiny limb buds are appearing, which will become the arms and legs. The next four weeks are

vitally important as development rapidly occurs.

At the End of Eight Weeks (Two Months)

The embryo is now about the size of your big toe, or a little over one inch long. All the major organs and systems are formed, yet some are not completely developed. The embryo clearly looks like a human. The long arm and leg bones are beginning to form and are visible under the embryo's thin skin. The brain has taken shape and the head makes up almost half of the embryo. The embryo now has a face. The embryo weighs only a quarter of an ounce!

At the End of Twelve Weeks (Three Months)

From the ninth week on, the embryo is now called a "fetus." The nails are developed and the fetus can suck its fingers and curl its hands into a fist. The kidneys are beginning to form urine and the tooth buds for all the baby teeth are appearing. The fetus is only about as long as your middle finger (three inches long) and weighs about one-and-a-half ounces.

Although you may be just starting to buy maternity clothes or to adjust your belt to the next notch, most of your baby's organs and tissues are already formed.

❓ Questions You May Have

Q: What if I skip meals— is that bad for the baby?

A: Yes, and for you too! During pregnancy, your baby depends entirely on you for energy. When you don't eat, your baby may not have the energy and nutrients it needs and will use up your own nutrient stores, which may leave you depleted. When you skip meals, you often eat much more food later to make up for it, and you may store those extra calories as fat. Try to avoid the "Feast or Famine" approach by taking the time to eat regular meals and snacks.

Q: I usually eat fast food for lunch every day. How can I eat more nutritiously?

A: Planning ahead and taking the time to shop and cook is the solution for too many meals eaten on the run. Eating "typical" fast food is costly–both in dollars and to your diet. Fast food provides lots of calories, but not too many nutrients. To improve on a typical fast-food meal, have fruit with it. On the other hand, fast food is improving, and eating nutritiously is getting easier, even when eating on the run. (See page 280 for "Meals in Minutes," and page 203 for "The Most Nutritious Fast Foods.")

Q: What if I just can't eat much at all? My "morning sickness" occurs all the time.

A: As noted earlier, extra calories aren't a priority in the first trimester. What is important is keeping your baby's environment safe, having an adequate intake of folic acid, and keeping well hydrated. Eat whatever you can to get through your nausea and make sure to drink plenty of fluids. The baby will draw on your stored nutrients if you aren't able to eat much. However, make your calories count. When you *are* able to eat, eat the most nutritious foods you can, and when your morning sickness has subsided, eat well to restock your body's nutrient stores.

▼ First-Trimester Menus

The menus and recipes in Chapter Thirteen were designed for the first trimester: the time in your pregnancy when eating can present the biggest problem. So, the menus are practical and realistic for what you may face.

Menus:

- Don't Feel Like Eating
- Don't Feel Like Cooking
- Don't Feel Like Eating or Cooking
- Feel Like Staying in Bed, but Can't
- Feel Great
- Blender Breakfasts (or, Snacks-to-Go)
- Snack Ideas
- High-Energy Mom Snack Ideas

The Second Trimester

You made it through the first trimester–congratulations! The second trimester includes the thirteenth through the twenty-sixth week and is usually when most women feel their best. During this time, you'll have lots of energy, especially if you're eating right and exercising. You'll mark the halfway point of your pregnancy and you'll feel your baby move!

Weight Gain/Energy Needs

During the last two trimesters of your pregnancy your body needs about three hundred more calories per day than you ate before you were pregnant. Eating at this level will result in a twenty-five- to thirty-five-pound weight gain–considered optimal for a healthy baby. However, many things will affect your energy needs, including prepregnant weight, activity level, and current weight. Some women are less active during the last half of pregnancy; others remain active and burn even more calories due to their increasing weight.

From now on, you should try to gain about one pound per week.[1] Remember that much of the extra calories and protein you are eating is working towards creating a healthy environment for your baby to live in until birth. The extra nutrients are required for increased blood volume, increase in placenta size, increase in fat storage, increase in breast tissue, and production of amniotic fluid. In addition, nutrients provide the building materials for your growing fetus!

In the next few weeks–usually between sixteen and twenty weeks gestation–you should feel a small fluttering in your uterus: this is your baby moving! It's a very exciting feeling and also a good reminder that during these special months you must take good care of yourself by eating right, exercising moderately, and trying to improve other lifestyle habits.

Protein Content of Common Foods

The RDA for pregnancy is 60 grams; for breastfeeding, 65 grams.[3]

Complete protein foods

Food	Serving sizes	Protein, in grams*
Beef, chuck arm roast	3 ounces	28
Pork, center loin	3 ounces	27
Turkey	3 ounces	27
Chicken breast	3 ounces	26
Flounder	3 ounces	25
Tuna fish, canned, drained	3 ounces	24
Beef, lean, ground	3 ounces	22
Scallops	3 ounces	16
Cottage cheese	½ cup	15
Ham	3 ounces	15
Eggs	2 large	12
Shrimp	3 ounces	11
Yogurt	1 cup	8
Milk, any type	1 cup	8
Cheddar cheese	1 ounce	7
Hormel Light & Lean hot dog	1	6
Frankfurter, beef	1	5
Quinoa (a high-quality grain)	½ cup	4

Incomplete protein foods

Food	Serving sizes	Protein, in grams*
Lentils, cooked	1 cup	18
Vegetarian chili, canned	⅔ cup	11
Tofu	½ cup	10
Turkee Slices (Worthington)	2 slices	9
Split pea soup	1 cup	9
Green peas	1 cup	9
Bulgur, cooked	1 cup	8
Peanut butter	2 tablespoons	8
Vega Link (Worthington)	2	8
Egg noodles	1 cup	7
Soy milk	1 cup	7
Brown rice, cooked	1 cup	5
White rice, cooked	1 cup	4
Bread, whole-wheat	1 slice	3

*Numbers rounded off to nearest whole number

Sources: *Value of Foods Commonly Used*, 15th edition, by Jean Pennington, *The Complete Book of Food Counts*, by Corrine T. Netzer, and manufacturer labels.

Now is a good time to take a personal inventory of diet and health habits. Later in this chapter you will find a diet and health survey and you will also find a few more in this book to help keep you on your toes!

▼

Protein Needs

Protein is very important during the second trimester for the growing tissue of the fetus and placenta, your expanding blood volume, as well as the growing breast and uterine tissues in your body.

All protein is not equal. Proteins are made of amino acids and, to be used most efficiently, all the essential amino acids must be present in a food in certain amounts and proportions. The term "complete protein" describes protein that has all the "essential" amino acids (amino acids that your body can't produce) in the amounts needed to build proteins. "Incomplete proteins" are missing one or more amino acids or they have small amounts of amino acids. This distinction is important for people who don't eat animal protein. In the past, we believed that we needed to "combine" incomplete proteins during the same meal to have all the needed amino acids. Now, we know that eating a variety of different protein sources through- out the day is adequate.[2]

Examples of foods that contain complete protein include beef, poultry, fish, milk, eggs, and cheese. Foods considered incomplete-protein sources include beans, rice, grains, peanut butter, nuts, pasta, and some vegetables. (Fruit contains very small amounts of protein.) Various protein sources supply different nutrients, so eat a variety of foods, both those that contain complete protein and those that contain incomplete protein. Even if you are not vegetarian, I encourage you to have more nonanimal protein sources, especially soy. Consider eating one or two meatless meals per week.

If you just aren't much of a meat eater, you can eat smaller amounts of the higher-protein meats or eat more vegetable sources of protein. (See Chapter Six, Vegetarian Eating, for more information.)

Other Nutrient Needs

Iron is important because the fetus will start storing iron for the future and you continue to need more iron for increased blood volume. Your body needs

potassium for nerve impulse transmission. If you vomited a lot during the first trimester, your body may be depleted of potassium. Vitamin C is necessary to produce collagen, a binding substance used in muscle, blood vessels, and nerves. Chromium is a trace mineral used in regulation of blood sugar. Inadequate intake may contribute to gestational diabetes, which often occurs during the second trimester.

The Power of Soy

Soy may just be the "health food" of the nineties. Several components of soy—protein, fiber, and phytochemicals (plant substances that are biologically active)—appear to have various benefits:

- Regular consumption of soy foods is linked to reduced risk of breast and rectal cancer.
- Soy protein seems to significantly lower serum cholesterol, LDL cholesterol, and triglycerides.[4] Soy-protein-based diet also significantly lowered cholesterol in children who had hereditary-type high cholesterol.[5] So, if high cholesterol runs in your

family, eating soy regularly could be helpful to keep your cholesterol level under control.

- Eating soy protein instead of animal protein may affect how much calcium is lost from bones—an important consideration for those who have such risk factors for osteoporosis as family history of osteoporosis and fair skin.[6]

So how do you get soy into your diet? First, leave all preconceived ideas about tofu behind. Tofu is a bit like plain yogurt—it hasn't a lot of taste on its own. However, tofu will pick up any flavor you decide to give it. TVP, or textured vegetable protein, is dehydrated and is a good substitute for hamburger in sloppy Joes, chilies, and soups. Be creative and try some soy in your diet! (See Chapter Six, Vegetarian Eating, and Chapter Fifteen, Menus and Recipes for the Third Trimester, for more ideas.)

Focus on Calcium

Calcium is a vital mineral for your baby's bone development. Unfortunately, it's a mineral that adults often delete from their diet when they cut down on dairy products. Although the RDA is 1,200 milligrams,[7] a recent National Institute of Health Consensus Conference on calcium intake recently recommended an intake range of 1,200 to 1,500 milligrams per day; four to five cups of milk contain this amount. Milk and dairy products also provide such important nutrients as protein, magnesium, vitamin D, and riboflavin. If you don't use dairy products, you should eat high-calcium vegetables—but you'll have to eat a lot of them! You should try to get your calcium from food first, before considering supplements.

Calcium Content of Foods and Beverages

The RDA for pregnancy and breastfeeding is 1,200 milligrams.

Animal Sources

Food	Serving sizes*	Calcium, in milligrams
Carnation Instant Breakfast, strawberry	1 serving with 1 cup 1% milk	500
McDonald's low-fat milkshake	1	350
Yogurt, fruit flavored, with nonfat dry milk	1 cup	314
Alba chocolate-flavored milk drink	1 cup	310
Low-fat milk, 1% fat	1 cup	300
Lactaid milk	1 cup	300
Frosty frozen dessert	small	300
Cheese pizza	2 slices	290
Whole milk, 3½% fat	1 cup	288
Buttermilk, cultured	1 cup	285
Chocolate milk, 2% fat	1 cup	284
Swiss cheese	1 ounce	272
Taco	1	200
Cheddar cheese	1 ounce	204
Macaroni and cheese	1 cup	200
Taco Bell Beefy Tostada	1	200
Cottage cheese, 2% fat	1 cup	155
Salmon, canned with bones	3 ounces	124
American cheese, processed	1 ounce	124
McDonald's frozen yogurt cone	1 cone	100

*1 cup = 8 ounces

Source: *Food Values of Portions Commonly Used*, 15th edition, by Jean Pennington.

(See page 226 for fast foods highest in calcium.)

Twelve Ways to Sneak Calcium into Your Diet

If you don't like milk, the following foods or recipes contain good sources of calcium, yet they don't taste like milk. If you think creatively, you can sneak calcium into your diet in dozens of ways. Here are just a few ways to increase the calcium in your diet. Recipes marked with an asterisk (*) and page number indicate the location of the recipe later in the book.

1. Make creamy soups (home-made or canned) with milk or evaporated milk.

2. Use evaporated milk (which has twice the calcium) when preparing such food as mashed potatoes, pudding, cream sauces, etc.

3. Eat dairy-based desserts such as pudding, frozen yogurt, milkshakes, and Berry Mousse Parfait* (page 273).

4. Add reduced-fat or fat-free cheese to your mashed potatoes, vegetables, pasta, sandwiches, and sauces. Instead of meat, use low-fat cheese or tofu made with calcium in your lasagna or Spinach-Stuffed Shells* (page 314).

5. Eat more corn tortillas! A meal of two bean tostadas contain almost four hundred milligrams of calcium.

6. Add molasses to homemade quick breads, cookies, and pancakes (or add to your mix). Sesame seeds and tahini (sesame seed butter) are also high in calcium and can be added to snack bars, cakes, vegetables, and dips. (See Favorite Snack Cake,* page 322, and Quick and Healthier Pancakes,* page 251.)

7. Add nonfat milk powder to prepared soups, prepared muffin and pancake mixes, milkshakes, and cream sauces.

8. Use plain yogurt as a base for salad dressing or veggie dip, or use fruit-flavored yogurt as a sauce for fruit salad or a dip for fresh fruit slices.

9. Eat fish with small bones. Salmon Paté* (page 221) contains both salmon and fat-free cream cheese (make sure to leave the skin off the salmon).

10. Prepare Broccoli Quiche* (page 296) or egg custard, both of which contain milk. Eat more vegetables that are good sources of calcium.

11. Instead of buying regular orange juice, buy Minute Maid Premium calcium-enriched orange juice. It contains three hundred milligrams of calcium in eight ounces.

12. Use silken tofu as a base for dips, puddings, and salad dressings, or use firm tofu as a meat substitute in lasagna and "meatloaf" (see Tofu Loaf,* page 315). (To make sure the tofu has calcium added, check the label.)

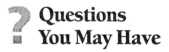

Questions You May Have

Q: I can't tolerate milk! What can I do?

A: Many African Americans, Asians, Native Americans, and

Calcium Content of Foods and Beverages		

The RDA for pregnancy and breastfeeding is 1,200 milligrams.

Vegetarian Sources

Food[1]	Serving sizes*	Calcium, in milligrams
American cheese, processed	1 ounce	124
Agar, dried	3½ ounces	625
Collard greens	1 cup	357
Rhubarb	1 cup	348
Spinach[2]	1 cup	278
Blackstrap molasses	2 tablespoons	274
Firm tofu made with calcium sulfate[3]	4 ounces	250–765
Turnip greens	1 cup	249
Tortillas, corn	2	196
Okra	1 cup	176
Sesame seeds	2 tablespoons	176
Kombu, raw	3½ ounces	168
Wakame, raw	3½ ounces	150
Regular tofu made with calcium sulfate[3]	4 ounces	120–392
Tofu made with nijari[3]	4 ounces	80–146
Kale	1 cup	79
Nori, raw	3½ ounces	58

[1] Foods are cooked unless otherwise noted.

[2] Spinach contains oxalates, which can significantly cut down on calcium absorption.

[3] Calcium sulfate and nijari are processing agents.

Sources: *Simply Vegan,* by Debra Wasserman and Reed Mangels, The Vegetarian Resource Group, and *Food Values of Portions Commonly Used,* 15th edition, by Jean Pennington.

Hispanics have lactose intolerance, meaning they have trouble absorbing and digesting lactose, or milk sugar. The result is uncomfortable gas, stomachaches and, in some cases, diarrhea. However, don't throw out the milk bottle forever! Research shows that as pregnancy progresses, especially in the third trimester, women who are lactose intolerant can break down much more lactose. This may be a compensatory effect since the body needs large amounts of calcium in the third trimester.[8]

Lactase, the enzyme that is lacking in lactose-intolerant people, can be purchased in drop form (to put into milk) or in pill form (to take directly before drinking milk). Lactase is sold over the counter in pharmacies under such names as "Lactaid," "Lactrace," and "Dairy Ease." You can also purchase Lactaid milk, which is 2% milk that has reduced lactose content.

Some people can tolerate milk with food, especially with food that contains fiber, such as milk over raisin bran at breakfast.[9] Cocoa may stimulate the body to produce more lactase, thereby increasing the tolerance of chocolate milk or hot cocoa.[10] I've found that some women tolerate whole milk better than skim or low-fat. This may be because the fat slows digestion of the milk and improves diges-

tion of the lactose. For those who can use the extra calories and sugar, chocolate milk is an option that will increase calcium in the diet. Other low-lactose dairy options are yogurt, buttermilk, sweet acidophilus milk, and cheese.

If none of the above solutions work for you, the last resort is to take a calcium supplement. (See page 34 for more about calcium supplements.)

Q: What about drinking chocolate milk?

A: Until recently, it was thought that the calcium in chocolate milk was not absorbed well because of another element in the milk, oxalate. However, now we know that not only the amount of calcium found in chocolate milk is similar to that found in regular milk (284 milligrams in eight ounces), but the amount of calcium absorbed from chocolate milk is also similar to that absorbed from whole milk, yogurt, and cheese.[11]

Another concern about drinking chocolate milk has been its caffeine content. You'll be happy to know that eight ounces of chocolate milk contains only five milligrams of caffeine—or about the amount found in five ounces of decaffeinated coffee. If you prefer chocolate milk to white milk, and can afford the calories

(179 for eight ounces of 2% low-fat chocolate milk compared to 120 calories for plain 2% milk), then drink and enjoy!

Q: Doesn't my prenatal vitamin have enough calcium?

A: No, though the pill seems big enough! If it did contain all the calcium needed, you really wouldn't be able to swallow it! Most prenatal vitamins contain only a small percentage of the RDA for calcium. You must obtain the majority of calcium you need from your diet.

▼

Focus on Iron

Some time during the twenty-fourth through the twenty-eighth week, your health care provider will probably have your blood tested again for anemia, a somewhat common occurrence during pregnancy. Because your blood volume expands up to 50 percent, you need twice as much iron than before you were pregnant. Knowing a few things about iron will help you prevent anemia and improve your iron status if you are anemic.

Iron is best absorbed from animal sources such as beef, eggs, and so on. If you are not a big meat eater, combine a small amount of animal protein with vegetable protein. This helps you absorb more iron from the vegetable foods. For example, mix a small amount of ham with your pinto beans, or chop a hard-boiled egg into your cooked spinach or spinach salad.

You can increase the amount of iron your body absorbs from food by eating a vitamin C food along with it. For example, have an orange, melon, or berries for dessert after a meal, or have raw or cooked tomatoes, tomato juice, broccoli, cabbage, greens, cauliflower, or bell pepper as your veggie. Or drink citrus juice, vegetable or tomato juice, or vitamin C-fortified apple juice with your meal.

Factors that inhibit the absorption of iron are:

- Coffee
- Tea
- Calcium supplements
- Antacids
- Dairy products
- Soy protein
- Wheat bran
- Fiber

Factors that aid in the absorption of iron are:

- Vitamin C. Other vitamin C foods include tomato, greens, cabbage, citrus, peppers, pineapple, mango, and papaya.

- Cooking with an iron skillet. The iron content of about three ounces of spaghetti sauce increases from three milligrams to eighty-seven milligrams of iron when cooked in an unenameled iron skillet.[12]

"How's Your Diet?" Quiz

First write down in the spaces provided on the next page everything you've eaten during the last day or on a typical day. Then,

Iron Content of Foods

The RDA for pregnancy is 30 milligrams; for breastfeeding, 15 milligrams.

Animal Sources

Food[1]	Serving sizes	Iron, in milligrams[2]
Clams	3 ounces	24
Pork liver	3 ounces	15
Oysters (also a great source of zinc)	3 ounces	11
Beef liver	3 ounces	6
Mussels	3 ounces	8
Canneloni with spinach and veal*	8 ounces	4
Roast beef sandwich	1	4
Chili*	1 cup	4
Stuffed green pepper with beef and crumbs*	1	4
Spaghetti and meatballs with tomato sauce*	1 cup	4
Shrimp	3 ounces	3
Egg McMuffin	1	3
Green pepper steak*	10 ounces	3
Beef and vegetable stew*	1 cup	3
Cheeseburger, fast food	1	3
Chicken á la king*	1 cup	2.5

[1]Foods are cooked, as applicable, unless otherwise noted.
[2]Numbers are rounded off.
*Also contains a significant amount of vitamin C, which helps absorption of iron.

Source: Food Values of Portions Commonly Used, 15th edition, by Jean Pennington.

using the recommended numbers of servings, make a tally for each serving eaten next to each food. Compare your totals for the day with those recommended.

Breakfast

_____

_____

_____

Lunch

_____

_____

_____

Snack

_____

_____

_____

Snack

_____

_____

_____

Dinner

_____

_____

_____

Snack

_____

_____

_____

Iron Content of Foods

The RDA for pregnancy is 30 milligrams; for breastfeeding, 15 milligrams.

Vegetarian Sources

Food[1]	Serving sizes	Iron, in milligrams[2]
Soy beans	1 cup	9
Tofu, firm	4 ounces	7–13
Blackstrap molasses	2 tablespoons	6
Chick peas	1 cup	5
Quinoa	1 cup	5
Pinto beans	1 cup	4
Prune juice	8 ounces	3
Spinach*	1 cup	3
Potato*	1 medium	3
Peas	1 cup	3
Soy yogurt, plain	1 cup	3
Figs	5 medium	2
Bulgur	1 cup	2
Watermelon*	⅛ medium	2
Bok choy*	1 cup	2
Green beans or broccoli*	1 cup	1
Tomato juice*	8 ounces	1

[1]Foods are cooked, as applicable, unless otherwise noted.

[2]Numbers are rounded off.

*Also contains a significant amount of vitamin C, which helps absorption of iron.

Numbers are rounded off.

Source: _Food Values of Portions Commonly Used,_ 15th edition, by Jean Pennington.

How Did You Do?

Your diet should contain at least the following:

10 servings of starches/grains (which should include three servings of whole grain)
Best choices: whole grains, whole-wheat bread and cereal, sweet potatoes, winter squash, potatoes, dried beans, peas, corn, wheat crackers, and popcorn.

3 servings of fruits
Best choices: papaya, mango, melon, berries, apricots, peaches, grapefruit, orange, and kiwi.

3 servings of vegetables

Best choices: broccoli, cauliflower, carrots, spinach, cabbage, leaf and romaine lettuce, greens, sweet peppers, and tomatoes.

Note: Don't forget to eat at least one vitamin C-rich and one vitamin A-rich fruit or vegetable every day!

6 ounces of protein (or equivalent)

Best choices: fish and shellfish, dried beans and legumes, tofu, poultry, lean beef, lamb, and pork. Be sure to eat a variety!

4 servings of dairy products (or high-calcium equivalent)

Best choices: skim and low-fat milk and yogurt, fat-free and low-fat cheeses, and tofu made with calcium.

3 to 5 servings of fat

Best choices: avocado, nuts, seeds, safflower oil, margarine, and salad dressing or mayonnaise made from safflower or canola oils. Remember that baked goods, fried foods, whole milk products, and desserts have many hidden fats. Fat has twice as many calories as carbohydrate or protein.

8 to 10 cups of fluid

You should be drinking to thirst, or at least eight cups of fluid per day, most of it from water.

▼

"Thrive on Five"

The National Cancer Institute is using the slogans "Thrive on Five" and "Five a Day for Better Health" to encourage Americans to eat more fruits and vegetables. Why? Fruits and vegetables are great sources of vitamins, minerals, and fiber. All plant foods also have other substances, called phytochemicals. These are biologically active substances that are very beneficial to health. We are just discovering their functions. An example of a phytochemical is beta-carotene—just one of hundreds of carotenoids found in food. Many studies show that eating more fruits and vegetables is correlated with reduced rates of cancer and heart disease.

The great thing about filling up on fruits and vegetables is that you are less likely to eat such things as chips, cookies, and other less-nutrient-dense foods. Try to eat a variety of fruits and vegetables from day to day.

Do you think that five fruits and vegetables a day sounds like a lot of food? Here are a few easy tips for adding fruits and vegetables to your meals.

Breakfast

▶ **Add mashed banana, dried fruit, or applesauce to pancake batter.**

Top pancakes and waffles with strawberries or other fresh fruit.

▶ **Whip up a fruit shake. (See pages 238–243 for recipes.)**

▶ **Add dried fruit, peaches, strawberries, blueberries, bananas, or other fresh fruit to your cereal.**

▶ **Eat a fruit or drink some juice before you have anything else.**

▶ **If you eat omelets, add tomatoes, mushrooms, and red or green peppers.**

Lunch

▶ **Add apple, raisins, pineapple, mango, or mandarin orange slices to your chicken, tuna, or tossed salad.**

▶ **Have a salad or raw veggies before your meal.**

Use darker greens, such as romaine or leaf lettuce or spinach, for your salads.

▶ Drink vegetable or tomato juice with your meal or as a premeal "cocktail."

▶ Add sprouts, leaf lettuce, thinly sliced cucumber, finely shredded cabbage, or spinach and tomatoes to your sandwiches.

▶ Stuff leftover veggies or salad in a pita pocket with cheese.

▶ To save time, buy the ready-to-eat salads, carrots, broccoli, etc. Talk about "fast food"!

Dinner

▶ Do a stir-fry for dinner. You can even buy the vegetables cleaned, chopped, and ready to go!

▶ Zip up your spaghetti sauce with bell pepper, zucchini, carrots, or eggplant.

Shred or chop these vegetables finely and they will cook quickly. If you have picky children at home, you can purée the cooked vegetables and the kids will never know the veggies are there!

▶ Use puréed roasted red pepper or other vegetable as the base for a sauce. (See page 316 for recipe.)

▶ Start dinner with a vegetable-based soup, such as minestrone or gaspacho. (See page 254 for recipe.)

▶ Make a fruit salsa to accompany your grilled chicken or seafood. (See page 299 for recipe.)

▶ Make an appetizer of oven-fried zucchini sticks or eggplant slices. (See page 222 for recipe.)

Dessert

▶ A mixed fresh fruit salad makes a great finish.

▶ Top angel food or pound cake with fresh or canned fruits.

▶ Make a fruit shake with frozen strawberries, raspberries, and milk. (See page 242 for recipe.)

▶ Try a fruit sorbet.

▶ Have a frozen yogurt layered with fruit.

▶ How about a frozen banana or frozen grapes?

▶ Grilled fruit kebobs to top off a grilled dinner.

▶ Dip strawberries in a yogurt dip or chocolate sauce. Everyone needs a splurge sometimes!

▼

Smart Snacking

When I ask my clients if they snack, they usually look embarrassed. You would think that "snack" is a four-letter word. Most people think of snacking as "eating foods they shouldn't" or "cheating." Actually, snacking can be healthy, and it's a must during pregnancy. Snacking helps you get all the nutrients you need when you can't eat much at a meal. It also gives you more energy during those times when baby seems to have sapped it all.

What Are the Best Snacks?

The best snacks are those that offer the most nutrition for the fewest calories. First are fruits and vegetables—they offer lots of nutrition, virtually no fat, and few calories. An added plus is their fiber and fluid content.

The Center for Science in the Public Interest, publisher of *Nutrition Action Healthletter,* recently published a list of the healthiest fruits, based on their nutrient and fiber content. Here are the top fifteen: papaya, cantaloupe, strawberries, oranges, tangerines, kiwis, mangos, apricots, persimmons, watermelon, raspberries, red or pink grapefruit, blackberries, dried apricots, and white grapefruit.[13] Don't despair if your favorite fruit isn't on this list—just try to include the above fruits more often to get the most nutrition.

Second on our list of good snacks would be other high-carbohydrate foods. They also provide energy, little fat, and contain fiber. Of course, they must also taste good! Lastly, we have the dairy and protein food combinations. Try to have a variety of snacks during the day—the following will give you some ideas.

Healthy Snack Options

- Dried or fresh fruit (Since dried fruits are concentrated, they are a great source of vitamins, minerals, and fiber. You can also keep them in your purse or desk drawer.)
- Raw vegetables (You can buy them ready to eat and keep them in your refrigerator.)
- Leftover vegetables (Heat them up for a healthy snack.)
- Fruit or vegetable juice, fruit juice mixed with club soda, or a fruit smoothie
- Health Valley Granola Bars (I like these because they are sweetened with fruit and are high in fiber.)
- Fibars (these contain added sugar and fat.)
- Raisin bran or other high-fiber cereal
- Rice or popcorn cakes (For a sweet tooth, Quaker Caramel Corn Popcorn Cakes are my favorite!)
- Popcorn (Choose the one with the least fat, or pop your own.)
- Rye or wheat crackers
- Graham crackers
- Fig Newtons
- Guiltless Gourmet No Oil Tortilla Chips, Baked Tostitos, or other baked chips with salsa

And don't forget the dairy foods!

- Milk
- Yogurt
- Low-fat cheese
- Dip made with cottage cheese or fat-free cream cheese
- Milkshake made with fresh fruit (See pages 238–243 for yogurt shakes.)

At Last, Low-Fat Chips

As I write this, I'm snacking on tortilla chips that aren't fried—and they taste great! Guiltless Gourmet Inc. did what was thought to be impossible: they made tortilla chips, as well as black bean and pinto bean dips, salsas, and queso dips, without added fat! One ounce of chips also provides eighty milligrams of calcium. Other baked chips are also available—Baked Tostitos, Baked Lay's, and many other brands. It is better to eat naturally low-fat chips than those made with Olestra (a fat substitute) while you are pregnant.

High-Protein Snacks

Add other protein foods for a hungry appetite. Eating a snack that contains protein before you go to bed at night can also prevent low blood sugar in the morning.

- Peanut butter on crackers or with banana or apple
- Whole-grain cereal with milk
- Cheese and apple
- Tortilla rolled up with ham and cheese or with refried beans and cheese

- Yogurt with grape nuts or granola
- Cottage cheese and fruit
- Fat-free cheese on celery, carrots, and broccoli
- Tortilla chips and fat-free refried beans

(See page 217 for other snack ideas.)

▼

Second-Trimester Challenges

Vaginal Discharge

Increased discharge is considered normal in pregnancy. It is usually whitish and is the result of an increased supply of blood and glucose to the vaginal walls and increased production of mucus by the endocervical glands. The acid level of your mucus changes in pregnancy, making you more susceptible to vaginal infections. If you have severe itching and irritation and a foul odor, contact your health care provider.

What you can do:

▶ Continue to bathe daily.

▶ Wear cotton underwear.

▶ Avoid feminine deodorants, powders, and bubble baths.

Constipation

Progesterone, a pregnancy hormone, slows down the movement of food in your intestine, causing more water and nutrients to be absorbed, and constipation is often the result. The pressure of the growing baby on your intestines and rectum can also cause this problem. An iron supplement can further worsen it.

What you can do:

▶ Drink plenty of fluids– at least eight to ten glasses daily, mostly from water.

▶ Eat high-fiber foods. Eating at least five fruits and vegetables a day will keep constipation away! (See page 47, "Focus on Fiber.")

▶ Exercise regularly.

▶ Avoid foods that cause constipation: some people are constipated when they eat certain foods, such as cheese and bananas.

▶ Avoid caffeine, since it can cause a loss of even more fluid, which can make the stools hard.

Hemorrhoids

Hemorrhoids are swollen or enlarged veins in the rectum. Hormones once again play a role in this problem, as does straining during a bowel movement. As the baby grows, greater pressure from the uterus displaces intestines, which can lead to constipation and then hemorrhoids.

What you can do:

▶ Prevent constipation.

▶ Discuss hemorrhoids with your health care provider.
Your health care provider may advise a stool softener or high-fiber laxative such as Metamucil. (If you do take a stool softener, keep in mind that it can take as long as three days to work. Don't take more than one type of stool softener at the same time.)

▶ DON'T take over-the-counter laxatives, stool softeners, or hemorrhoid treatments without your health care provider's approval.

▶ **Taking warm baths and sitting on soft pillows can relieve the pressure.**

▶ **Avoid heavy lifting, pushing, and standing for long periods of time.**

Stress

We all live with stress. If you don't manage your stress, it can lead to chronic medical problems such as ulcers and heart disease. Pregnancy offers its own special stresses. Just wondering whether you are doing "all the right things" for your baby is a stress. You may be debating about working after you have the baby or preparing another child for your "new arrival." You may be trying to figure out how you'll pay for the delivery or all those baby things you'll need to buy. The hormones of pregnancy can cause mood swings, and can cause you to cope less effectively with stress.

According to the March of Dimes, some studies show that extreme stress can play a role in low birth weight.

What you can do:

▶ **Make realistic goals.**

You probably can't physically do what you did before pregnancy. You must put yourself first; you need to take more time for rest,

time to exercise, time to plan and prepare healthy meals. This can put a time crunch on an already busy schedule. Try to plan for it.

▶ **Use relaxation techniques such as biofeedback and meditation.**

Many audio and video tapes with relaxing music and scenery are available—they can help you take a mental vacation. A daily walk can also help relieve stress and help put things in perspective.

▶ **Try to find support in your spouse, friends, and coworkers.**

Other new moms are especially empathetic to your needs. Remember that your spouse will be feeling his own stresses and probably needs your support too.

▼

How Baby Is Growing

At this time, all the major organs and systems are started or completely established. From now on, the fetus will start to gain more weight. Your body is producing more blood in order to nourish your baby. You need to be drinking plenty of fluids, preferably ten cups per day of

water, milk, juice, or soup. Anything with caffeine can cause you to lose your needed fluids.

At the End of Sixteen Weeks (Four Months)

Your baby is quite active, even though you might not feel it yet. Making facial expressions, swallowing, rotating feet, kicking, sleeping, waking, and even listening to you are all part of the daily routine. Fine downy "lanugo" hair, much like peach fuzz, is developing on the head. The fetus is now six to seven inches long and weighs six to seven ounces; the weight of a big, red apple.

At the End of Twenty Weeks (Five Months)

A growth spurt has occurred within the last month. The fetus now measures between eight and twelve inches long and weighs about one pound. Lanugo hair now covers the whole body, and the hair on the head is getting thicker. Eyebrows and eyelashes are developing. Mom is beginning to sense the baby's movements as the baby's muscles develop and the baby becomes stronger at turning and rolling.

At the End of Twenty-Four Weeks (Six Months)

Baby is now between eleven and fourteen inches long, averaging the length of a ruler, and weighs between one-and-a-half to one-and-three-quarters pounds. The fetus looks like a wrinkled old man, with its skin covered in vernix, a thick, creamy lotion that protects the skin while in the amniotic fluid. The eyes are opening and closing and baby can hear and respond to external noise and music. The distinct fingerprints and footprints are formed; even identical twins have different fingerprints. The alveoli in the lungs are just beginning to develop. If the baby is born at this time, it would need extremely specialized care.

Second-Trimester Menus

Most women feel their best during the second trimester, and the menus and recipes in Chapter Fourteen reflect this. Your appetite may be robust, so the menus are a little heavier. Some recipes will take a little more time in case you feel like spending more time in the kitchen.

Menus:

• A Month of Breakfast Ideas
• Menus for a Hungry Appetite
• I Could Cook All Day
• Company's Coming!

The Third Trimester

The third trimester is an important time for many reasons. It's the "home stretch," so to speak; a time when you will be making last-minute preparations for your baby's arrival. Likewise, your baby will be making strides in its growth to prepare for its birth into the world.

Weight Gain/Energy Needs

During the last three months of your pregnancy, you will probably gain a large proportion of your total weight. Just when you think you cannot gain another pound, or expand your stomach another inch, you do! Remember that as you prepare for the baby's arrival, you still need to eat and to make wise food choices.

You should continue to gain about a pound a week during this time. Remember that if you are overweight or underweight, your weight gain should be adjusted accordingly. If you find that you have exceeded your goal weight already, discuss this with your health care provider, who will still want you to continue gaining weight, but perhaps at a slower rate. Caution: never try to lose weight while pregnant, no matter how much weight you have gained. Your baby needs you to eat adequately so that it can grow and develop enough to survive on its own in our world!

Many women find that their "get up and go"…"got up and went"! Regular exercise (even a simple walk around the block) will improve your endurance and you won't feel like a couch potato! If you find that you are much less active than in previous months, you may not need the entire three hundred extra calories recommended earlier. However, you still need all the added nutrients, so if you do cut down on food intake, you must make your food choices with even more care!

On the other hand, you may find that with the thought of your baby's arrival just around the corner, you have renewed energy! You may need to increase your calories. (See page 218 for "High-Energy Moms" snack ideas.)

As your due date gets closer, you might consider getting more of your calories from complex carbohydrates. Competitive athletes often "carbohydrate load" before a big event. Labor and delivery could qualify as such an event! Building up your store of carbohydrate may give you a bit more energy needed for long labors.

Weighing In

Are you one of those weight-conscious women who weigh daily? Don't! Although being aware of your weight is a good idea, during the third trimester you are more prone to water retention and fluctuations in weight gain. So when you panic, thinking you've gained a pound in two days, the weight gain may simply be a result of water retention. Develop a healthy attitude about weight by weighing just once a week, and at the same time of day under the same conditions. This will give you a truer idea of how your weight is progressing.

Note: If you do find that you have gained two or more pounds

in two days, or if you notice extreme swelling in your hands, face, or feet, or have headaches or trouble with vision, notify your health care provider. This may be a sign of preeclampsia. (See page 114 for more information.)

▼

Other Nutrient Needs

Your need for vitamins and minerals during the third trimester remains essentially the same as during the second trimester. Calcium is important during the third trimester for the laying down of calcium in the baby's bones. Brain development during the third trimester makes zinc a key nutrient. Zinc is critical throughout pregnancy and a deficiency is related to premature delivery and many other problems. Vitamin B_6, essential for the use of protein, is necessary for the building of tissues, including brain and muscle tissue. B_6 is needed in proportion to the protein in your diet; the more you eat, the more you need. Also important for brain development are omega-3 fatty acids, primarily found in cold-water fish such as salmon and tuna. Try to eat fish at least once or twice a week.

Keep in mind that certain water-soluble vitamins such as thiamin, riboflavin, and niacin are required in amounts relative to your calorie intake. Thus, if you increase your calories, make sure your diet contains foods rich in these vitamins. Women who follow strict vegetarian diets (no animal protein) should take a supplement of vitamin B_{12}; 2.2 micrograms per day.[1]

Research data shows that pregnant women's diets contain less than the RDA for vitamin B_6, vitamin D, vitamin E, folate, iron, zinc, calcium, and magnesium.[2] How does your diet stack up? Take the following diet analysis to find out. Answer "yes" or "no":

1. I eat a variety of foods daily.
2. I eat a dark-green or orange vegetable daily.
3. I eat a citrus fruit or a fruit or vegetable high in vitamin C daily.
4. I eat two to three servings of protein food daily.
5. I eat a variety of protein sources, including plant proteins.
6. I eat three servings of whole grains almost every day.
7. I eat six fruits and vegetables on most days.
8. I eat four servings of dairy products or high-calcium food daily.

9. I am gaining about one pound per week.
10. I avoid caffeine, alcohol, and drugs.

If you answered yes to seven or more questions, you're doing pretty well. Less than that? Well, you know what you need to work on.

▼

Focus on Vitamin B₆ and Zinc

Vitamin B₆ is necessary for many reactions in the body; namely building protein from amino acids and forming hemoglobin and neurotransmitters in the brain. Women usually don't have enough B₆ in their diets. Most recently, however, vitamin B₆ has made the news with the information that adequate amounts help decrease blood levels of homocysteine, an amino acid that increases the risk of heart disease.

The more protein in your diet, the more B₆ you need, which shouldn't be a problem since high-protein foods are good sources of vitamin B₆. Also, women who take birth control pills seem to need more of the vitamin, so if you have recently been taking birth control pills,

try to have extra B₆ in your diet. Vitamin B₆ is water soluble and can be destroyed by cooking and processing.

Zinc has many functions during pregnancy; it is necessary for conception, for every phase of growth, and for the immune system. Zinc even helps to ensure that your baby is not premature. Low zinc intake has been related to neural tube defects and

Good Sources of B₆

The RDA for pregnancy is 15 milligrams; for breastfeeding, 19 milligrams.

Animal Sources

Food	Serving sizes*	B₆ in milligrams
Beef liver	3 ounces	.77
Chicken, light meat	3 ounces	.51
Pork loin	3 ounces	.40
Ham	3 ounces	.39
Halibut	3 ounces	.34
Tuna, light	3 ounces	.32

Vegetable Sources

Food	Serving sizes*	B₆ in milligrams
Mustard greens	1 cup	1.62
Soybeans	1 cup	.85
Potato, baked with skin	1 medium	.70
Banana	1 medium	.70
Bran flakes	¾ cup	.60
Prune juice	1 cup	.60
Lentils	1 cup	.57
Chickpeas	1 cup	.54
Sweet potato	1 cup	.51
Pinto beans	1 cup	.50
Brown rice	1 cup	.50
Dates, dried	10	.42
Wheat germ	¼ cup	.30

*Values represent cooked foods, as applicable.

Sources: *Food Values of Portions Commonly Used*, 15th edition, by Jean Pennington, and *The Nutrition Challenge for Women*, by Louise Lambert-Lagacé.

other birth defects. Unfortunately, zinc is a mineral that non-pregnant women often don't get enough of. High-fiber diets can interfere with absorption of zinc. Beef and shellfish are generally rich in zinc; vegetarian women need to eat plenty of zinc-rich legumes and whole grains.

▼

What about Sugar?

Sugar has gotten knocked around a lot in the past ten years. Many myths are still circulating about sugar. Here are "just the facts":

- Sugar doesn't cause diabetes, though it does cause the body to produce more insulin in order to use the sugar. This happens with any carbohydrate food, but the effect is more pronounced with simple sugars.
- Sugar doesn't appear to cause hyperactivity. Studies have shown just the opposite—sugar actually has a calming effect when given to children.[3,4] Often, the increased activity in children after eating a sugary food may be from the caffeine, as in a cola. Another explanation may be the activities that generally surround the eating of a lot of sweets, such as a birthday party or Halloween. However, individual reactions to any food are possible.
- Sugar does cause tooth decay, as do many other carbohydrate foods.
- High-sugar foods are often low-nutrient foods. They can also be high in fat, so if your diet has a lot of sweets in it, your diet may be too high in fat and calories and lacking in important nutrients.
- Sugar in moderation helps your food taste good, though many of us have too much sugar in our diets. Estimates show that total sweetener consumption in the U.S.

Good Sources of Zinc

The RDA for pregnancy is 15 milligrams; for breastfeeding, 19 milligrams.

Animal Sources

Food	Serving sizes*	Zinc, in milligrams
Oysters	3 ounces	74
Crab, Alaskan	3 ounces	6.4
Pork or beef liver	3 ounces	6.0
Beef, top round	3 ounces	4.7
Veal roast	3 ounces	3.7
Lamb chop, lean	3 ounces	3.0
Pork roast	3 ounces	2.6
Lobster	3 ounces	2.5
Clams	3 ounces	2.3
Shrimp	3 ounces	1.3
Trout	3 ounces	1.2

Vegetable Sources

Food	Serving sizes*	Zinc, in milligrams
Wheat germ, toasted	¼ cup	4.7
Green peas	1 cup	2.0
Bran flakes	¾ cup	1.9
Spinach	1 cup	1.4
Bran muffin	1 medium	1.1

*Values represent cooked foods, as applicable.

Sources: *Food Values of Portions Commonly Used*, 15th edition, by Jean Pennington, and *The Nutrition Challenge for Women*, by Louise Lambert-Lagacé.

is 18 percent of the diet; the American Dietetic Association recommends limiting sugar in the diet to 10 to 15 percent of total calories.[5]

Tips for Keeping Your Energy Up!

You may have heard that the third trimester, and especially the last month, is a real challenge. You feel as though you can't possibly get bigger. Getting out of your chair or bed (especially if you have a waterbed!) is sometimes tough, and your energy level may need a boost. On the other hand, many women feel energetic and get sudden bursts of energy (often called the nesting syndrome) when they want to get everything done! The following tips will help you feel at your best during the last months of pregnancy.

▶ Put up your feet from time to time.

Some swelling in the feet and legs is considered normal these last few months. Keep in mind that the extra twenty to thirty pounds you are now carrying are putting a lot of pressure on legs, knees, and feet. Wear flat, supportive shoes; support hose may also be a good idea.

▶ Take catnaps at lunch if you can, but *after* you've eaten!

(I remember several times taking naps on my boss's couch during lunch.)

▶ Let the housework go!

It's good practice for the first few months with baby. Start putting your feelings first and the housework second. Do only what has to be done (laundry, for example), or enlist the help of your spouse or other children.

▶ Don't forget those in-between snacks–they help boost your energy.

Keep a "snack stash" in your drawer–peanut butter crackers, raisins, dried figs, prunes, apricots, graham crackers, and granola bars.

▶ Keep up with your exercise program.

Exercise is probably the last thing you want to do when you feel tired, but it really will help in the long run. I don't really like to swim, but when I attended a water exercise class for pregnant women, I loved it. You see, you feel weightless in the water and that is a nice feeling! After a long work day, being in the water can be very refreshing.

"Baby Pick Me Up" A High-Energy Drink
(Two Servings)

1 frozen peach or nectarine or ½ cup canned (freeze for 45 minutes or more)

½ banana

½ cup frozen strawberries

1 cup plain yogurt or 1 cup milk

2 tablespoons nonfat dry milk

Honey, molasses, or sweetener, to taste

Blend all ingredients in blender. Makes approximately 2 cups. If you don't have frozen fruit, adding ice for desired consistency will increase the volume.

Nutrient analysis per serving:

141 calories

9 grams protein

6 grams fiber

0 grams fat

Percentage of RDA for pregnancy:

Vitamin C–47%

Vitamin B$_{12}$–39%

Potassium–31%

Third-Trimester Challenges

Backache

As pregnancy progresses and the uterus enlarges, the curvature in the spine increases. Hormones also cause the pelvic joints to loosen and relax. You may notice that the way you walk is a bit different than before you were pregnant. This may be due to expansion of joints and an adjustment in posture to compensate for carrying a big "front load."

What you can do:

▶ Practice good body mechanics and posture.

▶ Avoid bending over and lifting heavy objects (including older children, if possible).

Bend at the knees and keep your back straight.

▶ Wear low-heeled shoes.

▶ Learn to do pelvic tilts–they will relieve pressure on the back and stretch and tone muscles.

Ask your health care provider or childbirth educator for instructions or see page 164.

▶ Bend your knees slightly when standing in place.

Edema/Swelling

Many women experience ankle swelling in the last trimester because blood and fluid circulation (between the heart and the lower extremities) becomes more and more difficult. Let your health care provider know if you have swelling in your hands or face; this could be a sign of pre-eclampsia.

What you can do:

▶ Elevate your legs to the level of your hips as often as possible.

▶ Avoid standing for long periods of time.

▶ If you must sit for long periods, try to stand up, stretch, and move around a bit to improve circulation.

▶ Avoid anything that will restrict circulation: stockings with tight bands, tight slips or pants, tight knee highs, and so on.

▶ Don't restrict fluid intake!

Heartburn

As the baby grows, it compresses your stomach, leaving minimal space for food. The hormones that slow down your digestion also relax the sphincter that keeps food in your stomach. These changes cause stomach acid to back up into your esophagus, causing a burning sensation that feels as though it's around your heart.

What you can do:

▶ Eat small, frequent meals.

▶ Stay away from gassy, spicy, and greasy foods.

▶ Don't overeat.

▶ Stand or walk around after eating, instead of lying down immediately after a meal.

▶ Keep your head slightly elevated when you're in bed.

Sleepless Nights

As your body gets larger, you may find that getting comfortable in bed is quite a chore. The baby kicking, heartburn, and anxiety about the arrival of the new person in your life can add to sleeplessness.

What you can do:

▶ **Try a bedtime ritual: warm bath, decaffeinated mint tea or warm milk, and soft jazz or easy-listening music.**

▶ **Support yourself with pillows.**

One new mom says, "Our bed was a virtual oasis of pillows! I used two behind me to support my back, one between my knees to relieve back pressure and one for my head."

▶ **Practice the relaxation and breathing techniques that you learned in childbirth class.**

▶ **Continue regular exercise; it has a calming effect and can help with insomnia.**

As another new mom shares, "My husband and I enjoyed a leisurely walk every evening after dinner. It gave us quiet time to talk and helped me to sleep better at night. Of course we always had other things we could do, such as cleaning house or paying bills, but we made our walk together a priority."

▼

How Baby Is Growing

Your baby is now rapidly filling your uterus. The baby will be turning flips less often, yet you might feel rhythmic movements that are hiccups!

At the End of Twenty-Eight Weeks (Seven Months)

A baby born at this time is considered able to live outside the uterus, though its lungs are still not mature. Your baby did a lot of growing in the last month and should weigh between two-and-a-half and three pounds and is fourteen to seventeen inches long. Baby is now storing calcium and its bones are hardening. Many babies now find they fit better upside down and start to position themselves for birth. Your health care provider can determine if the baby is positioned head down.

At the End of Thirty-Two Weeks (Eight Months)

All your baby needs to do now is develop lung surfactant (which enables the lungs to inflate and deflate properly) and store some fat. Baby is beginning to store minerals such as iron, calcium, and phosphorus. The kicks are strong and vigorous and many women can feel a heel, fist, or elbow through their abdomen. Your baby now weighs between four-and-a-half and five pounds and is between sixteen-and-a-half and eighteen inches long.

At the End of Thirty-Six Weeks (Nine Months)

Baby is now making great strides in growth and is gaining close to half a pound per week. The bones in the head are soft and ready for delivery. Lanugo hair and vernix are disappearing. Fat deposits under the skin help fill out the body and eliminate the wrinkling of the skin. Baby will settle lower into your pelvis and often seems to slow down in activity level. No day should ever pass without your noticing baby's presence. You should feel your baby move at least ten times in a twelve-hour period. If you don't—contact your health care provider.

At the End of Forty Weeks (Ten Months)

Your baby is not considered "full term" until thirty-eight weeks. At this time, the baby has a well established sleeping pattern and individual styles of responses. The baby will continue to gain weight until the time of delivery. These last few weeks can be tiring as you wait for the arrival and meeting of your new little one.

Congratulations!

Third-Trimester Menus

The main problems with eating during the last months of pregnancy are:

1. You get full quickly.

2. Fatigue may prevent you from wanting to cook.

3. Heartburn may restrict the variety or amount of food you eat.

4. You may be so busy getting ready for the baby that you neglect your own nutrition needs.

The third trimester menus are designed with the above in mind. Now is also a good time to prepare some foods to freeze for those first few days or weeks with your new baby. You may be trying to cut food expenses since you are buying many expensive necessities for the baby. So, the following list includes some budget menus too.

Menus:

- Menus from the Grocery Deli
- Using Leftovers with Flair
- Meals in Minutes
- Feel Full
- Vegetarian Budget

Vegetarian Eating

This chapter answers such questions as:

- *How can I get enough calcium in my diet if I'm vegetarian?*
- *I'm diabetic, how do vegetarian foods fit into my diet?*
- *How can I get vitamin B$_{12}$ in my diet if it is only found in animal foods?*
- *Must I buy special vegetarian foods to have a good diet?*

Vegetarian eating is on the rise! Going meatless is becoming a growing trend as more people realize the benefits of eating more plant proteins. (See Chapter Four for more on soy protein.) Even if you just "lean" toward vegetarian eating, you can receive many of the same healthful benefits.

Most people eat vegetarian to a certain extent, without even thinking about it. The teen who picks up a bean burrito is doing it, the mom who makes pasta with marinara sauce and cheese is doing it, and, of course, the practicing vegan who eats no animal products is doing it too. They all do it for a variety of reasons; because eating vegetarian is healthier, because they're concerned about the environment or animal rights, or simply because it's cheaper.

The Food Guide Pyramid is a guideline for a healthy eating pattern for everyone. However, it exemplifies the pattern of a vegetarian diet–based on grains, fruits, and vegetables, with smaller amounts of protein, dairy, fat, and sugar.

Food Pyramid Guide
Suggested Daily Servings

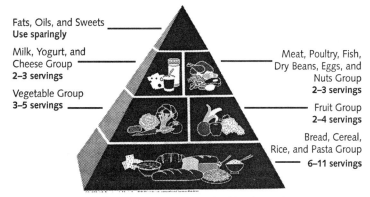

Fats, Oils, and Sweets
Use sparingly

Milk, Yogurt, and Cheese Group
2–3 servings

Vegetable Group
3–5 servings

Meat, Poultry, Fish, Dry Beans, Eggs, and Nuts Group
2–3 servings

Fruit Group
2–4 servings

Bread, Cereal, Rice, and Pasta Group
6–11 servings

Source: U.S. Department of Agriculture/U.S. Department of Health and Human Services.

Vegetarians– The Healthy Minority?

Many people would like to have the health record that vegetarians do. Fewer vegetarians die from heart disease than do meat eaters.[1,2] Total serum cholesterol is generally lower too.[3,4] Vegetarians generally have lower blood pressures and lower rates of Type II diabetes than do non-vegetarians.[5] Recent research shows that a low-fat vegetarian diet along with stress management and exercise can actually reverse coronary heart disease.[6] Vegetarians are generally closer to their ideal body weights than are nonvegetarians. Some studies show that vegetarians have lower rates of osteoporosis, cancer, kidney stones, gallstones, and diverticular disease.[7,8,9,10]

Good genes? Not necessarily. Most vegetarian diets are low in saturated fat, and so can prevent high cholesterol levels and heart disease. Vegetarians eat many fruits and vegetables; this increases their intake of beta-carotene and fiber–both of which are thought to be cancer fighting. Lacto-ovo vegetarians have adequate calcium in their diet, which may be protective against colon cancer. Vegetarians may also have beneficial lifestyle habits that contribute to good health, such as regular exercise and abstinence from tobacco and alcohol. Maintaining ideal body weight can reduce the risk of heart disease, high blood pressure, and diabetes. But is a vegetarian diet healthy? The position of the American Dietetic Association states, "Vegetarian diets are healthful and nutritionally adequate when appropriately planned."[11] The key word here is "planned." Even a vegetarian diet can be un-healthy if it has too much fat and sugar, or if it doesn't have enough of a variety of foods, including protein sources. If you are currently a vegetarian to some degree, your diet is probably on its way to meeting the dietary guidelines. If you are contemplating becoming vegetarian, or leaning toward it, you can become part of the "healthy minority" too!

The Pregnant Vegetarian

Some women turn to vegetarian foods because they don't tolerate meat very well during pregnancy. Sometimes eggs and cheese, or black beans go down a lot easier than a steak! Of course, many women are practicing vegetarians before they become pregnant. Vegetarianism has several levels:

Lacto-ovo vegetarian

This person eats no meat, poultry, or fish, but does eat dairy products and eggs. These vegetarians have little trouble meeting nutrient needs for iron, calcium, B_{12}, or vitamin D.

Vegan

This person is the "true" vegetarian. Since she eats no animal products whatsoever, she should be sure to include reliable sources of vitamin B_{12}, which is found only in animal products or fortified foods. The vegan's need for calcium is actually less than that of meat eaters who consume larger amounts of protein. However, the vegan may have to make an effort to consume enough vegetable sources of calcium. Similar to meat-eating pregnant women, vegan women may also have a problem with iron. Women living in northern latitudes and those who have very little exposure to the sun in winter may have a problem producing enough vitamin D, which is made in the skin after exposure to sunlight, and is also found in dairy products.

No-red-meat "vegetarian."

This person is someone who avoids red meat but does eat dairy products, fish, and/or chicken. Although people who eat no red meat may call themselves vegetarians, vegetarian organizations do not regard them as vegetarians. These types of "vegetarians" generally will have no problem meeting nutrient needs, except for possibly iron, which is found in lesser amounts in the white meats.

▼

Nutrients of Special Concern

How does pregnancy impact vegetarians? Except for a few exceptions, pregnant vegetarians can expect to meet or exceed their nutritional needs. In fact, a study that compared the diets of health-conscious vegetarian women vs. nonvegetarian women showed that vegetarian nonpregnant women ate more of most nutrients than meat-eaters except for vitamin B_{12}, calcium, and zinc.[12] This is a cause for concern since B_{12}, calcium, and zinc are very important during pregnancy. The table above right shows the results.

Vegetarians who eat a variety of foods should pay particular attention to just a handful of nu-

Comparison of Vegetarian (Vegan) and Nonvegetarian Diets of Women Aged Twenty to Forty.		
Expressed in percentage of the RDAs.		
Nutrient	Vegetarians (Vegan)	Nonvegetarians
Calcium	72	119
Folic Acid	231	49
Iron	118	102
Magnesium	141	108
Vitamin B_6	117	101
Vitamin C	310	193
Vitamin A	336	205
Vitamin B_{12}	25	189
Zinc	71	92

trients: vitamin B_{12}, iron, calcium, and vitamin D. Since vitamin B_6 and zinc are nutrients lacking in all women's diets, we'll address them too.

Vitamin B_{12}

Since vitamin B_{12} is only found in animal products and fortified foods such as commercial breakfast cereals, you should make sure that you have a source of vitamin B_{12} in your diet while you are pregnant and breastfeeding. Because formulations often change, be sure to check the nutrient label.

According to Suzanne Havala, M.S., R.D., Nutrition Adviser to the Vegetarian Resource Group, "Some vegetarian specialty foods thought by many to be good sources of vitamin B_{12}, such as

tempeh and spirulina, are in fact not reliable sources. Food labels listing the vitamin B_{12} content of these foods include forms of the vitamin that are not active for humans and may compete for absorption with cyanocobalamin, the form we use."

If your diet contains neither animal products nor foods fortified with vitamin B_{12}, you probably need a vitamin supplement. Ask your health care provider.

Vitamin B_{12}-Fortified Foods

These cereals are currently fortified with at least 2.2 milligrams of vitamin B_{12} per serving. However, since formulations often change, read the label to make sure the product still contains added vitamin B_{12}.

Product 19
Total
100% Bran
Post Grape Nuts
C.W. Post (raisin, plain,
   and granola)
Post Raisin Bran
Maypo hot cereal
Ralston Bran Flakes
Multibran Chex
Post Bran Flakes
Wheat Chex
Team
Nutri-Grain Wheat
Nutri-Grain Corn

Source: Nutritionist III, Version 7.2

Iron

Even though intakes for iron are about the same for vegetarians and nonvegetarians, the type of iron that vegetarians eat may be not be absorbed as well as the iron in meat. However, vitamin C consumed with nonheme iron (the form of iron found in plant foods) helps increase the absorption of the mineral. Vegetarian diets are usually high in vitamin C.

Although anemia is no more common among vegetarians than meat-eaters, anemia can occur in any woman due to the high requirement for iron during pregnancy.[13,14] Thus, a supplement of thirty milligrams of ferrous iron is recommended for all pregnant women. (See page 62 for vegetarian sources of iron.)

Calcium

Calcium won't be a problem for you unless you are a vegan, are lactose intolerant, or just don't like milk! Since vegetarians generally have less protein in their diet, they might lose less calcium through their urine than people with a high-protein diet. Although the RDA for calcium is 1,200 milligrams, the vegan's need for calcium is less than average; the World Health Organization's guideline of 1,000 to 1,200 milligrams may be a more appropriate estimate.[13] The calcium content tables on page 59 will give you an idea of other foods high in calcium besides dairy products. If you are lactose intolerant, see page 59 for information. If you don't like milk by itself, but do eat other dairy products, see page 58 for tips on "sneaking calcium into your diet."

Some sea vegetables are good sources of calcium and other minerals. If you eat sea vegetables regularly, be aware that if they come from polluted waters, they could contain heavy metal pollutants. You should make sure your seaweed comes from a controlled source, such as a sea vegetable farm in the U.S.

Substances in green leafy vegetables and in whole grains (oxalates and phytates) have been thought to decrease absorption of some minerals including calcium. Research in this area is ongoing, but it seems as though the amount of oxalate and phytate in the American diet is not significant enough to change calcium absorption dramatically.[14] However, if vegetables are your main calcium source, you might want to concentrate on eating those low in oxalates: broccoli, collard greens, kale, and mustard and turnip greens.

Another option is to take a calcium supplement. Talk to a registered dietitian about increasing the calcium in your diet or ask your health care provider about a supplement.

Vitamin D

The need for supplemental vitamin D is rare because the body can usually produce all that it needs from exposure to sunlight. Few foods are naturally high in vitamin D; dairy products are fortified with it in the U.S. If you are strictly vegan and you either live in a northern latitude or have very limited exposure to the sun, you may need a supplement of not more than 100 percent of the RDA.

Brief, casual exposure of the face and hands to sunlight is thought to be equivalent to 200 IU of vitamin D (the RDA for pregnancy is 400 IU). The location, time of year, atmospheric conditions, clothing, amount of melanin in the skin, use of sunscreen, and blockage of light by window glass can all affect the production of vitamin D.[15]

Vitamin B$_6$

All women seem to have a problem getting enough vitamin B$_6$. Your body needs this vitamin in proportion to your protein in-take, so if your diet is especially high in protein foods, you may need even more B$_6$. (See page 71 for a list of vegetarian sources of B$_6$.)

Zinc

Zinc is a very important nutrient in the developing fetus. It is widespread in such foods as legumes, shellfish, whole grains, and cheese. Many people don't have enough zinc in their diet.

One study that evaluated the diets of vegans and of lacto-ovo vegetarians found that neither group met the RDA for zinc. The mean intake for vegan women was only 13 percent of the RDA, while lacto-ovo vegetarian women's average intake was 71 percent of the RDA. The women's food choices in this study were mostly low-zinc foods such as fruits, salads, and vegetables.[16]

Factors that may affect absorption of zinc include fiber, phytates, and some minerals. To obtain an adequate amount of zinc, vegetarians and especially vegans, must make careful food choices. Consult the list on page 72 to see how much zinc your diet supplies.

Protein

Protein is important during pregnancy, and although vegetarians have just a little less protein in their diets than do nonvegetarians, their intake still exceeds the RDA. The list of foods below will give you an idea of foods that will supply you with the ten extra grams of protein needed daily during your pregnancy. Keep in mind that eating a variety of protein foods throughout the day is important so that your body can utilize the protein for building material.

Vegetarian foods that contain ten grams of protein:

Black beans (or any legume), ¾ cup
Brown rice, 2 cups
Cashews, ½ cup
Peas, 1¼ cup
Peanut butter, 2¼ tablespoons
Quinoa, 1 cup
Soy yogurt, 1 cup
Tofu (firm), 2 ounces

The Eating Expectantly Vegetarian Diet

This diet covers both vegan and lacto-ovo vegetarians and is meant as a guideline only–eating a variety of high-nutrient foods will provide the nutrition you need without following a structured diet.

8 to 10 or more servings of starches or grains
1 serving is 1 slice of any type bread, 1 flour tortilla, or ½ cup pasta, potato, rice, or corn.

4 or more servings of milk or soymilk products
1 serving is 1 cup of any type milk, soy milk, or yogurt, preferably skim or low-fat.

Note: If you don't drink soy or cow's milk, you will need to make sure you get enough calcium from other food sources or a supplement.

4 or more servings of fruits
1 serving is 1 medium piece of fresh fruit, ½ banana, ½ cup canned fruit in its own juice, 1 cup melon or berries, ½ cup juice, or 2 plums or nectarines.

4 or more servings of vegetables

(1 serving is ½ cup cooked non-starchy vegetable or 1 cup lettuce.

Note: Be sure to include at least 1 fruit or vegetable that is a good source of vitamin A and 1 serving that is high in vitamin C.

3 to 5 or more servings of fat

1 serving is 1 teaspoon oil, ⅛ avocado, 10 peanuts, 5 olives, 1 teaspoon margarine, mayonnaise or butter, or 2 teaspoons reduced-fat margarine, mayonnaise or butter, ½ ounce cream cheese, or 1 tablespoon sour cream.

Note: It is best to have a balance of the essential fats–omega-6 (safflower oil is rich in omega-6) and omega-3 (the vegetable precursor is alpha-linoleic, found in canola, soybean, and olive oils.)

6 protein equivalents

1 protein equivalent is ½ cup of tofu, 2 tablespoons peanut butter, ½ cup cooked dried beans, ¼ cup tempeh, 1 ounce cheese (preferably reduced-fat or fat-free), ¼ cup cottage cheese, 1 egg, or 2 egg whites.

Sample Vegan Menu

This menu contains about 2,400 calories and exceeds the RDA for all major nutrients except vitamin D (it contains 0 percent of vitamin D). Vitamin D can be produced in the skin with sufficient sunshine.

Breakfast

1 cup oatmeal with 1½ tablespoons molasses and 2 tablespoons raisins

1 piece whole-wheat bread with 1 tablespoon peanut butter

1 cup soymilk

Snack

1 cup Minute Maid Premium calcium-enriched orange juice

Lunch

1 cup navy bean soup with 1 piece of whole-wheat bread

Broccoli and tofu stir-fry with 1 cup tofu, ½ cup broccoli, and 1 cup brown rice

1 cup soymilk

Snack

1 apple

Dinner

Salad with 1 cup romaine lettuce, ½ tomato, ¼ avocado, and vinaigrette dressing with 2 teaspoons canola oil

Stuffed bell pepper with ½ cup bulgur, 1 cup black beans, and ½ tomato

½ cup corn

1 cup soymilk

Snack

Shake with 1 cup soymilk and ¾ cup frozen strawberries

Sample Lacto-Ovo Vegetarian Menu

This menu, which contains eggs and dairy products, contains approximately 2,400 calories and exceeds all of the RDAs for pregnancy.

Breakfast

1½ cups Bran Chex with 2 tablespoons raisins and ½ banana

1 cup skim milk

1 piece toast with 2 teaspoons peanut butter

Snack

1 ounce string cheese

1 apple

1 ounce baked tortilla chips

Lunch

1½ cups split pea soup

1 cup spinach salad with ½ tomato, mushrooms, ¼ avocado, 1 ounce grated reduced-fat Cheddar cheese, croutons, and vinaigrette dressing with 2 teaspoons canola oil

1 piece whole-wheat bread

1 orange

8 ounces low-fat yogurt

Snack

1 cup milk

2 cups popcorn

Celery sticks

Dinner

1 cup Black Bean and Corn Salad (page 224)

1 serving Broccoli Quiche (page 296)

Whole-wheat roll with
1 teaspoon reduced-fat
butter or margarine
1 cup skim milk

Snack

Strawberry Shake (page 242)

▼

Vegetarian Shopping List

Now that you are pregnant, you are probably much more aware of what you buy at the store. This handy shopping list can be reproduced and used weekly. (See page 169 for more information about shopping and label reading.)

Produce/Tofu

tofu

vegetables: asparagus, artichokes, broccoli, Brussels sprouts, beets, cabbage, carrots, cauliflower, celery, corn, eggplant, garlic, green beans, lettuce (romaine, leaf, Boston), mushrooms, onions (white, red), peppers (green, red, yellow), potato (sweet, white, new), rhubarb, rutabaga, spinach, summer squash, Swiss chard, tomatoes, turnips, winter squash, zucchini squash

fruit: apples, avocados, bananas, blueberries, canteloupe, cherries, grapes, grapefruit, honeydew melon, lemons, oranges, pears, peaches, plums, pineapple, raspberries, strawberries, watermelon

other:_____

_____

_____

Note: Foods that aren't in season fresh, should be bought frozen.

Dry Staples

grains/flour/etc.: barley, bulgur, nutritional yeast, oats, quinoa, wheat germ, wheat pastry flour, whole-wheat flour

rice: basmati, brown, instant, long- and short-grain, wild

dried fruit: apricots, dates, prunes, raisins

nuts and seeds: almonds, cashews, peanuts, sesame seeds walnuts

sweeteners: honey, molasses, sugar (brown, white)

pasta: cous cous, wheat, white

other:_____

_____

_____

Canned Goods/Jar Goods/ Packaged Items

beans: adzuki, black, chickpeas, garbanzo, kidney, navy, pinto, refried

nonfat evaporated milk

fruit: peaches, pears, pineapple

spreads/dips: chutney, fruit spread, peanut butter, tahini spread, tempeh

soups

tomatoes: paste, sauce, spaghetti sauce, whole

vegetarian specialty foods: veggie burger mix seaweed

other:_____

_____

_____

Breads

bagels, crackers, English muffins, pita, popcorn cakes pretzels, rye, tortillas (corn, flour), whole-wheat

other:_____

_____

_____

Dairy Case

cheeses: American, low-fat Cheddar, low-fat cottage cheese, mozzarella, soy, Swiss

other:_____

_____

milk: low-fat, skim, soy

soy yogurt

eggs

fresh pasta

biscuits

spreads: butter, margarine

other:_____

_____

_____

Oils/Condiments

flavored vinegar

low-fat salad dressings

**low-sodium soy sauce,
    tamari sauce, mayonnaise,
    mustard**

oils: olive, canola, walnut

spices: _____

_____

_____

Frozen Foods

frozen dinners _____

_____

frozen meals_____

_____

fruits _____

_____

meat substitutes _____

_____

pancakes, waffles _____

_____

**sorbet, tofutti, frozen
    yogurt, sherbet**_____

_____

vegetables_____

_____

veggie burgers _____

_____

seitan

tempeh

Snack Foods

rice cakes, crackers,

pretzels, graham crackers,

granola bars, cookies

other:_____

_____

Drinks

juices: frozen, vegetable,
    bottled

sparkling water

**decaffeinated coffee, tea,
    Cafix**

other:_____

_____

Nonfood Items

paper goods

soaps

toiletries

other:_____

_____

Complementary Proteins– An Old Myth

A myth has been passed down for years about complementary proteins. Even recently, vegetarians have been advised to eat the traditional legume with grain, grain with dairy, or nut and grain to have a "complete protein." Current thinking is that as long as a vegetarian eats a variety of foods with enough calories, she will have enough of all the amino acids. According to a position paper of the American Dietetic Association, "Mixtures of proteins from grains, vegetables, legumes, seeds, and nuts eaten over the course of the day complement each other in their amino acid profiles without the necessity of precise planning and complementation of proteins with each meal, as the recently popular "combined proteins theory" has urged."[17]

Vegetarian Menus

In Chapter Fifteen, you will find two weeks of budget menus, modified to fit pregnancy needs.

Vegetarian Fast-Food Choices

Since more people are going meatlesss, even if only occasionally, more restaurants are catering to vegetarian needs. The Vegetarian Resource Group recently released a book that lists natural-food restaurants across the country: *Guide to Natural Foods Restaurants in the U.S. and Canada* (Avery Publishing Group, 1995).

The following list of fast-food restaurants is an excerpt from *The Vegetarian Journal,* which summarizes the availability of vegetarian items at chain restaurants. *The Journal* is published by Vegetarian Resource Group, a nonprofit group devoted to vegetarianism. You can call them at (410) 366-VEGE. (See Chapter Twelve for more information on vegetarian menus at fast-food restaurants.)

An Update of Fast-Food Vegetarian Items

We hope this survey will help provide some answers to your questions about vegetarian foods available in fast-food restaurants. Please let us know if you hear of any new vegetarian items being sold in these establishments.

Au Bon Pain: Au Bon Pain has a variety of vegetarian choices and even has suggestions for healthy, low-fat meals. Nutritional information is available at each location. Four types of vegan bagels are available–plain, cinnamon, onion, and sesame. They also have several types of breads, none of which appear to be vegan. For breakfast a variety of muffins and Danishes are available, all of which are vegetarian. Lunch and dinner options include two vegan salads, the large garden and the small garden, both of which are made with two types of lettuce, red cabbage, carrots, tomatoes, cucumber, and red or green pepper. They also make a spinach and cheese croissant. Vegetarian soups include garden vegetarian, vegetarian chili, cream of broccoli, and tomato Florentine. When I last spoke to a consumer

advisor, she said that the company is expanding its menu and might include some new vegetarian soups.

Auntie Anne's: Auntie Anne's is a chain found in many food courts in shopping malls. They offer a variety of hand-rolled pretzels. The flavored pretzels and dips contain butter. However, although most of their pretzels are flavored with butter, upon request they will make one without butter. A pretzel ordered here without butter is vegan and low-fat.

Arby's: Arby's is now using vegetable oil for its fried foods. Their buns contain eggs or milk derivatives. Arby's offers the Garden Salad, which contains cheese, and a small vegan side salad. Arby's also offers a baked potato, and is presently testing vegetable pita pockets that contain broccoli, carrots, cauliflower, and celery. Their milkshakes contain animal gelatin, and the cheese contains animal rennet (as most cheese does). Arby's is working to improve its selection of healthy alternatives and confirmed that they are investigating other meatless options. They have typically offered low-fat products and are phasing out the use of MSG in all their products.

Baskin Robbins: Most Baskin Robbins' desserts are vegetarian and some are even vegan. Flavors made with marshmallow, however, contain animal gelatin. Dairy-free products include ices and sorbet. Most of their products are also egg-free with the exception of egg nog, French vanilla, vanilla, and custard flavors, and those with cookie and cake pieces. Baskin Robbins has put together a pamphlet that offers suggestions for individuals watching their cholesterol, fat, sugar, sulfite, and/or gluten intake.

Bob's Big Boy: Bob's Big Boy, part of Marriott Corporation's family of restaurants division, contains a decent selection for vegetarians, though options for vegans are limited. Breakfast options include cereal, potatoes, pancakes, French toast, bagels, toast, muffins, and a wide selection of fresh fruit. Bob's has just recently switched from instant oatmeal to old-fashioned, hearty kettle oatmeal from Quaker. Another pleasant surprise at Bob's is the Garden Lasagna, which is a vegetarian lasagna containing cheese, spinach, carrots, and onions. Bob's has offered a vegetable stir-fry in the past, but it did not sell well enough, so they decided upon the chicken stir-fry presently on their menu. This is a good example of how support by vegetarians could influence whether vegetarian options are offered. Other vegetarian items on Bob's menu are French fries, onion rings,

baked potatoes, and coleslaw. The Marriott Corporation certainly seems open to offering more vegetarian options if the demand is present.

Burger King: Burger King uses only vegetable oil for their fried products. Their national headquarters stated that it is standard procedure for fries, French toast, onion rings, and hash browns to be fried in oil separate from the "food" products, meaning the chicken and fish. However, a letter we received from a Burger King employee stated that the French fries are the only fried foods cooked in a separate vat. To be sure, ask at the restaurant you are visiting. Other vegetarian options at Burger King include the garden and side salads, croissants, bagels, blueberry muffins, and lemon pie. The cherry and apple pies contain casein (a milk derivative), and Snickers Ice Cream Bar contains gelatin. Burger King actually has a Veggie Whopper, which is cheese on a bun with whatever condiments and toppings you'd like. They will also make it without cheese. The Whopper buns may contain animal shortening, but the hamburger buns are purchased locally; so ask when you go in. The oat bran bun contains dairy products. Their bagels are made with vegetable shortening, but contain egg whites. Onion rings contain whey, but their

hash browns and French fries appear to be vegan. Burger King probably has the best quality salad dressings of the fast-food chains, since they use Paul Newman's dressings, which avoid using preservatives and artificial ingredients. The French, reduced-calorie Italian, and oil and vinegar dressings are all vegan. Their garden salad contains cheese, while the side salad lists only lettuce, tomatoes, cucumber, celery, and radishes. Burger King is successfully marketing a Spicy Bean Burger in the United Kingdom.

Carl's Jr.: French fries, onion rings, zucchini, and other fried foods at Carl's Jr. are cooked in vegetable oil. Their onion rings and zucchini contain dairy derivatives. Bread products that contain no animal shortening, eggs, or dairy derivatives include breadsticks, hot dog bun, flour tortilla, English muffin, and Kaiser bun. None of their baked goods contain animal shortening. They have an all-you-can-eat salad bar, as well as macaroni, potato, and pasta salads in some stores. They also offer a Lite Potato, with margarine on the side. Carl's Jr. is making efforts to remove MSG from all their foods.

Chi-Chi's: Chi-Chi's restaurants use soybean oil to prepare their refried beans and other deep-fried items. They list the following items as being vegetarian: Chips and Salsa (vegan), Vegetable Chajita (vegan), Cheese Nachos, Guacamole, Chili Con Queso, Vegetable and Spinach Quesadillas, Cheese and Onion Enchiladas, Mexican Fried Ice Cream, and Mexican Salad. However, most of their cheeses do contain rennet, which is an enzyme from the stomach of calves. You can request their pepperjack cheese, which we were told does not contain animal rennet. Although they use vegetable oil for all their fried foods, meat and vegetable products are fried in the same oil.

Church's Fried Chicken: Vegetarian options at Church's include coleslaw, French fries, okra, and mashed potatoes without gravy. They said that they fry their products in an all-vegetable shortening, but they fry their chicken nuggets in same oil.

Cracker Barrel: Vegetarian items available at Cracker Barrel include grits, coleslaw, French fries, onion rings, fried okra, and fried apples. The fried foods are not prepared in separate oil from the meat products, although all products are cooked in vegetable oil. The menu offers a variety of cooked vegetables, including corn on the cob, baked potatoes, and baked sweet potatoes. The sourdough bread is their only bread that does not contain dairy derivatives. Salads are available and can be modified to omit meat and dairy products.

Dairy Queen: Dairy Queen/Brazier stores use only vegetable shortening to prepare their foods, and the only food they fry is French fries. Ingredients in buns and onion rings depend upon the local supplier. They offer a garden salad, which contains eggs, and a side salad, which is apparently vegan.

Del Taco: Bean burritos, quesadillas, and tostadas are all vegetarian, and if the cheese is left out, they are vegan. Refried beans are prepared with 100 percent soybean oil and all sauces are meat-free.

Denny's: Denny's has a variety of choices for each meal. For breakfast, buttermilk biscuits, hash browns, French toast, and waffles are all available, along with seasonal fresh fruits. For dinner and lunch they offer a garden salad with eggs as a garnish, but the eggs can be omitted. There are a variety of side dishes, including French fries and onion rings, both of which appear to be vegan, as well as mozzarella sticks and cream of broccoli soup, which contains dairy but does not have an animal base. All fried foods are prepared in vegetable oil, but vegetarian items are cooked in the same oil as meat products. Two vegetarian sandwiches are available–grilled cheese and a veggie cheese melt. Breads are purchased locally and may contain dairy derivatives, and many of their cheeses contain animal rennet.

Domino's: Domino's has four ingredient groupings for their pizza crust, and your local unit might be using any one of them. Only one of the recipes is apparently vegan. The rest contain whey, and may contain egg, butter, buttermilk, cheese, and other dairy derivatives. None of these recipes contain lard. Their sauce appears to be vegan. The enzymes in their cheese are listed as being either of vegetable or animal origin.

El Chico's: El Chico's uses only vegetable oil for frying. Their refried beans reportedly do not contain lard, but you may want to check at your local restaurant.

Eat'n Park: Vegetarian options at Eat'n Park include the Gardenburger and a vegetarian stir-fry, as well as a salad bar.

El Pollo Loco: They offer a vegetarian burrito, which is basically a bean burrito prepared with beans that are cooked in olive oil. The vegetarian burrito, like other items, is made to order; so it can be ordered without cheese for a vegan burrito. The tortillas, both corn and flour, are vegan. Other vegetarian items include corn, potato salad, and a side salad. For dessert they have churros.

Hardee's: Hardee's uses vegetable oil to cook all fried products. They offer premade salads, including a garden salad (which contains cheese) and a side salad (which is vegan). Other vegetarian possibilities at Hardee's include pancakes, hash rounds, egg and cheese biscuit, cinnamon raisin biscuit, coleslaw, mashed potatoes, yogurt, and fries. Hardee's biscuits contain buttermilk and their gravy is sausage-based. Their Crispy Curls and French fries are fried separately from their fried meat products. Their mashed potatoes are instant and appear to be vegan except for the natural flavoring, which is questionable. Hardee's is also willing to make a cheese sandwich with toppings on a roll, but the cheese contains animal rennet.

Jack in the Box: They have a pamphlet that lists the ingredients for all their products. They cook with a griddle shortening that is a 100 percent vegetable oil blend, but the ingredients for this blend include natural butter flavor. The shortening blend for the fryers contains no animal products. As a rule, they fry French fries and onion rings separately from the meats, but this is not strictly enforced. Bread products that appear to be vegan include their English muffins, hamburger buns, sesame breadsticks, tortilla bowl (wheat), pita bread, and gyro bread. The croissants contain nonfat dry milk and butter, and the sourdough bread is grilled with shortening. The onion rings contain whey and egg yolk solids, and the apple turnover contains vegetable shortening. Hash browns, French fries, and guacamole appear to be vegan. The seasoned curly fries contain nonfat dry milk. Jack in the Box offers a side salad that is vegan. Their reduced-calorie French dressing contains nonfat yogurt, but the low-calorie Italian dressing appears to be vegan, with the possible exception of the "natural ingredients." Their "secret sauce" contains egg yolks and Worcestershire sauce (which contains anchovies). The cinnamon churritos contain dairy products and the cheesecake contains gelatin, but the apple turnover is vegan (although it is fried in the same oil used to fry animal products).

Kentucky Fried Chicken: KFC, as they prefer to be called these days, uses only vegetable shortening in all frying procedures, but their potato wedges are fried in the same oil as the chicken. The three breads they offer contain no animal shortening or dairy, but all contain egg products. Some stores carry a garden salad, which is vegan. Other vegetarian options include corn on the cob, coleslaw, fries, plain buttermilk biscuits, mashed potatoes (which contain butter and milk), Italian pasta salad, macaroni and cheese, and vegetable medley. The garden rice, green beans, mean greens, red beans and rice, and BBQ baked beans all contain meat or meat flavoring. Side dishes differ from store to store, but the ones mentioned here are found in 95 percent of the American KFC restaurants.

Little Caesars: No one can accuse Little Caesars of not being veggie-veggie. In their new "Vegetarian Guide" (available by writing to Corporate Communication, 2211 Woodward Avenue, Detroit, MI 48201-3400), Little Caesars discusses vegetarianism, vegetarian options available, and even what to get if you mean vegan!! Most Little Caesars use microbial or vegetable rennet in their cheese, but the Dallas, Greensboro, Atlanta, and Chicago area Little Caesars use calf rennet; so your best bet is to ask at each location. Their dough and tomato sauce are vegan, so order a pizza without cheese for a vegan meal. Other vegan items include Crazy Sauce and Crazy Bread, without Parmesan cheese. The Veggie Sub Sandwich is vegetarian.

Long John Silver's: All their fried foods have always been prepared in partially hydrogenated soybean oil. They offer prepared salads, corn on the cob, hush puppies, French fries, and green beans. The fries and hush puppies are prepared in the same oil as the meats. They also offer coleslaw, but at this time it is in the midst of being reformulated; so check the ingredients of this item during your next visit.

McDonald's: Fries and hash browns are both cooked in 100 percent vegetable oil, and are supposed to be prepared in vats separate from those used for meat. McDonald's offers a garden salad, which includes eggs, and a side salad, which is vegan. Beware that their Red French Reduced-Calorie dressing lists Worcestershire sauce, which contains anchovies. Their only dressing that appears to be vegan is the Lite Vinaigrette. For breakfast, vegetarian options include hash browns, apple bran muffins, and cereal. All three Danishes available contain gelatin. The Egg McMuffin can be ordered without meat, and so can the egg and cheese biscuit. McDonald's cookies appear to be vegan; the lecithin used is soy-derived. The chocolate chip cookies contain dairy products and the apple pie (which contains lecithin) is vegetarian.

Many McDonald's also prepare the Big Mac Sandwich without meat if requested. (The buns are vegan; however, the special sauce contains egg yolk.) McDonald's appears to be very interested in educating consumers as to what is in the food they are eating and provides information on ingredients, calories, fat, cholesterol, and sodium. Call 1-800-524-5900 if you want to receive any of this information.

Nathan's: Their thick French fries are cooked in corn oil. Corn on the cob is often available.

Pizza Hut: Pizza Hut Pan crust contains whey, but the Thin 'n Crispy and Hand-Tossed crusts are vegan. Whey is also an ingredient in the breadsticks. Pizza sauce contains MSG and cheese flavor, which is made with animal enzymes. A meat base is used for the pasta sauce. The cheese used on the pizzas is made with synthetic rennet.

Ponderosa: Ponderosa has a large food bar that typically contains plain vegetables as well as a salad bar, fruit, and fried foods. Ingredient listings were not available, but it seems possible to come up with a decent vegan meal at Ponderosa. People in the new-product testing department for Ponderosa did state that they are working on some vegetarian options!

Popeye's: Vegetarian items include corn on the cob, coleslaw, onion rings, and apple pies.

Rax: Rax is now using only Crisco, an all-vegetable shortening, for their fried foods. However, their beans are first cooked with lard. Their crackers and croutons may contain animal shortening, and their buns contain milk powder. Some of their pasta is vegan, but the rainbow rotini contains egg whites. Their spaghetti noodles appear to be vegan, but their sauce contains Parmesan cheese. The Rax salad bar has the regular salad bar offerings, plus macaroni salad, and, occasionally, a three-bean salad that appears to be vegan.

Round Table Pizza: The cheese used on Round Table Pizza is made with microbial enzymes, which have replaced animal rennet. Round Table has a variety of vegetable toppings, including black olives, garlic, mushrooms, pineapple tidbits, green peppers, tomatoes, onions, and jalapeño peppers. Their dough and tomato sauce are vegan. They use vegetable shortening.

Sbarro: This Italian fast-food chain is often located at travel rest areas and inside shopping malls. Their pizza crust is made with vegetable oil, and their marinara sauce contains cheese. The baked ziti and mostaccioli are made with egg pasta.

Shakey's: Shakey's uses vegetable oil for frying, and all of their dough contains vegetable shortening. Deep-fried vegetarian items are sometimes cooked in the same oil as the deep-fried meats, depending on the number of fryers available. We were unable to determine whether their dough contains dairy products or if their cheese contains animal rennet. They have a salad bar.

Shoney's: Shoney's has a breakfast bar with fruit, cake, bagels, and muffins. Other breakfast items include cereals, home fries, pancakes, hash browns, grits, and toast. Shoney's also has various prepared salads, a salad bar, and soups.

Skipper's: While the employees of many eating establishments seem to have little or no knowledge about ingredients in their foods, the Quality Assurance Manager at Skipper's was an exception. She definitively answered questions and had access to the sources of ingredients in their foods. Skipper's uses soybean oil for frying all their menu items. Their bread and breadsticks contain dairy products, but their crackers do not contain any animal products. They offer a garden salad that includes mixed greens, cucumbers, tomatoes, and carrots. Other vegetarian foods include baked potatoes,

zucchini slices, and coleslaw made with mayonnaise. They also have onion rings made with a beer-based batter that is vegan. They seemed very open to suggestions for new items. With a little encouragement and support, more vegetarian options might be offered.

Subway: Subway offers a veggies and cheese sub, which is a combination of vegetables including lettuce, tomatoes, green peppers, hot peppers, black olives, onions, and/or pickles. These are placed on a vegan sub roll, either white or wheat, and can be accompanied by cheese, mayo, oil, and/or vinegar. The cheese Subway uses is made with vegetable rennet. A salad with the same choice of vegetables is also available. Many locations are now offering Gardenburger subs and select stores are selling White Wave soy turkey subs. The Gardenburger sub is vegetarian, the "turkey" sub is vegan, but the soy cheese used in the "turkey" sub contains casein. These sandwiches are approved for "local sandwich status," meaning that individual Subway owners can choose to sell the product if they think the demand is big enough. Speak to your local Subway manager if you'd like to try to have either of these subs sold at the shop you frequent.

Taco Bell: Taco Bell has added a new line of low-fat dishes, which have some vegetarian differences. For example, on the regular menu, both the corn tortillas (hard tacos) and wheat tortillas (soft tacos) are vegan, but the heat-pressed flour tortillas used for burritos do contain nonfat dry milk. However, on the low-fat menu, the corn and wheat tortillas are vegan, as well as the light heat-pressed tortillas used for the low-fat burritos. Corn or soy oil is used in all frying processes. Both the regular and low-fat refried beans are vegan. Cheeses in the regular and low-fat dishes may contain animal rennet or vegetable enzymes; this differs from store to store. Taco Bell's guacamole contains sour cream. For dessert, the Cinnamon Twists and Border Ice products are vegan.

Taco John's International: Available vegetarian items include bean burritos made with refried beans cooked in canola oil. No lard or tropical oils are used in any products or food preparation. Both the nachos and Potato Olés are also vegetarian, but are fried in the same oil as the meat products. The tortillas contain no animal shortening, but may contain dairy products. The guacamole is vegan. Any item on the menu can be made vegetarian by substituting beans for meat. If you are vegan, request no cheese or sour cream. The cheese Taco John's uses contains no animal rennet.

TacoTime: TacoTime uses vegetable oil for their deep fryers, and wanted to make it clear that they have never used lard in thirty-three years of business. Their refritos are made with vegetable shortening. Tortillas are vegan. Vegetarian dishes available at TacoTime include soft bean burrito, crisp bean burrito, refritos (bean, sauce, and cheese), tostados, nachos, and Mexi-fries. They could not tell me for sure whether vegetarian fried items, such as the Mexi-fries, are cooked in separate oil from the meat products. When I last spoke with them, they were in the midst of hiring a person who would deal with questions pertaining to ingredients and nutrition; so if you have further questions for this company, call them.

T.G.I. Friday's: Though T.G.I. Friday's is more of a "regular" versus "fast-food" restaurant, we included it here because this chain presently has several "real" vegetarian options on the menu, including a vegetarian burger called a Garden Burger. Apparently, public response has been overwhelmingly positive, and they are very interested in expanding their vegetarian selections. The Garden Burger does have some dairy in it. Other op-

tions include a Fresh Vegetable Baguette, which contains cheese and is served with yogurt, and the Garden Cob, their number-one-selling salad, contains artichokes, green peppers, yellow squash, and other veggies. They also have a Vegetable Med-ley, which is steamed vegetables served with rice and a dinner salad. Beware that the brown rice pilaf served with the Medley contains chicken base. Order a baked potato as a substitute, and you'll have a filling, vegan meal.

Wendy's: Over the last couple of years Wendy's has made some definitely provegetarian changes. Wendy's SuperBar has one of the best salad bars in the fast-food arena, and they are constantly striving to make it better. They have removed the "natural beef flavor" from the spaghetti sauce, making it vegan; the sauce can be placed over the rotini, which is also vegan. They also offer an alfredo sauce, which is vegetarian, and macaroni and cheese. At the Mexican Fiesta, the refried beans no longer contain lard. The only questionable ingredient in the Spanish rice is the natural flavoring, which may be animal-derived. The flour tortillas contain whey, but Wendy's taco chips, taco sauce, and taco shells are vegan. Also available are several salads made to-go—the deluxe garden salad and the side salad are both vegetarian, but do

list imitation cheese as an ingredient. Besides the salads-to-go, the Garden Spot salad bar offers the makings for a salad. Vegetables include alfalfa sprouts, broccoli, carrots, cauliflower, cucumbers, chives, green peppers, lettuce, mushrooms, onions, and tomatoes. Vegan dressings include French, Sweet Red French, Golden Italian, and Reduced-Calorie Italian, none of which contain questionable ingredients; Wendy's has informed us that the natural flavor found in these dressings is not animal-derived. Their fat-free French contains white honey, and the Italian caesar dressing contains anchovy paste, as well as egg and cheese. The croutons contain cheese and egg whites. Other vegetarian items found at the salad bar include breadsticks, Cheddar chips, coleslaw, cottage cheese, potato salad, pudding, and fruit. All Wendy's locations have the Garden Spot salad bar, but unfortunately only some locations have the SuperBar. Hot vegetarian items at all Wendy's locations include a baked potato with choice of toppings and French fries. The French fries are cooked in separate oil from the meat products; however, there is the possibility that oil used to cook the chicken could be rotated into the French fry vat! They also offer a vegetarian sandwich, which is a choice of toppings on

Food	Calories	Protein*	Carbo-hydrate*	Fat*	Fiber*
Nutrient Information for Some Products Currently Available at Large Natural-Food Stores					
Amy's Shepherd's Pie	160	5	27	4	5
Amy's Tofu Vegetable Lasagna	300	13	41	10	6
Boca Burger	97	13	9	1	4
Cascadian Farm Indian Vegetarian Meal	250	9	46	4	7
Cascadian Farm Oriental Vegetarian Meal	260	13	40	7	10
Celentano Lasagne Primavera	210	11	32	4	5
Garden Chef Garden Burger	140	8	21	2.5	5
Garden Chef Garden Dog	120	19	4	2.5	1
Natural Touch Garden Vege Pattie	110	10	8	4	3
Natural Touch Vegetarian Dinner Entree	220	19	2	15	2
Señor Felix's Spinach & Ricotta Empanada	260	10	41	10	6
Soy Rice Tempeh	140	12	13	5	5
Traditionally Seasoned Tempeh	140	31	4	0	1
Turkey Style Sandwich Slices	80	13	7	0	1
Veggie Pockets Bar-B-Q Style	290	10	45	8	5
Veggie Pockets Greek Style	250	10	37	8	4
White Wave Vegetarian Sloppy Joe	320	36	21	10	9

*In grams

Source: Manufacturers' labels.

a bun (which contains whey) without meat. They say that all their cheeses are made with microbial enzymes. Wendy's has reportedly tested a grainburger and they are looking into other vegetarian possibilities. Their consumer department was very helpful, and they definitely seem open to new ideas. Let's encourage them to follow up on a veggie burger!

Mrs. Winner's: Their potatoes are fried only in vegetable oil.

Source: "What's In Fast Food," by Michael Keevican, 1996, Vegetarian Resource Group, Baltimore, Maryland.

▼

Vegetarian Convenience-Food Choices

Going meatless is now catching on, and vegetarian foods are now widely available at your neighborhood grocery store. The fat in some products is still surprisingly high, so be sure to read the label if fat is a concern for you. To the left is a table that lists the nutrient information for some products currently available at large natural-food stores. Nutrient content is per serving listed on label.

Following are just some of the frozen entrees, either vegetarian (containing cheese or milk) or vegan, found in most grocery stores. To make a complete meal, add milk or yogurt, vegetable, fruit, and, in some cases, beans, or other source of protein.

Budget Gourmet Macaroni and Cheese with Cheddar and Parmesan
Budget Gourmet Three-Cheese Lasagna
Healthy Choice Manicotti with Three Cheeses
Healthy Choice Pasta Shells Marinara
Lean Cuisine Angel Hair Pasta
Lean Cuisine Cheese Ravioli
Lean Cuisine Fettucini Primavera
Lean Cuisine Macaroni and Cheese with Broccoli
Michelina's Spaghetti Marinara
Weight Watchers Kung Pao Noodles and Vegetables
Weight Watchers Parisian-Style White Beans with Vegetables
Weight Watchers Pasta and Spinach Romano
Weight Watchers Paella Rice and Vegetables
Weight Watchers Peking-Style Rice and Vegetables
Weight Watchers Pilaf Florentine
Weight Watchers Risotto with Cheese and Mushrooms
Weight Watchers Santa Fe-Style Rice and Beans

Here are some ideas for convenience foods you can buy at the grocery store to form the basis of a vegetarian meal.

Bird's Eye Meal Starter Oriental Stir Fry
Bird's Eye Meal Starter Primavera
Bird's Eye Meal Starter Teriyaki Stir Fry
Green Giant Create-A-Meal Garlic Herb
Green Giant Create-A-Meal Szechuan Stir Fry
Green Giant Harvest Burgers
Healthy Choice Split Pea, Garden Vegetable, or Country Vegetable Soup
Health Valley Vegetarian Chili
Morning Star Farms Veggie Burgers
Progresso Lentil or Black Bean Soup
Rosarita or Kuner's Vegetarian Refried Beans

▼

Eating after Delivery

Your doctor must order the diet, or type of meal, that you receive in the hospital. Make sure your doctor understands that you want a vegetarian meal and specify which type. Many hospitals have options for vegetarians, but they usually aren't vegan.

In addition, a dietary technician or registered dietitian may visit you to see if you have specific likes or dislikes or if you are having any problems eating. Make your preferences known, and also try to select your own menu, if possible. Be polite, but persistent!

(See page 147 for more information about eating after delivery. You can also read *Hospital Survival Guide,* by Suzanne Havala, M.S., R.D., and *Vegetarian Journal Reports,* by Vegetarian Resource Group, 1990.)

Eating after Surgery

If you have a cesarean section, you may not eat solid food for a day or so, depending on which type of anesthesia you receive. The progression from "nothing by mouth" to "regular diet" usually starts with clear liquids such as clear juices, broth, gelatin, coffee, tea, and soda. As your tolerance increases, your diet will progress to a full-liquid diet, which includes such foods as thinned hot cereals, cream soups, and dairy products, in addition to clear liquids.

You should be able to omit the nonvegetarian foods and eat double portions of the other foods. Again, make sure that your doctor has left instructions for you to have a vegetarian diet once you can eat solid food.

? Questions You May Have

Q: I just found out I have gestational diabetes; how can I fit vegetarian foods into my meal plan?

A: Actually, a vegetarian diet fits very well into the guidelines of a diabetic diet. Depending on your blood sugar, your dietitian may want you to eat less carbo- hydrate and more fat. To do this you could increase your intake of nuts, avocado, peanut butter, and cheese. Visiting with a reg- istered dietitian would be help- ful in planning a vegetarian diet to meet your specific needs. On this page you will find a table of some typical vegetarian foods with their exchanges.

Q: Is a vegetarian diet lower in fat than a diet containing meat?

A: Generally, yes. However, a vegetarian diet can be as high in fat as a meat-containing diet. For example, lacto-ovo vegetarians may eat a lot of cheese, eggs, and low-fat or regular dairy products, which raise the fat content of the diet. A diet that is not well plan- ned can have as much fat (in- cluding saturated fat) as the typ- ical American diet!

A vegan diet can also be high in fat, although most of the fat would be unsaturated (unless you regularly use coconut prod- ucts and palm or palm kernel oil). For example, nuts, tahini, avocado, and nut butters, staples for some vegetarians, are very high in fat. Other hidden fats can find their way into the diet through such goodies as tofu ice cream and carob.

The important feature for any type of diet is that high-fat foods (especially those high in saturat- ed fat), be eaten in moderation.

Q: I've heard a lot about the RDAs. Can a vegetarian meet the RDAs?

A: Many people think that RDA stands for Recommended Daily Allowances, when it really stands for Recommended Dietary Allowances. The RDAs are de- signed for the maintenance of good nutrition of practically all healthy people in the United States. They have a built-in safe- ty margin.[14]

Exchanges for Special Vegetarian Foods		
Food	**Serving Sizes**	**Exchanges**
Beans, dried, cooked	1/2 cup	1 starch + 1 very lean meat
Brewer's yeast	3 tablespoons	1 starch
Bulgur, cooked	½ cup	1 starch
Carob flour	⅛ cup	1 starch
Kefir	1 cup	1 milk + 1 fat
Loma Linda Veggie Links	1 ounce	1 high-fat meat
Morningstar Farms Grillers	1 ounce	1 high-fat meat
Miso	3 tablespoons	1 vegetable
Seaweed, cooked	½ cup	1 vegetable
Soy flour	¼ cup	1 lean meat + ½ bread
Soy grits, raw	⅛ cup	1 lean meat
Soymilk	1 cup	1 milk + 1 fat
Tahini	1 teaspoon	1 fat
Tempeh	4 ounces	1 starch + 2 lean meats
Tofu, soft	½ cup	1 medium-fat meat
Tofu, firm	½ cup	2 medium-fat meats
Wheat germ	3 tablespoons	1 starch

Source: Modified from *Vegetarian Journal Reports,* Vegetarian Resource Group.

Some sources say that the World Health Organization's RDIs (Reference Daily Intake) are closer to the needs of the vegetarian population. For example, the RDAs for calcium are 1,200 milligrams; the RDIs for calcium are 1,000 to 1,200 milligrams.[14] Which is correct? Both. The RDAs are based on the typical U.S. diet, which contains meat, while the RDIs take into account the needs of populations that don't eat meat.

How will you know whether you are getting enough of all the nutrients? Eat a variety of many foods as outlined in one of the vegetarian meal plans listed previously. Eat as many unrefined foods as possible, and enough calories, and the rest of your diet will fall into place. Your weight gain and your baby's size (as checked by fundal height and ultrasound) will also show that your diet meets the mark.

Q: I'm worried about being in the hospital and not being able to eat vegetarian... any advice?

A: First of all, if you preregister at your hospital, you might be able to request a vegetarian diet then. When you go to the hospital in labor, you will probably be allowed to eat only ice chips or perhaps clear liquid, such as apple juice. This is because if you need anesthesia, your stomach should be empty. During this time, you might want to remind your doctor that when you *can* eat, you would like a vegetarian diet. You might even want to write down your request before you go to the hospital.

After you have your baby, you will probably be allowed to eat a "real meal." Your meal may depend on what's left in the kitchen—which, in turn, depends on what time your baby was born! Babies seem to love arriving off hours, and that may mean "slim pickings" for a very hungry new mom! A simple meal would be just a cheese sandwich, fruit, and juice. For vegans, the selection may be very limited if after hours. You may want to bring in some nonperishable snacks from home as options for after delivery.

Special Care for High-Risk Pregnancies

Expect the Unexpected

The unknown can be awfully scary—especially when you're pregnant. This chapter tells you about special conditions, how they may affect you and baby, and what you can do. Although other complications may be associated with pregnancy, this chapter will discuss only the conditions that can affect or can be affected by your diet. Being informed is the key to taking charge of your health and having the healthiest pregnancy possible!

Dealing with Your Emotions

When you discover that you have a high-risk condition, you will probably find yourself on a rollercoaster ride of emotions. Guilt, fear, anger, denial, depression, loneliness—you may experience some or all of these emotions. Some emotions are helpful in getting you through the rough times. On the other hand, emotions can be unhealthy if they prevent you from taking care of yourself.

For example, guilt and fear may motivate you to make changes in your lifestyle to protect your baby and denial may give you a cushion of time to get used to the idea of a high-risk condition. However, depression and loneliness can sometimes alienate us from people who can help us the most. Recognizing these feelings for what they are can help you adjust and seek support from others. If you experience any of these feelings to the point where they hinder your dealing with your situation or significantly affect your sleeping or eating patterns, speak with your physician.

When I was put on bed rest for eleven weeks with my second child, I too had many of the emotions you are feeling right now.

I got so upset at one point, that I was just going to walk out the front door and walk away from my problems. Of course, that wasn't possible, but it did give me an emotional release. (And looking back, the idea of trying to walk away from your own stomach is pretty funny!)

What helped me the most was the support I received from others and reading about the experiences of other women on bed rest. Whatever happens and whatever you have to do to get to the end of your pregnancy, it will be worth it when you see your healthy baby!

You Are Not Alone

One of the hardest things about having a high-risk pregnancy is that you may feel as though you are the only person with your problem. However, many women have experienced or are now going through the same challenges you are. Sidelines National Support Network is a network of local support groups for women experiencing high-risk pregnancies and for their families. Call to find a local support group or a listening ear. Send your own thoughts, poems, jokes, and anecdotes to share with others.

You can contact the network by writing to Sidelines National Support Network, c/o Candace Hurley; 2805 Park Place, Laguna Beach, CA 92651, or by calling 714-497-2265.

The Confinement Line will find a woman to act as your support line while you are on bed rest. You can write to them at The Confinement Line Childbirth Education Association; P.O. Box 1609, Springfield, VA 22151, or call 703-941-7183.

▼

Preexisting Diabetes

If you are currently diabetic, you probably already know the importance of managing your diabetes. Before conception and during pregnancy are critical times to control your blood sugar. Before you think about becoming pregnant, consult your physician, who will want you to be in "tight control" and will want to closely monitor you.

The Importance of Tight Control

High blood sugar in the first six to ten weeks of gestation is related to birth defects. Consequently, babies of women who have diabetes are at a higher risk of birth defects. However, moms who maintain acceptable blood sugar control are no more at risk for having babies with birth defects than the general population.[1]

The American Diabetes Association suggests that, *before* conception, diabetic moms-to-be keep fasting (over-night fast) and pre-meal (just before a meal) blood sugars between 70 and 100 milligrams, one-hour-after-meals blood sugars less than 140 milligrams and two-hours-after-meal blood sugars under 120 milligrams. Be sure to work out your individual goals with your health care provider.[2]

The Health Care Team

Before we go further, we should talk about a group of people who are very important to the health of your baby—the health care team. You will need some specialized medical professionals to help in your care. If you are not already working with these health professionals, you can find them by calling a local medical society, asking your family physician, or calling a local chapter of the American Dietetic Association or the American Diabetes Association.

A diabetologist, endocrinologist, or physician who specializes in the care of diabetics is someone you should talk to before you become pregnant, to make sure you are in good control of your diabetes.

A **perinatologist** is an obstetrician who specializes in high-risk pregnancies, or one who has experience working with pregnant diabetics. Some women consult with a perinatologist before they get pregnant if they have had previous problems in pregnancy.

An endocrinologist is a physician who specializes in caring for people with diabetes and also treats other conditions that involve hormones. You may be under an endocrinologist's care already or your obstetrician may refer you to one to help manage your diabetes during pregnancy.

A certified diabetes educator (C.D.E.) will probably be a registered nurse, but dietitians and physicians can also hold the designation of C.D.E., which refers to someone who has many hours of experience working with people who have diabetes and who has also passed a certification exam. The nurse educator, or nurse practitioner, is a registered nurse who has more education and/or experience in a specialized field. This will probably be the person you work closely with for day-to-day management of your diabetes.

A registered dietitian (R.D.) is someone who will develop an individual eating plan for you. An individual meal plan is important since it can be specifically designed with your activity level,

work schedule, lifestyle, and favorite foods in mind. The dietician usually works closely with the nurse educator. Your dietitian can also work with you after you have your baby to help with diet for breastfeeding and weight loss.

A pediatrician or neonatologist is someone who provides medical care for your baby after it's born. Since babies of diabetics sometimes have problems, a specialist such as a neonatologist (who specializes in newborns up to six weeks old) might be needed.

You are the most important member of the health care team. You are responsible for the day-to-day management of your diabetes, including contacting other members of the team to let them know how you are doing or when you need help.

What to Expect

If you are taking insulin, you will probably have to adjust your doses, with the help of your health care team. Some women need to adjust their insulin dosage as often as every five days because of increased need.[3] If you were controlled with diet or oral medications (Type II diabetic, or noninsulin-dependent) before pregnancy, there is a good chance you will be put on insulin during pregnancy. However, after you have your baby,

you will most likely return to your prior mode of treatment, especially if you return to your ideal body weight and exercise regularly.

Some women take injections before every meal to keep their sugar in control. Others use a pump. Be prepared to take more shots if needed. Taking more shots will most likely mean checking your blood sugar more often.

Possible Effects on Mom

Pregnant diabetics have a greater chance of having a miscarriage, hypertension, preeclampsia, and excess amniotic fluid.[4]

What to watch out for:

Some "normal" conditions of pregnancy can be a real challenge for diabetics. And, some "normal" conditions for diabetic women are also more challenging during pregnancy.

Insulin resistance: As pregnancy progresses, especially around the twenty-fourth to twenty-eighth weeks, a hormone produced by the placenta resists insulin. Therefore, the body needs much more insulin. Diabetic moms-to-be may need twice the insulin they usually take.

Sign of insulin resistance:

increased blood sugar

Ketoacidosis: Ketones are by-products of fat breakdown and are a sign that glucose is not available and the body is breaking down fat stores for energy. As ketones increase in the bloodstream (usually as a result of high blood sugar from not having an adequate dose of insulin), the pH level of the blood changes and ketoacidosis occurs. Because of changing insulin needs and energy requirements during pregnancy, ketoacidosis can occur more quickly and, if not treated, can eventually lead to a coma.

Signs of ketoacidosis:
If you have any of these signs, seek medical attention fast! (Some symptoms are similar to signs of hyperglycemia, but are much more intense.)

  excessive urination
  excessive thirst
  fruity, acetone, or alcohol
    breath
  listlessness; total lack
    of energy
  nausea
  abdominal pains
  vomiting
  labored breathing

Morning sickness: If you have this common symptom of pregnancy, it can throw off your usual intake of food. Vomiting can cause dehydration and upset insulin needs. Both can result in low blood sugar. Follow the guidelines for morning sickness

in Chapter One and "sick-day rules" guidelines later in this chapter.

Signs of morning sickness:
  nausea
  vomiting

Hypoglycemia (low blood sugar): Low blood sugar can occur because of increased activity, energy demands of baby, and from increased insulin dosage. Always have glucose tablets or glucose gel with you, or keep in your purse a food that is a quick source of energy, such as chewable candy, fruit juice, or nondiet soda. Be sure to have a more substantial snack, such as half a sandwich or cheese and crackers, about a half hour later. Add milk for a more substantial snack.

If you have low blood sugar more than once a week, report this to your health care provider. If you can pinpoint the cause of your low blood sugar, try to remedy it with the guidance of your health care team. Preventing the low blood sugar is often just a matter of eating before exercise, eating a bigger meal, or adding a snack, or you may need a different insulin schedule. Many people are surprised to find that they have been giving their injections incorrectly, even though they may have been taking shots for years. This could also affect your blood sugar.

Signs of hypoglycemia:
(These signs may develop very quickly.)

  nervousness
  shakiness
  dizziness
  perspiration
  cold, clammy skin
  blurred vision
  headache
  disorientation, difficulty
    paying attention
  irritability, sudden mood
    changes
  pale skin

Hyperglycemia (high blood sugar): Hyperglycemia is elevated blood sugar. It can be caused by changes in how your insulin is being used (see insulin resistance); by being less active, by being under mental or physical stress (such as illness); by eating more food, or different types of foods, than usual; or by a combination of any of these factors. Elevated blood sugars can cause your baby to grow larger and fatter than normal (macrosomia), which may lead to a difficult delivery.

Signs of hyperglycemia:
(These signs occur gradually.)

  hunger
  frequent urination
  increased thirst
  headaches
  fatigue

Infections: Even minor infections can increase blood sugar and change insulin requirements. This can cause a breakdown of fat and lead to ketoacidosis (see definition on page 100). If you have the symptoms of ketoacidosis, seek medical attention immediately.

Sick-Day Rules

During illness, follow these rules. If you are sick with a virus or infection, your blood sugar will increase, even though you may not be eating much. The following rules are important to remember:

▶ **Contact a member of your health care team.**

This is the first sick-day rule during pregnancy, especially if you are vomiting or have diarrhea.

▶ **Continue to take your insulin.**

Talk to your physician to see if you should take the same dose. You may actually need more.

▶ **Check blood sugar more frequently.**

Your doctor or diabetes educator will let you know how often. This will prevent any potential problems of high blood sugar and ketoacidosis. Your doctor may also want you to check your urine for ketones more frequently.

▶ **Prevent dehydration.**

Do this by drinking at least half a cup of fluid per hour. If you can't keep much food down, and you are taking insulin, you must have carbohydrate in liquid form–this will give your body energy and will prevent dehydration. Examples of liquids (as well as some easy-to-digest solid foods) that contain ten to fifteen grams of carbohydrate are:

Fruit Juice or Sweetened Drinks
   ⅓ to ½ cup apple juice
   ½ cup orange juice
   ⅓ to ½ cup soda or fruit
      punch (not diet)
   ¼ to ⅓ cup lemonade

Solid Foods Easy to Digest
   4 saltine crackers
   ¼ cup sherbet
   ½ popsicle (these vary from
      brand to brand)
   ¼ cup regular Jell-O
   10 ounces chicken noodle
      soup
   10 ounces chicken and rice
      soup
   8 ounces cream of
      mushroom soup
      (prepared with water)

▶ **If you can eat solids, drink plenty of calorie-free drinks to avoid dehydration.**

Good examples are water, broth or bouillon, decaffeinated tea, sugar-free and caffeine-free soda, sugar-free fruit drinks or popsicles, etc.

▶ **Replenish lost sodium or potassium.**

If you are losing a lot of fluid through vomiting or diarrhea, you will need to replenish your body with these important minerals. Here are good sources:

Sodium: Bouillon, canned soups, salted crackers, and Gatorade (choose regular or sugar-free, depending on your ability to eat other solids).

Potassium: Orange juice, melon, papaya, banana, orange-pineapple-banana juice, pineapple juice, tomato juice, vegetable juice, and dried fruits.

How Diabetes May Affect Your Baby

Blood sugar crosses the placenta from you to your baby. High blood sugar causes the baby to produce more insulin. The effects of large amounts of sugar and insulin can cause serious risks, including a greater chance of stillbirth. However, stillbirth is not common.

Birth defects occur more often in babies of mothers who are diabetic. Fortunately, pre-conception planning, early prenatal care, and keeping blood sugars in a narrow range can dramatically decrease that risk. If possible, seek medical counseling before you consider pregnancy.

Women with diabetes are prone to having bigger babies (macrosomia). High levels of blood glucose in mom, especially during late pregnancy, are thought to be responsible. After thirteen weeks gestation, your baby can start producing its own insulin in response to high blood glucose levels. Insulin acts as a growth hormone, causing baby to deposit excess fat, and the increased size may make a C-section necessary.

Babies of diabetics sometimes have hypoglycemia (low blood sugar) immediately after delivery and they must take glucose or sugar water. They are also prone to having higher bilirubin levels, or jaundice, which is easily treated with special lights in the hospital. Babies of diabetic moms can have a higher chance of having respiratory distress syndrome.[5]

If your diabetes is advanced and you have some blood vessel damage, you may have restricted blood flow to the placenta, so your baby may have problems growing and may be small for gestational age.

What can you do:

To keep your diabetes under good control during pregnancy:

▶ See your doctor before you become pregnant.

You may also want to see a registered dietitian to get a handle on dietary management.

▶ Eat more high-fiber foods and whole grains.

Soluble fiber helps keep blood sugar in control by slowing digestion. Foods high in soluble fiber include oatmeal, legumes and peas, barley, fruits, and vegetables. The antioxidants and insoluble fiber found in whole grains have additional benefits, such as preventing constipation.

▶ Monitor your blood sugar.

Your physician will give you the blood sugar range within which you should stay. The blood sugar range during pregnancy is much stricter than when you are not pregnant. Remember that blood glucose values reflect what has happened in the last one to three hours.

▶ Eat regular meals and snacks.

You will want to eat balanced meals at regular intervals. Most women need 2,000 to 2,400 cal-

ories, divided between carbohydrate (45 to 50 percent), fat (30 to 35 percent), and protein (20 percent). Your calories will be divided between meals and snacks. Especially important is the bedtime snack, which should contain carbohydrate, fat, and protein. Eating a snack before bedtime (especially one that contains protein) can prevent hypoglycemia in the middle of the night. Some women even need a snack in the middle of the night (such as a glass of milk) to keep their blood sugar up.

▶ Exercise.

You should ask your physician about specific guidelines for frequency and duration of exercise and when NOT to exercise (such as when blood sugar is too low or too high). Regular exercise can decrease your need for insulin and also make you feel more energetic! When you exercise, always take glucose gel or tablets, fruit juice, or hard candy with you, and eat a snack or meal before you exercise. Never exercise when you know your blood sugar is low or when ketones are present. Also, don't give your insulin injection in an area that you will use immediately in exercise. For example, don't give it in the leg if you will take a brisk walk im-mediately afterwards. (See page 103, "Gestational Diabetes," for other tips on exercising.)

Labor and Delivery

Many doctors will induce labor for pregnant women who are diabetic. With all the high-tech equipment available, your physician can tell just when the baby is developed enough to enter our world. About one-half of all diabetics will need a cesarean delivery because the baby is too big to fit through the birth canal, or because of other complications.[6]

During the first twenty-four to forty-eight hours postpartum, your insulin requirements can drop dramatically. You may need to watch for signs of hypoglycemia. Within a week after delivery, your insulin needs should return to prepregnant levels.

How to Cope

▶ **Keep stress low.**

Remember that stress can also raise blood sugar. Learn some new techniques to handle your stress, such as relaxation, visualization, and advanced planning. Again, seek cooperation from others to help reduce your stress.

▶ **Remember that the extra time and discomfort you experience now will only last nine months.**

When you have your healthy baby, it will all be worth it.

▶ **Seek out a diabetes support group, preferably one for pregnant women.**

Research shows that women who have more social support can follow their dietary and self-monitoring regimens better.[7]

▶ **You and your family need to be committed to your pregnancy and to the unborn child.**

Everyone should learn how insulin works, the importance of dietary management, and what to do in case of hypo- or hyperglycemia. You'll also need your family's emotional support and understanding.

"It was really tough to put myself first," says Cindy, a woman who has been diabetic for fifteen years. "When I was pregnant with my second child, I felt guilty when I had to stop whatever I was doing to get myself something to eat because of low blood sugar. But I learned that I had to put myself first for the sake of my baby."

▶ **Learn to recognize the early warning signs of hypoglycemia, hyperglycemia, and ketoacidosis so you can take action.**

▶ **Always be prepared to handle a low blood sugar reaction.**

(See page 100 on how to treat hypoglycemia.)

Gestational Diabetes

Almost 3 percent of all pregnant women will have diabetes of pregnancy, or gestational diabetes mellitus (GDM).[8] Diabetes mellitus is a disorder that prevents the body from using a simple sugar called glucose. GDM is a type of diabetes that occurs only during pregnancy and usually disappears after delivery.

Glucose is a simple sugar that is the final product of carbohydrate digestion. Carbohydrate is found in all starchy foods, such as bread, potatoes, and corn, and is also in milk, fruits, and vegetables. Forms of simple carbohydrate that enter the bloodstream more quickly are found in candy, jam, syrup, honey, and table sugar. Your body can also make glucose from protein and stored carbohydrates. Every cell in the body uses glucose for energy.

Insulin is the hormone produced by the pancreas that allows glucose to enter your body's cells. A trace mineral called chromium is necessary for insulin to work.

Evidence shows that inadequate dietary chromium could lead to GDM. Chromium is found in whole-grain cereals and breads, wheat germ, meat, and brewer's yeast—foods that are in short supply in many women's diets. It can't hurt to try to include more of those foods in yours.

During pregnancy, women need two to three times more insulin for the body to use glucose. This increase is due to increased body weight and increased levels of hormones that work against insulin; these hormones peak during the twenty-fourth to twenty-eighth week. When the body cannot produce the insulin it needs, high blood sugar and diabetes are the result.

Effects on Mom

Many women have no signs that they have GDM. Some of the symptoms of GDM are also the typical signs of pregnancy, such as fatigue and frequent urination, so you may not be able to tell them apart. Some women have the symptoms of high blood sugar or low blood sugar, listed on page 100. Women with GDM have increased risk of preeclampsia (a type of hypertensive disorder of pregnancy) and urinary tract infections. Symptoms of urinary tract infections include burning during urination and frequent urination.[9]

Effects on Baby

The most common problem is delivering a large baby (macrosomia), which may produce a difficult delivery, trauma to the baby during delivery, and/or increased need for a C-section.

Less common problems sometimes seen in babies of mothers with GDM include greater risk of premature delivery, hypoglycemia (low blood sugar) at birth, increased bilirubin in the blood (jaundice), and respiratory distress syndrome.[10]

A recent study shows that intensified management of blood glucose resulted in similar rates of macrosomia, C-section, stillbirth, and respiratory complications in diabetic and nondiabetic women.[11]

Who is at risk?

For Gestational Diabetes

Risk factors for gestational diabetes include a previous stillbirth, history of miscarriages, family history of diabetes, previous delivery of an infant weighing over nine pounds, previous gestational diabetes, urinary tract infections, hydramnios, sugar in the urine, and more-than-ideal body weight. Evidence also shows that the risk of GDM goes up with each subsequent pregnancy, and as you get older.[12]

For Adult Onset (Type II) Diabetes

As opposed to Type I Diabetes, which generally has an onset in childhood and requires insulin from then on, Type II Diabetes is usually diagnosed in adulthood and, as a rule, does not require insulin injections.

It is estimated that half of all diabetics in the U.S. haven't even been diagnosed. Your chances of becoming diabetic are greater if you—

- have a close relative who is diabetic.
- were diagnosed with GDM in a previous pregnancy.
- are overweight.
- have had a baby that weighed nine pounds or more.
- are African American, Native American or Mexican American.
- are over forty years old.

Testing for Diabetes

When you are between the twenty-fourth and twenty-eighth week of pregnancy, your health care provider will ask you to take a glucose screening test that tests for sugar in the blood. This test is done without special preparations such as fasting or eating certain foods. First you will be asked to drink a very sweet drink called glucose (it tastes like cola syrup before the carbonated water is added). One hour later, your blood will be drawn and the amount of sugar (or glucose) in your blood will be tested. If your blood sugar is over 140 milligrams, this is considered a positive, or "abnormal," test. You may be asked to–

• see a registered dietitian (R.D.) for meal-planning guidance

OR

• take a glucose tolerance test, which is similar to the glucose screenig test but lasts three hours. You will need to follow a special high-carbohydrate diet for three days prior to the test. Your health care provider will give you the specific instructions. After drinking the glucose, a health professional will draw your blood every hour for three hours.[13]

Once your physician diagnoses you with GDM, you may be referred to a specialist, such as an endocrinologist or a perinatologist, who probably works with a staff of diabetes educators. However, your physician may decide to treat the diabetes aspect of your pregnancy by working closely with an R.D., who will give you a diabetic meal plan, and a Nurse Educator, who will teach you about

monitoring your blood sugar. (If you aren't referred to an R.D., you should request a referral!)

▼

The Diabetic Eating Plan

Many people think that going on a diabetic diet means they must give up all their favorite foods. This is just not true!

The diabetic eating plan is simply a way of eating that includes balanced amounts of carbohydrate, fat, and protein at each meal. All foods are allowed except simple sugars such as table sugar (sucrose), honey, jam, syrup, and foods that contain a lot of sugar, such as cakes, pies, cookies, and candy. However, foods with a small amount of sugar are allowed in moderation, when "counted" into your meal plan. For example, graham crackers, animal crackers, and angel food cake are foods allowed in moderation when your blood sugar is in good control.

The goal in managing your diabetes is to keep your blood sugar within a certain range. General guidelines are listed on page 98 under "Preexisting Diabetes." However, your doctor or nurse educator may have individual recommendations for you. You can control your blood

sugar by not eating too many carbohydrates at one time and "balancing" your meals with protein and fat. The protein and fat slow digestion and cause a slow, gradual rise in blood sugar, instead of a fast rise that would occur if you ate a carbohydrate food by itself.

Carbohydrate is found in starchy foods such as bread, crackers, cookies, rice, potatoes, corn, milk, yogurt, dried beans, fruit, and fruit juice. Carbohydrate is found in smaller amounts in nonstarchy vegetables such as green beans, carrots, and squash. The Sweet Success Program in California recommends staying away from fruit juices and processed and refined starch products such as instant potatoes, instant noodles, instant hot cereals, and cold processed cereals. They also recommend avoiding sugar-containing sauces such as teriyaki and barbecue. On the other hand, they encourage the use of whole-grain breads, non-instant oatmeal, legumes, and lentils because of their small effect on blood glucose.[14] Of course, any food containing concentrated sugars also provides concentrated sources of carbohydrates and should be avoided.

Your meal plan will be arranged with your current eating pattern, individual lifestyle, and activity level in mind. The calories, carbohydrate, protein, and fat that you need in a day will be calculated and then divided between your meals and snacks. Snacks are important because they allow you to eat smaller meals and prevent your blood sugar from dropping too low. (See page 108 for snack ideas.) Following up with the dietitian is important because assessing the energy needs and eating patterns of a person is difficult in just one visit. Your meal plan may need adjusting as your activity level increases or decreases.

Your Meal Plan

The frequently used type of meal pattern is one that distributes your calories as 40 to 50 percent carbohydrate, 15 to 20 percent protein and 30 to 40 percent fat. Commonly, some women have high blood sugar in the morning. This is due to hormones from the placenta, which cause the body to be resistant to insulin. A reduced-carbohydrate, higher-fat morning meal that does not contain simple-carbohydrate foods (such as milk, fruit, or fruit juice) has successfully controlled the higher blood sugar for many women.

Bev Spears, R.D., of The Diabetes Center of New Mexico, starts their gestational diabetic patients with just one serving of a starchy food (such as one piece of toast) at breakfast. If the blood

sugar testing shows that the amount is well tolerated, the carbohydrate will be increased. The preliminary diet also doesn't include milk or juice, because many women's blood sugar is sensitive to the simple carbohydrates found in those foods. Milk may be added back into the diet as tolerated.[15] Generally, fruit juices (even ones with no added sugar) should be avoided, since they can increase blood sugar at any time. Vegetable juice and tomato juice are okay.

Your diet will probably be based on the Exchange Lists for Meal Planning 1995, from the American Diabetes Association and The American Dietetic Association. This eating plan uses a combination of foods from six food groups—starch, fat, milk, meat, fruit, and vegetable. Each food in a group has approximately the same number of calories and other nutrients, so they can be "exchanged" for each other. For example, one serving of starch has eighty calories and fifteen grams of carbohydrate. You won't have to worry about all those numbers, but do get to know the serving sizes. (See page 107 for "Exchange List.")

Your dietitian will give you a complete list of exchanges from the American Diabetes Association.

The following meal plan has about 2,200 calories and is an

example of a meal plan that your dietitian might develop for you. Your calorie needs will vary depending on your size, your ideal body weight, and your activity level. An individualized diet developed just for you is very important. The sample below is an example only and is not intended to replace individual counseling by a diabetes educator.

Breakfast

1 medium-fat meat = 1 egg

2 starch = 1 piece whole-wheat toast, ½ cup old-fashioned oatmeal

1 fat = 1 teaspoon tub margarine or butter

1 milk = 8 ounces sugar-free or ¾ cup plain yogurt

Snack

1 starch = ¾ ounce whole-grain crackers

1 fruit = 1 small apple

1 medium-fat meat = 1 ounce string cheese

1 skim/very low-fat milk = 1 cup sugar-free low-fat fruit yogurt

Lunch

3 starch = 2 slices whole-wheat bread, 1 ounce pretzels

2 very-lean meat = 2 ounces tuna packed in water

1 fat = 1 tablespoon reduced-fat mayonnaise

2 vegetable = 1 sliced tomato, raw veggies, romaine lettuce

1 skim/very low-fat milk = 1 cup 1% milk

Exchange List

1 starch =	1 piece bread; 1 tortilla; 6 crackers; ½ cup pasta, bulgur, corn, potatoes, or hot cereal; ⅓ cup rice; ½ cup beans, peas, or lentils (also counts as 1 very lean meat); or ¾ cup flaked cereal
1 fat =	1 teaspoon margarine, oil, mayonnaise, or butter; 1 tablespoon diet margarine (30 to 50 percent oil) or lowfat mayonnaise; 1 tablespoon salad dressing or 2 tablespoons low-fat dressing; ⅛ of an avocado; 20 small peanuts; 8 large olives; 2 tablespoons sour cream; or 1 slice bacon
1 milk =	*Skim/very low-fat:* 1 cup skim milk; ½% or 1%-fat milk or buttermilk; 1 cup nonfat or low-fat sugar-free yogurt; or ¾ cup plain nonfat yogurt
	Low-fat: 1 cup 2%-fat milk or ¾ cup plain low-fat yogurt
	Whole: 1 cup whole milk or 1 cup kefir
1 meat/meat substitute =	(1 ounce unless specified)
	Very lean: fish; shellfish; chicken or turkey breast; fat-free cheese; sandwich meats with 1 gram or less fat per ounce; ¼ cup nonfat or low-fat cottage cheese; or ½ cup cooked dried beans, peas, or lentils (also counts as 1 starch)
	Lean: round, sirloin, or flank steak; pork tenderloin; ham; veal; leg of lamb; dark meat of chicken (no skin); cheese and lunch meats with 3 grams of fat or less per ounce
	Medium fat: most other beef; mozarella cheese; cheese with less than 5 grams of fat per ounce; 1 egg; dark-meat chicken with skin; salmon; tuna in oil (drained); ground turkey; or ½ cup tofu
	High fat: spareribs, sausage, regular cheese, hot dogs, or sandwich meats with 8 grams of fat or less per ounce
1 fruit =	1 medium fresh; ½ banana; 12 cherries; 15 grapes; or ½ cup canned, unsweetened
1 vegetable =	½ cup cooked vegetables; ½ cup vegetable juice; or 1 cup raw vegetables

Source: *Exchange Lists for Meal Planning,* The American Diabetics Association and The American Dietetic Association, 1995.

Snack

1 starch + 1 very lean meat = ½ cup low-fat refried pinto beans

1 starch = ¾ ounce baked corn tortilla chips

1 fruit = 1 orange

Dinner

3 lean meat = 3 ounces grilled tenderloin steak

2 vegetable = ½ cup each broccoli and carrots

2 starch = 1 small baked potato, 1 whole-wheat roll

2 fat = 1 teaspoon tub margarine or butter, 2 tablespoons sour cream

1 skim/very low-fat milk = 1 cup 1% milk

1 fruit = ½ frozen banana

Snack

1 starch = ½ whole-wheat bagel

1 very lean meat = 1 ounce fat-free cream cheese

1 fruit = 1¼ cup berries

After You Start a Diabetic Diet

Don't be alarmed if you have a small weight loss after you start a diet to control your blood sugar. This is fairly common, especially if you are now eating fewer carbohydrate foods than you did previously. Just remember that it should be temporary—lasting no more than about five days. If the weight loss continues, talk to your doctor or dietitian.

You may be asked to monitor your blood glucose yourself to find out how much sugar is in your blood. On the other hand, some physicians will randomly test your blood sugar during your office visits.

Blood sugar monitoring involves pricking your finger and letting a drop of blood fall on a "test strip." The test strip will be placed in a tiny machine that will "read" your blood glucose level and display it on a panel. Your blood sugar and ketone testing records are good tools to see if you are eating enough food. Go over these records with your health care team.

If you find that your blood sugars are consistently low at certain times of the day, try to figure out why. Some possibilities are:

- Not enough food at the previous meal or snack.
- Need to add a snack two hours or so before your sugar is low.
- Not the right kind of snack. (Read on for good snack ideas.)
- You are more active, are exercising close to this time, and need more food.

Healthy Snacks

A diabetic snack should contain some carbohydrate, fat, and protein. However, you can have just a carbohydrate snack alone, as long as it is not juice. Your own lifestyle, activity level, and weight gain will dictate the type of snacks you need. Again, your individual snack needs should be discussed with your dietitian, diabetes educator, or physician.

Balanced Snacks

Each snack equals one starch or one fruit, one meat, and one fat exchange. To add a milk exchange, add one cup milk or one cup plain or sugar-free yogurt.

1 ounce Swiss cheese and 6 rye crackers
2 tablespoons peanut butter and 2 popcorn cakes
1 piece whole-wheat bread and 1 ounce light cream cheese
1 small bran muffin and ¼ cup cottage cheese
1 pear and 1 ounce string cheese
½ ham sandwich on rye bread with 1 teaspoon mayonnaise
1 apple with Caramel Dip (see recipe on page 321)
⅓ cup refried beans with 1 ounce cheese
9 Wheat Thins and 1 ounce turkey

2 tablespoons peanut butter and ½ small banana
Raw veggies, 1 ounce cheese dip, and 6 crackers

Starchy Snacks

Each snack is equal to one serving of starch.

½ whole-wheat pita bread
6 rye rackers
15 cheese nips
2 rice cakes
1 granola bar, sweetened with fruit (the ones from Health Valley are recommended)
3 graham crackers
4 Triscuit crackers
½ cup black beans
1 ounce baked tortilla chips

"Free" Snacks

These foods have very few calories so they can be eaten as desired when you don't have any "exchanges" left from your meal plan. Do not eat these snacks alone before exercise since they will not affect your blood sugar:

Raw vegetables with 2 tablespoons of fat-free dressing
Sugar-free Jell-O or sugar-free popsicles (if your doctor allows artificial sweeteners)
Vegetable broth
Lettuce and raw greens
Cucumbers, celery

Exercise– A "Shot in the Arm" for Women with Diabetes

Imagine that there was something that made you feel more energetic and relaxed, made your legs muscular instead of flabby, allowed you to eat more without gaining too much weight, and reduced your long-term risk of heart disease. This "something" also helped you avoid taking insulin or reduced your dose. Would you go out and buy "it" by the bucket-full? "It" turns out to be exercise, and it is strongly recommended for women who have gestational diabetes.

Health care providers generally recommend that you exercise twenty to thirty minutes daily, and at least three times per week; some suggest a daily walk. However, you should talk to your health care provider to see what specific guidelines he or she has for you. Regular exercise improves the efficiency of your own insulin, which can help control blood sugar levels so that you don't have to take insulin.

A study done at the Sansum Medical Research Foundation in Santa Barbara found that regular exercise normalized fasting and post-prandial (after-meal) glucose levels, which prevented the use of insulin. The women worked out on arm ergometers

(stationary bicycles that use the arms to pedal) three times per week for six weeks.[16] According to Lois Jovanovic-Peterson, M.D., in her book, *Managing Your Gestational Diabetes,* "If your doctor tells you to restrict physical activity due to premature labor, you may still be able to do upper-arm exercises–such as lifting two-pound weights while sitting in a chair." You can do this while watching the news or your favorite soap! You can do such exercises on a daily basis, split between two ten-to-twenty-minute sessions.[17]

We would all "like" to exercise regularly, but may have a problem fitting regular exercise into a busy schedule. The solution is learning to make exercise a priority and finding the time for it regularly. (See Chapter Eleven, Fitting Fitness In, to learn how to exercise without thinking about it. Also found in Chapter Eleven are exercise guidelines for pregnancy, which are different than before pregnancy.)

If you start exercising when your blood sugar level is normal, you could have low blood sugar when you finish. Here are some tips for avoiding low blood sugar during exercise:

- If you know your blood sugar is low, delay exercise until you have had a meal or snack.

- If your blood sugar is within normal range, eat one serving of fruit before a thirty-minute activity.
- If your blood sugar is within normal range, eat one serving of starch and one serving of fruit before an activity that lasts an hour or more.
- If your activity is more strenuous, you may need to increase the amount of food for your snack.
- If your activity is longer than two hours, such as a hike, eat before you go and also bring snacks to eat along the way.
- Always carry hard candy or glucose tablets with you in case you have low blood sugar or an insulin reaction. Packaged peanut butter or cheese crackers are also good to keep in your purse.

Sources: *Guidelines for Making Food Adjustments for Exercise for People,* Nutrition Guide for Professionals and *Diabetic Education and Meal Planning,* edited by Margaret Powers, The American Dietetic Association and American Diabetes Association, 1988, p. 41.

Gestational Diabetes in a Nutshell: Keys to Control

▶ **Eat balanced meals at regular intervals.**

See a registered dietitian to make a personal meal plan for you.

▶ **Keep your activity level up!**

Try to do some daily activity. Talk to your doctor about recomending an exercise program; most physicians approve of walking or swimming.

Note: DON'T exercise if your blood sugar is elevated or if ketones are present in your urine—contact your physician. (See Chapter Eleven, Fitting Fitness In, for more information on exercise during pregnancy.)

▶ **Divide the food you eat daily into three meals and two to three snacks.**

Especially important is the bedtime snack, which should include some starch, protein, and fat.

▶ **Keep a handle on weight gain by making wise food choices.**

Choose foods that are low in saturated fat.

▶ **Avoid emotional eating, such as eating when you are sad, angry, or stressed out.**

▶ **Eat more whole-grain foods and legumes.**

Avoid concentrated sweets such as cookies, candy, pie, sugar, honey, and chocolate. Also limit or avoid fruit juices, even unsweetened ones. They contain concentrated amounts of fruit sugar, which can raise your blood sugar.

▶ **Expect to monitor your blood sugar; your diabetes educator will teach you how to do this.**

Your blood sugar level will show you how your diet is affecting the amount of glucose in your blood and will be used to adjust your diet and exercise regimen.

At first, your health care provider will ask you to test your blood sugar as much as four to five times a day for the first week. This could include testing in the middle of the night, when blood sugar sometimes drops. When your blood sugar is in good control, you will probably test less often.

▶ **Keep your diet high in fiber.**

Fiber helps stabilize blood sugar. So stay away from foods made with white flour as much as possible. Try to eat raw, instead of cooked, fruits and vegetables. Eat high-fiber cereal with milk as a snack. (See page 47, "Focus on Fiber.")

▶ **Smile!**

You have a unique opportunity to improve your own and your family's diet! Try to make the changes permanent.

About Artificial Sweeteners

Should you use artificial (nonnutritive) sweeteners while you are pregnant? The answer to that question varies. Many physicians allow their patients to have sweeteners in moderation. Some physicians ask their patients to avoid them totally. The position of the American Dietetic Association is that aspartame (NutraSweet) is safe for use during pregnancy, with the exception of women with phenylketonuria (PKU), a rare genetic disorder in which phenylalanine cannot be metabolized and builds up in the body in toxic amounts. Because saccharin (Sweet'n Low, Sugar Twin) can cross the placenta, excessive use should be avoided, while acesulfame K (Sweet One) is safe for use during pregnancy.[18] The American Diabetes Association also discourages heavy use of saccharin during pregnancy.[19] Use of saccharin has also been discouraged immediately prior to pregnancy.[20] Meanwhile, the American Academy of Pediatrics Committee on Nutrition concluded that the blood levels of phenylalanine (an amino acid) resulting from aspartame ingestion would not be harmful to an individual or fetus during pregnancy.[21]

The Center for Science in the Public Interest (CSPI, a consumer "watchdog" group) has saccharin (Sugar Twin, SweeTen, Sweet'n Low), aspartame (NutraSweet, Equal) and acesulfame K (Sweet One, Sunette) on their "top-ten additives to subtract from your diet" list.[22] One concern CSPI has about aspartame, which agrees with the concern of the American Dietetic Association, is that the breakdown products (aspartic acid, phenylalanine, and methanol) could be hazardous to the fetus, particularly if the fetus had phenylketonuria (PKU). Women who have PKU should not consume any products containing aspartame.

On the other hand, Dr. Richard Black from the University of Toronto, who has done extensive research on sweeteners, says: "The amount of breakdown products from drinking diet soda made with NutraSweet is negligible compared to the amount of the same products metabolized from eating almost any food. You'd get more methanol from eating an apple than from drinking a few cans of diet pop. However, like anything, there could be danger to the mother and fetus if she went overboard and drank two or three liters of diet soda a day, not necessarily from the sweetener, but because of other things found in soda."[23]

With more sweeteners such as cyclamates and alitame awaiting FDA approval, choices of sugar-free sweeteners will undoubtedly soon increase.

Diet Foods

It's not just sugar and calories that dietetic products may be lacking, some are also missing vitamins and minerals, which are so important for you and your baby. One mineral that diet sodas do have is phosphorus, which can be a problem in large amounts. It is thought that a high proportion of phosphorus to calcium in the diet is what causes leg cramps during pregnancy.

If you choose to use artificially sweetened products, moderation is the key. What's moderation? Most professionals consider one to two servings a day moderate— a serving being one diet soda (caf-

feine-free!), one serving of diet gelatin, pudding, or hot cocoa.

For more information on sweeteners, contact the International Food and Information Council: brochures about artificial sweeteners, additives, and food safety; 1100 Connecticut Avenue NW, Suite 430; Washington, D.C., 20036; 1-202-296-6540. You can also call NutraSweet Consumer Affairs at 1-800-321-7254.

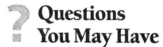

Questions You May Have

Q: Will I have to take insulin?

A: If your blood sugar can't be controlled by diet and exercise alone, you will probably take insulin, in the form of a self-administered shot. You may take one or several insulin shots daily. If you do take insulin, and even if you don't, you will probably be asked to monitor your blood sugar.

Blood glucose monitoring is a great way of seeing how you are doing with your diet. You may be following your meal plan closely, yet seeing high blood sugars. This is because some foods affect your blood glucose quite differently, even though they are similar in carbohydrate value and calories. Also, some women can tolerate carbohydrates better than others.

Q: I've seen diabetic candy sweetened with mannitol. What is that?

A: Some "diabetic" products contain sugar alcohols. These have names ending with "ol" such as mannitol, sorbitol, and xylitol, and are primarily used in candy and chewing gum. These substances have the same number of calories as table sugar or sucrose, but are broken down in the body differently. They are usually fine if eaten in moderation, such as two pieces of hard candy; too much at one time can cause diarrhea.

Q: What else can affect my blood glucose?

A: Many other factors can affect your blood glucose or blood sugar level:

- The combination of foods you eat at a meal (how much protein, fat, carbohydrate, fiber).
- How much fiber is in your diet. Fiber slows down digestion, and release of glucose into the bloodstream is slower.
- Your activity level. Exercise uses up extra glucose and

causes insulin to work more efficiently, thus keeping your blood sugar down and reducing the likelihood that you will have to take insulin.
- Your overall health. Infection and illness can increase blood sugar levels. (See page 101 for "Sick Day Rules.")
- Your stress level. Emotional stress can also increase your blood sugar level.

Q: Can hypoglycemia harm my baby?

A: One animal study indicates hypoglycemia in mom does cause hypoglycemia in baby, and that baby will produce glucose from other sources, such as fat, for his needs. Continued bouts of hypoglycemia could cause poor growth in the baby.[24]

If you taking insulin, some doctors recommend having a glucagon kit available for severe hypoglycemic reactions (glucagon is a hormone that increases blood sugar). Make sure that relatives, friends, and coworkers know what to do for you if you start having the symptoms of hypoglycemia, including knowing how to use the glucagon kit. Also, be sure to wear a necklace or bracelet that identifies you as diabetic.

Q: Will I still have diabetes after I have my baby?

A: Most women's blood sugar levels go back to normal shortly after delivery. Only a small number of women continue to have glucose intolerance.

However, over half of the women who have gestational diabetes will be diagnosed with Type II, or Adult-Onset Diabetes, ten to fifteen years after their child is born. Women who have GDM with one pregnancy are very likely to have it with other pregnancies too. The American Diabetes Association recommends having your blood sugar tested three months after delivery and then once a year to make sure your blood sugars are normal.[25] Can you avoid post-pregnancy diabetes? Very possibly, if you maintain your ideal body weight and exercise regularly. Eating a balanced diet is also beneficial.

Q: What about my next pregnancy?

A: You have a very high chance of having GDM with subsequent pregnancies. Losing excess weight between pregnancies, exercising regularly, and eating well can cut your risk.

Q: What if I get sick and can't eat?

A: If you get ill and don't feel like eating, or can't keep food down, you should first contact your health care provider. Women are usually instructed to continue to take insulin (if you are on insulin) because illness can raise blood sugar levels. You must also continue drinking fluids, so that you don't become dehydrated. (See page 101 for "Sick Day Rules.")

Q: Will my baby be diabetic?

A: Not at birth. The only effect your baby may experience from your diabetes is low blood sugar, which is easily taken care of with a dose of sugar water. However, diabetes tends to run in families. By raising your child with healthy eating and exercise habits, you could possibly prevent your child from having diabetes as an adult. What a nice gift!

Q: The week before I had my blood sugar checked, I was eating a lot of candy and soda. Is that what caused my diabetes?

A: No. However, you may have craved sweets because of the diabetes. When your blood sugar is high, but you don't have enough insulin to use the glucose, your body sends out the signal that you need energy.

Sugar does not cause diabetes. However, excess simple sugar and starches in the diet cause the pancreas to secrete more insulin; and if your body cannot produce the amount of insulin needed, the result is high blood sugar.

▼

High Blood Pressure/ Pregnancy-Induced Hypertension (PIH)

Sarah was surprised when she went to her doctor's office and found that her blood pressure was elevated. She felt fine! No one in her family had high blood pressure (or hypertension), and she had never had a problem with it. Sarah's condition, called Pregnancy-Induced Hypertension (PIH), is diagnosed in 10 to 20 percent of women expecting their first child.

Sarah was asked to take time to rest. Because she was a salesperson at a local department store, "resting" was virtually impossible while she was at work. However, she did try to put her feet up for a few minutes when she could and rested a lot in the evenings.

After closely monitoring her blood pressure for several weeks, Sarah's doctor decided she should be on strict bed rest to prevent the blood pressure from getting worse. She took a temporary disability leave, which allowed her to keep receiving some income. After two months on bed rest, Sarah delivered a healthy, blue-eyed boy who weighed seven pounds.

For Sarah, following the doctor's orders paid off! Keeping her doctor's appointments and staying in bed kept her blood pressure from going up any more and improved her circulation. The improved circulation allowed adequate blood flow and nutrients to her baby so he could grow adequately.

Had Sarah not taken such good care of herself, the PIH might have escalated into more serious conditions called preeclampsia and eclampsia. PIH, preeclampsia, and eclampsia are all forms of hypertensive disorders of pregnancy. They are all a progression of the same disease, which includes high blood pressure. These disorders are also known as the toxemias of pregnancy, or simply toxemia. Because the term "toxemia" has been used to describe the hypertensive disorders of pregnancy in the past, some people may still use the term.

The following list of definitions will help you understand high blood pressure during pregnancy:[26]

Pregnancy-Induced Hypertension (PIH) or Transient Hypertension refers to high blood pressure caused by pregnancy. PIH may also be called gestational hypertension. Women with PIH usually have no symptoms and their blood pressure generally goes back to normal after delivery. They are at risk for developing PIH again in subsequent pregnancies and may also develop chronic hypertension later in life.

Preeclampsia refers to several complications, including high blood pressure, protein in the urine, and excessive fluid retention. Kidney and liver damage can occur if untreated.

Eclampsia is a potentially fatal condition in which the mother can go into convulsions or a coma.

Chronic Hypertension is high blood pressure that existed before pregnancy, or that is diagnosed before the twentieth week of pregnancy.

If preeclampsia is superimposed upon chronic hypertension, the woman would have high blood pressure and the symptoms charcteristic of preeclampsia: protein in the urine and edema.

What Happens to Blood Pressure during Pregnancy

Blood pressure usually drops during the first half of pregnancy and then rises to normal rates. Women with mild hypertension may also experience that drop and may have normal blood pressure by mid-pregnancy. Not until the third trimester does blood pressure increase to the point where some type of treatment (such as bed rest or medication) may be necessary. Once blood pressure increases, it may not drop back down to normal levels until after delivery.

Though the causes of PIH are not fully understood, poor nutritional status is one risk factor. It appears to occur at a higher rate when a woman has a combination of poor nutritional intake and no prenatal care.

Your overall food intake, including adequate calories, protein, and certain minerals, appears to be important in preventing high blood pressure. If you don't have enough energy or calories from carbohydrate or fat in your diet, your body will use dietary or tissue protein for energy. This can reduce protein needed for tissue growth and can also limit the protein used in fluid balance. Underweight women who fail to gain weight

properly have a higher risk of developing PIH.

You are more likely to develop hypertension during pregnancy if you fall into one or more of these categories:[27,28]

- You are pregnant for the first time.
- You are expecting multiple fetuses.
- You are diabetic.
- You have kidney disease.
- You were overweight before your pregnancy.
- Your mother had preeclampsia.

The information below applies to women with PIH and those with chronic hypertension.

Risk to Mom

The biggest danger of increased blood pressure during pregnancy is the development of preeclampsia. Restricted activity and bed rest are two treatments to ensure that your blood pressure is controlled and your baby has an adequate circulation of blood and nutrients.

Risks to Baby

While you may have no symptoms of high blood pressure, it can reduce blood flow—and thus oxygen supply and nutrients to the baby. So your baby may not grow properly and may have IUGR (intrauterine growth retardation). Your physician will probably monitor your baby's heart rate and growth with ultrasound tests. Women with hypertension are also more likely to have a miscarriage or stillbirth. If your blood pressure cannot be controlled, your baby may be delivered prematurely.

What Can You Do?

If you have chronic high blood pressure before pregnancy:

▶ **See your physician before you become pregnant.**

Establish good blood pressure control and a "baseline" reading of your blood pressure.

▶ **Lose weight and start a regular exercise program before pregnancy.**

Both can help reduce your blood pressure.

▶ **When you become pregnant, see your physician as soon as possible to start your prenatal care.**

Be sure to keep your appointments with your health care provider so that you and your baby can be monitored.

If you are diagnosed with high blood pressure during pregnancy:

▶ **Get plenty of rest– at least eight hours of sleep per night.**

Also, try to lie down a few hours during the day on your left side to increase blood flow to your baby. When sitting, elevate your legs above your hips to improve circulation.

▶ **Monitor your blood pressure.**

You may go to your doctor's office more often for a blood pressure check, or you may check it at home. Keeping track of your blood pressure will give you and your physician a better idea of your average blood pressure over time.

▶ **Be aware of your sodium intake.**

Because your need for sodium increases during pregnancy, restricting sodium in your diet is not necessary. However, women who are "salt sensitive" before pregnancy and follow a sodium-restricted diet may want to continue to watch their sodium during pregnancy. Ask your physician about your specific sodium needs. Foods with excess sodium include pickles, regular canned soups, smoked and cured

meats such as bacon, sausage, and ham, and many frozen and ready-to-eat foods. Sodium information can be found on the nutrition label.

▶ **Eat plenty of calcium-rich foods.**

Research has shown that calcium plays a role in reducing blood pressure and may also reduce the risk of preeclampsia and premature birth.[29,30] Though the evidence isn't conclusive enough to recommend supplementary calcium over the RDA, getting plenty of calcium through your diet can only help! Try to have at least four servings of calcium-rich foods every day. If you are intolerant or allergic to milk, a supplement from your physician may be warranted. If you don't like dairy products, see page 58 for tips on "sneaking" calcium into your diet.

▶ **Eat balanced, healthy meals.**

Follow the Eating Expectantly Diet!

▶ **Watch your activity level.**

Because you will want to restrict your activity or may be on bed rest, you'll need super-speedy meals. (See page 280 for "Meals in Minutes" and page 121 for eating tips for women on bed rest.)

▶ **Avoide caffeine, alcohol, and cigarettes–these substances can increase blood pressure.**

▶ **Keep your stress level low. Cut down on commitments and chores. If you're a "Type A" person, learn to slow down!**

▶ **Continue drinking plenty of fluids, even if you are retaining fluid.**

▶ **Avoid prolonged vigorous exercise, including lifting.**

This is especially important for women with other children at home. Instead of picking up your other children, squat (don't bend over with straight knees!) to their level. Your physician will have more specific exercise guidelines for you.

What Can You Expect?

There is a possibility that if your blood pressure does increase, you may be asked to restrict your activity, be on bed rest or be hospitalized. Rest has been shown to reduce premature labor, lower blood pressure, and help your body get rid of excess water.[31]

Even if you aren't given special instructions for rest, you should set aside time every day to be off your feet. Making rest a priority on your own may prevent imposed restricted activity and medications from your doctor! (See page 121 for "Coping With Bed Rest" if bed rest or hospitalization becomes necessary.)

Elevated blood pressure and preeclampsia may warrant an early delivery of your baby, preferably through induced vaginal delivery. However, in cases where a speedy delivery is necessary, a C-section may be done.

In some cases, even if you comply with bed rest or restricted activity orders, your blood pressure may still not be adequately controlled, and you may need to be hospitalized, put on medication, or deliver prematurely. For women who have chronic high blood pressure before pregnancy, hospitalization is not uncommon.

Rest during Pregnancy

Tell the typical woman to "rest" and she'll say "Oh, okay," and proceed to take a fifteen-minute "catnap," but will continue to go about her very busy lifestyle. Most people don't realize how vital rest is for pregnant women with high blood pressure.

Kathy said her doctor told her to rest and she did lay down for a rest "every so often." She

didn't realize exactly what he meant. Eventually, she was put on strict bed rest and when she went into labor, her blood pressure became very elevated and she had to have an emergency C-section. She wished that someone had explained what "rest" meant!

If you're told to rest, this is what you should do:

▶ **Rest one to two hours off your feet in the morning and afternoon every day. Ask your doctor for specifics.**

▶ **Arrange with your supervisor to have some type of rest period at work or arrange for a reduced work schedule.**

▶ **Enlist the help of older children to help with household duties, or you may need some extra help with child care.**

▶ **Avoid stressful situations that could further increase your blood pressure.**

❓ Questions You May Have

Q: How will I know if I am developing preeclampsia?

A: These are specific signs and symptoms of preeclampsia:

- Swelling of hands, face, feet, and legs. Some water retention during the last months of pregnancy is normal. However, if the swelling moves to the upper part of your body, it may be a sign of preeclampsia.
- Sudden increased weight gain. If weight gain is not explained by increased food or fluid intake and occurs over a short period of time, this may also be a symptom. If you gain several pounds over a few days or in less than a week, check with your physician.
- Persistent, violent headache. If you have a severe headache that just won't go away, contact your physician immediately. This may be a warning sign of a convulsion.
- Visual difficulties. Blurred vision or partial-to-complete blindness are signs of preeclampsia. Again, seek medical attention immediately.

- Stomach pain. This can also be a sign of preeclampsia.[32]

Q: Will I still have high blood pressure after delivery?

A: Probably not immediately after delivery, unless you have chronic hypertension. Women who have pregnancy-induced hypertension are very likely to have high blood pressure later in life. You might reduce your risk of hypertension by going back to your ideal body weight after pregnancy, exercising regularly, and eating a nutritious diet containing adequate high-calcium foods. (See page 151 for more information on losing weight after delivery.)

Women with preeclampsia have about the same risk of developing hypertension later in life as those who never had the disease.[33]

Q: What about my next pregnancy?

A: If you have PIH, you have about an 80 percent chance of developing it again in later pregnancies. If you have preeclampsia along with chronic hypertension, your risk of having the same problem with other pregnancies can be as high as 70 percent.[34]

On the bright side, if you do have the same problem with your next pregnancy, you will be a pro at handling it! You will

know how to take it easy and relax, how to monitor your blood pressure, and what to expect during your pregnancy.

For more information on coping with chronic disease during pregnancy, I recommend an excellent book called *Intensive Caring* by Diane Hales and Timothy Johnson, M.D., Crown Books.

▼

Expecting Twins or More

One way to have a ready-made family is to have twins, triplets, or more! And with suggested weight-gain guidelines, you may indeed feel as though you are feeding a houseful during your pregnancy.

Weight Gain

The Subcommittee on Nutritional Status and Weight Gain during Pregnancy has concluded that a weight gain of thirty-five to forty-five pounds produces the healthiest twins.[35] A study done in Washington state found a weight gain of about forty-four pounds was associated with optimum outcome of pregnancies lasting at least thirty-seven weeks and babies weighing over five-and-a-half pounds.[36] Diane Dimperio, M.S., R.D., Associate in Obstetrics and Gynecology at the University of Florida, has devised a suggested weight gain chart for multiple pregnancies. (See chart below.)

The pattern of your weight gain is also important. The pattern of early low weight gain (less than 0.85 pounds per week before twenty-four weeks) and late, low weight gain (less than 1 pound per week after twenty-four weeks) has been associated with poor growth and adverse outcomes.[37]

Once you find out you are carrying multiple fetuses, you should make an effort to eat more and eat the best foods you possibly can. Diane Dimperio suggests that fetal growth has critical points, during which time you should make sure that your intake is adequate. The critical point for twins occurs at twenty-eight to thirty weeks; for triplets, at twenty-four weeks; for quadruplets, at twenty to twenty-two weeks.[38]

You and your health care provider will probably work out an individual goal for you.

What Affects the Weight of Your Twins?

- Your diet and weight gain
- Length of gestation
- Sex of your babies
  (same sex vs. mixed sex)
- Type of twins
  (identical vs. fraternal)

Low birth weight is a concern for any multiple pregnancy. Although twin pregnancies accounted for only 2 percent of all births in 1986, 16 percent of all low-birth-weight infants were twins.[40] Low birth weight is a problem because it increases the risk of sickness and death in babies. Single babies and twins grow at about the same rate until about the thirty-second week, when growth in twin pregnancies appears to slow down. Also, multiple pregnancies are often shorter than the usual forty weeks. Twin pregnancies average thirty-seven weeks. A shortage of only three weeks doesn't seem as though it would make much of a difference, but it does. Since babies often increase their weight by up to one-third pound per week in the last weeks of pregnancy, three weeks can make a big difference![41]

Several factors affect the weight of your babies, one of them being your diet. Besides adding the calories and nutrients that your babies need, diet can actually lower your risk of prema-

Weight Gain Recommendations in Multiple Gestation for Second and Third Trimester[39]

Recommended Gain (in pounds)

Pre-Pregnant Weight	Weight Gain	Twins	Triplets	Quads	Quints
Low					
	Total	40–50	50–60	60–70	70–80
	Month*	6–7.5	7.5–9.25	9–11	10.5–12.5
	Week*	1.5–1.75	1.75–2.25	2.0–2.5	2.5–3.0
Standard					
	Total	35–45	45–55	55–65	65–75
	Month*	5–7	6.5–8.5	8.25–10	10–12
	Week*	1.25–1.75	1.75–2.0	1.75–2.5	2.25–3.0
High					
	Total	25–35	35–45	45–55	55–65
	Month*	3.23–5.0	5–7	6.5–8.5	8.25–10
	Week*	0.75–1.25	1.25–1.75	1.75–2.0	1.75–2.5

*Recommended gain is for second and third trimester and assumes a five-pound gain in first trimester.

ture delivery and babies' low birth rate.

At the Montreal Diet Dispensary, a special program called the Higgins Nutrition Intervention Program was used to try to decrease some of the risks apparent in disadvantaged mothers of twins. The program consisted of individualized risk assessment, determination of dietary needs, nutrition education based on clients' eating patterns, and regular follow-up. Women not able to afford the prescribed diet were given a supplement of milk and eggs.

The program, which had previously been proven successful with mothers expecting one baby, also produced positive results with mothers of twins. The twin infants of mothers who participated in the program weighed almost three ounces more than the infants of nonparticipating mothers. The program infants had a 25-percent-lower rate of low birth weight and a 50-percent-lower rate of very low birth weight (babies with very low birth weight are usually the sickest babies who require intensive care). Also, the preterm delivery rate was 30 percent less. Some of the specifics of this intervention program included eating one thousand extra calories and fifty extra grams of protein above non-

pregnant needs after twenty weeks. Women who were underweight before pregnancy and those with special risk conditions, such as the poor outcome of a prior pregnancy, received further instructions.[42]

What Can the Higgins Program Do for You?

One researcher has found that women who have multiple gestations ate about the same amount as those pregnant with just one fetus.[43] That means you probably need to take a close look at what you're eating. Better yet, have your diet analyzed by computer (see form at back of book) and seek the services of a registered dietitian, who can give you individualized dietary advice. Increased calories and protein seem to be a significant factor in preventing low birth weight and prematurity in certain groups of women.

To achieve the thirty-five to forty-five-pound weight gain, you will need to gain about one-and-a-half pounds per week during the second and third trimesters. This may require an additional five hundred to six hundred calories per day more than your prepregnant diet. Based on the Higgins research, you could need up to a thousand extra calories per day.

How Can I Possibly Eat More Food?

You probably feel that you can't really eat much more. The answer is to eat concentrated foods.

First, make sure your diet has all the essentials—especially protein, fruits, and vegetables. (See page 44, "The Eating Expectantly Diet.") Then add "extra" foods to boost your calorie intake. The foods most concentrated in calories are fat and sugar—the usual "no-nos." However, to get all the calories you need with what seems to be an ever-shrinking stomach, you must give yourself permission to eat "extras." (See page 45, "Protein Needs," to ensure you are receiving adequate protein.)

The easiest "extra" to add is fat—concentrate on adding vegetable fat. You may need to eat as much as 40 percent of your calories as fat to gain enough weight. Put nuts, olives, and avocado in your salads and sandwiches. Eat guacamole! Add butter to your vegetables, more salad dressing to your salads, use extra oil when cooking, etc. Eat more salmon—it has more fat and the fat is important for your babies' brain and eye development. Another way to add more calories to your diet is by eating high-sugar foods. By that I don't mean you should drink a soda and eat a candy bar every day! Instead, turn to the category of foods I call the "good extras," which include milk shakes, puddings, peanut butter cookies, and other foods that are high-calorie, but will also provide nutritional basics to your diet. (See page 218, "High-Energy Mom Snack Ideas," for healthy snack choices.)

Vitamins and Minerals

You will need increased amounts of some vitamins relative to your calorie and protein intake, because of your babies' increased growth. The increased amount of food, a well-selected diet, and a vitamin/mineral supplement prescribed by your health care provider should take care of the extra needs. Diane Dimperio suggests one extra serving of a dairy product for each extra fetus you are carrying, to meet the need for calcium. Nutrients that you may need in greater amounts than are in the typical prenatal supplement are folic acid, zinc, iron, copper, and beta-carotene.[44]

If you cannot meet your calcium needs through food, please take a supplement. (See pages 27–33 for examples of foods high in the nutrients listed above.)

What about Triplet and Quadruplet Pregnancies?

Since triplet and quadruplet births are rare, little research is available pertaining to them. There is also little consensus of advice regarding nutritional needs and weight gain. Triplet and quadruplet pregnancies are usually managed by a specialist, and you will be given very individualized advice according to your prepregnant weight, weight gained so far, and the size of your babies. You should seek help from a registered dietitian to ensure that you are meeting your nutrient needs. Here are a few observations:

Triplets

You should expect preterm delivery weights of each of your babies to be less than the weight of a baby from a twin or single pregnancy. One study showed that, on average, triplets weighed a little over three and three-quarters pounds. The average hospital stay for triplets was twenty-nine days, and, generally, more triplets required intensive care than other babies.

The good news is that the risk of sickness among moms or serious complications among trip-

lets is not higher than between twins. And the odds are on your side if you can follow most of the above information about nutrition for twins.[45]

Quadruplets

If you can imagine four babies growing inside you, you probably suspect that your pregnancy will require extra-special care! In one study of seventy moms who were pregnant with quadruplets, bed rest was introduced at about seventeen weeks. (See the next topic, "Coping with Bed Rest.") Tocolytic agents–drugs that stop the labor contractions–were used in 83 percent of the women beginning at twenty-five weeks. The mean age of the babies at delivery was 31.4 weeks, or at about seven-months gestation. Because of the shortened length of pregnancy, and other factors, the mean weight of the babies was about three and one-quarter pounds.

The average weight gain was only forty-six pounds, which is close to the amount of weight gain recommended for twin pregnancies. Complications found in nearly one-third of the women were: bleeding in the first trimester, pregnancy-induced hypertension, and anemia.[46]

Coping with Bed Rest

We all dream of just one day in bed, to sleep, watch TV, or catch up on our reading. Wishes do come true but, unfortunately, when it rains, it sometimes pours.

Bed rest is prescribed for multiple reasons, including hypertension or preeclampsia, multiple gestation (twins or more), premature labor, or poor growth of baby (also called intrauterine growth retardation, or IUGR). Some women are put on bed rest for several months, which can give a person "cabin fever."

Following is a guide to help you make the most of your stay. This information was developed by talking with others and also by personal experience. I was on bed rest for eleven weeks for preterm labor. It was all worth it in the end. Robert was healthy and weighed seven pounds, seven ounces, and even my labor had to be helped along a little!

At first, the time seemed to go on forever. But once I got into a routine, and my doctor gave me the okay to get up a little more, time became much more bearable. I wrote most of the following information before I was on bed rest, so I was able to follow

my own advice. And it worked! I hope it helps you too!

Welcome to "Club Bed"

Setting Up the Room

You will probably want to set up a makeshift bedroom near the place where your family gathers. A family room off the kitchen works nicely. Here are the basic living supplies with which you'll want to furnish your new room:

- Bed with plenty of pillows (or rent a hospital bed).
- Phone that will reach to the bed or a portable (think of it as your link to the outside world); and don't forget the phone book.
- Ice chest or mini-fridge for your bedside.
- Microwave (not a necessity, depending how strict your bed rest is).
- Large bedside table or a hospital-type table that can be raised or lowered to your level. This can be rented from a medical supply company (several TV trays work well too).
- Any medicines you are taking, including those you might rarely take for heartburn, constipation, etc.
- Large pitcher, filled with fresh water daily, and an ice bucket.

- Soup cans for doing arm exercises (if your physician approves).
- An intercom system. Invest early in one for the baby—this will save your voice and save your family lots of trips back and forth fetching for you.

Bed rest joke: The best and worst thing about bed rest: You aren't the cook and you aren't the cook! (From *Sidelines* newsletter, Winter 1992.)

Eating and Dietary Considerations

Yes, eating takes on a whole new challenge when you spend your time on a six-by-four-foot mattress or couch! Keep in mind that you will need fewer calories than usual since you'll be using very little energy for activity. If you are taking medication to stop your contractions, it may increase your metabolism and you may need to eat about the same as you did before. Another potential problem is that the lack of activity may increase blood sugar and lead to gestational diabetes. To help control your risk, avoid concentrated sweets and fruit juices. (See page 103 for more about gestational diabetes and, if your appetite isn't good, see page 119, "How Can I Possibly Eat More Food?," for tips on adding calories. Following is a guide to "Bedroom Cuisine:"

▶ **Make lists and menus so your family or friends can shop for you.**

▶ **Keep snacks next to you:**
- A fruit bowl filled with fresh and dried fruit such as figs and prunes
- A jar of peanut butter
- Individually wrapped string cheese
- Wheat and rye crackers, graham crackers, rice cakes, baked tortilla chips
- Raw veggie sticks in plastic container with ice
- Cheese food that doesn't need refrigeration
- Nuts

Note: Beware that convenience foods that need no refrigeration are often high in fat and salt. Eat accordingly!

If you have a microwave next to you:

- Low-fat popcorn
- Decaffeinated tea bags, decaffeinated coffee, hot chocolate mix, and mugs
- Cans of hearty single-serving soups such as split pea, chunky chicken vegetable, and beans with ham
- Shelf-stable meals and stews (See page 197 for examples.)

If you are allowed to get up briefly to make a meal, the fol-

lowing can be prepared in six to seven minutes.
- Scrambled eggs with toast
- Frozen microwave dinners (See page 198 for healthy choices.)
- Refried vegetarian beans, corn tortilla toasted in oven, cheese, lettuce, and tomato
- Chef salad with prepared lettuce in the bag–you just add the tomato, cheese, ham, turkey, etc.
- Bean soups in a cup

Quick leftover meals:

From baked chicken:

- Chicken salad with pineapple
- Chicken fajitas, burritos
- Chicken curry over bulgur
- Chicken taco
- Chicken-English-muffin melt
- Chicken sandwich

From pasta:

- Pasta with tomato sauce (bottled)
- Pasta salad with tuna
- Pasta primavera
- Turkey tetrazzini
- Quick tuna casserole

Other ideas:

- Chinese takeout or delivery
- Pizza delivery (also delivered sandwiches, pastas, etc.)
- Supermarket deli (ready-made meals and snacks)
- Have friends or church take turns making meals for the family.

Entertainment to Keep Handy

You may have to be creative with this one!

- Radio or stereo
- TV and VCR, with remote control (thank goodness for modern technology!) Be sure you have a *TV Guide*.
- Minilibrary set up with magazines, books, stationery, photo albums, etc.
- Diary to keep track of your days
- Calendar
- Computer with which to play games, keep track of finances, write letters. A modem can really connect you to the rest of the world, especially if you're "connected" on the Internet. The first laptop computer was probably invented by a woman on maternity bed rest! You can also borrow your kid's Nintendo or Game Boy!
- Large notebook for making all kinds of lists–things to do, things for others to do, things to buy, things to make, bills to pay, what's on sale where, etc.
- Puzzles and crossword puzzles
- Crafts such as cross-stitch, embroidery, knitting, etc.
- Books on tape for when you get tired of reading

Ten Things to Do to Keep Your Mind Alive

1. *Volunteer by phone.* Have you always wanted to volunteer, but never had the time? Here's your chance. You could do fund-raising, or check on latchkey kids or elderly shut-ins. Or you could create your own network of other bed-bound moms. A good place to start would be the Red Cross, or check the local paper for volunteer opportunities.

2. *Enhance your skills.* Take a correspondence course, or a class on TV. Learn a new computer program (desktop publishing seems to be a winner).

3. *Increase your vocabulary.* Several good books are available, such as *30 Days to a More Powerful Vocabulary.* Crossword puzzles and other word games can also help. Keep a dictionary nearby.

4. *Learn a language. Parlez vous Français?* Many language courses are available by mail. Your new language could be the start of a dream trip to Monte Carlo or Madrid.

5. *Shop without dropping!* By computer and modem, you can hook into Prodigy, Compuserve, and many other multi-service databases. Several home shopping networks are on TV, too. Just be sure to stick to a budget; shopping binges could be hazardous to your financial future! If you're worried about getting furniture and clothes for the baby, Sears, Penney's, and other department stores still sell through a catalog and can deliver to your door.

6. *Have a makeover.* You may not feel like putting on makeup but, just for a change, you might have someone come over and give you a new hairstyle or makeup look.

7. *Become a financial wizard.* Plan your retirement. Send for information on all those great-sounding mutual funds, etc. Keep up with the stock market. Plan how you'll pay for your baby's college.

8. *Make a quilt, afghan, or rug.* You can order kits by mail.

9. *Start your Christmas shopping, even if it's March.* Use TV shopping, catalogs, or start making the presents with crafts.

10. *Create new recipes.* No kidding! Recently, I met a soldier who was in a National Cooking Contest. It turns out he developed his recipe while he was stationed in Saudi Arabia during Operation Desert Storm. I was wondering how he ever found access to a kitchen, or found time to cook. He thought about cooking and wrote down all his ideas for ingredients. When he got back home, he experimented with a few and sent them to the contest.

Exercise/Activity

Your activity level is a very individual matter that should be discussed with your doctor. However, you should ask about doing isometric exercises, and/or arm exercises using light weights or twelve-ounce cans. Such exercises will help you keep some muscle tone and avoid feeling sore from lack of movement. Remember that you can always practice your kegels!

Also ask about turning from side to side often during the day. This will help prevent soreness in muscles and skin.

Other Survival Tips

▶ **Make a "work" schedule of what you'll do during the day.**

This will make the day seem shorter and less monotonous.

▶ **Enlist others' help. If you have other children, make a poster of chores for them to do.**

It may be a good time for them to learn to do laundry, dishes, even cooking, depending on their ages. If you don't have children, you'll need to depend on your spouse, significant other, family (if they live close by), or friends. Although asking others to do things for you will be tough, make a list of all the little things that need doing and delegate them to different people. Hire a maid service if necessary.

► **Remember it's okay to let the housework go. (In this case, it's a must!)**

You have only one priority; for your little one to grow as much as possible for as long as possible. Whether the floor is mopped or the carpet is vacuumed really has little importance. Investigate getting household help from a home-care agency. My insurance covered this benefit, which improved the quality of our life immensely. A home-care assistant can take care of your other children, cook, clean, run errands, and so forth.

► **Think positively.**

You might want to invest in a "positive thought for the day" type of book. Though the time in bed might be rough, having a premature or sick baby would be much worse. Make the most of your time.

► **Find other women in the same boat.**

Ask your doctor, hospital, or Childbirth Education Association for names of other "at home" moms. Start a support group, or at least find a person that you can

chat with. Call the numbers on page 98 for more support.

► **You would be surprised at the number of services that will come to your home!**

I had a massage therapist visit my home weekly because I had a lot of soreness from "laying around." I think this also improved my circulation and pampered me. You can also find someone who will cut your hair in your home, and so forth. Though these are really "splurges," it's the little things that often help you make it through the tough times.

▼

Age and Pregnancy

In the past, most women started their families in their early twenties. Now many women are waiting until they are over thirty-five years old or into their forties. At the same time, teenage pregnancies are on the rise. Becoming a mom at both ends of the age spectrum offers different challenges.

Waiting to start a family can have both advantages and disadvantages. Some women find that "thirty-something" is the perfect time for them. They are financially more stable, have spent time developing a career,

and are ready to start on the "Mommy Track." On the other hand, they may be more set in their ways and may be less physically ready for pregnancy and motherhood. If you are in this last group, you are part of a growing group of women who want to have it all, but not all at once.

Barbara never really thought about having children until she was thirty-five years old. Then her biological clock started ticking and suddenly Barbara wanted to join the ranks of "moms." She had heard that older moms-to-be had a few more risks compared to their younger counterparts, so she visited her physician, who assured her she was in great physical shape. She worked out five times a week, didn't smoke, had no chronic diseases, and had already cut out caffeine. She did, however, skip meals, and often ate on the run.

Her doctor explained that she was on the right track in improving her lifestyle, but that she should work on her diet. He told her that slight nutrient deficits could affect fertility. She then consulted a registered dietitian who, after looking at a three-day food diary, made some suggestions to Barbara about how she could improve her diet.

The dietician suggested Barbara continue taking her mulitvitamins (which contained folic acid) and advised her to add other supplements containing nutrients that were missing in her diet.

Barbara worked a few months to improve her diet and then became pregnant eight months later. She delivered a healthy baby boy weighing seven-and-a-half pounds! She was so thrilled with motherhood, that she became pregnant again when Brian was eighteen months old.

Stories such as Barbara's are common, though a few years ago pregnant women over thirty-five sent up a red flag in the minds of health care providers. A recent study done at Cornell University Medical Center revealed that important maternal complications did not occur with higher frequency in women over thirty-five than in women twenty to thirty-four years old. The babies of the older women also had lower rates of perinatal death (death during pregnancy or within the first twenty-eight days after delivery).[47]

An even larger study from Mount Sinai School of Medicine found that women between thirty and thirty-four and over forty years old had slightly lower rates of small-for-gestational-age babies and the frequency of fetal and infant death was slightly lower in women over thirty-five. Women over thirty-five did have a slightly higher risk of having a low-birth-weight infant. However, there was no evidence they

had more premature deliveries.[48] The consensus seems to be that, with early prenatal care, vigilance, and commitment to their pregnancy, older women can have excellent pregnancy outcomes.[49]

What Can You Expect?

Women over thirty-five can have a higher risk of certain complications of pregnancy, such as gestational bleeding, placental abruption, and placenta previa. Other problems, such as gestational diabetes and pregnancy-induced hypertension, which occur more frequently with older moms, are due to the fact that these problems occur more often in all people as they age.

As women get older, they have higher risks of having a baby with Down's syndrome or other genetic defects. They may also need more time to become pregnant. C-sections are more common too, though a specific reason is not known. One speculation is that physicians are more vigilant and conservative in their treatment of older women who are pregnant for the first time. Prolonged second stage of labor appears to occur more often in women over thirty.[50]

Also, by waiting to start your family, you could end up with an instant family of four! The time frame within which women

conceive twins peaks from age thirty-five to thirty-nine. After forty, the odds of having twins go down.[51] Additionally, many treatments for fertility, such as GIFT and ZIFT, result in multiple fetuses.

▼

Adolescent Pregnancy

Adolescent pregnancy, besides being psychologically stressful to the teen and her parents, is also physically stressful since the mom-to-be is often still growing herself.

Some evidence shows that in young mothers who are still growing, mother and baby compete for nutrients. This is especially true in teens aged twelve to fifteen, whose infants are more likely to be born with lower birth weights. Other research shows that teens who are still growing do not use fat stores for the growth of the fetus, but for their own growth.[52]

One thing is certain; whether mom is growing or not, teens are nutritionally at risk due to skipping meals, eating away from home, and making poor food choices. In the 1990 Rand Youth Poll, two-thirds of the teens polled ate little or no breakfast.[53] In another study, 61 percent reported snacking on foods high in fat and sugar, such as chips, ice cream, candy, and cake.[54]

The typical teen diet tends to be low in calcium and iron. In addition, the percentage of overweight teens is higher now than ever before, and many are turning to unsafe weight-loss measures, which further puts them at risk for nutrient deficits.

Add the "normal" nutritional challenge of a pregnancy on top of the above factors, and you may have someone who needs a nutrition overhaul.

One study found that 59 percent of pregnant teens with limited incomes were anemic on their first prenatal visit. The average diet consisted of just three servings of milk, three servings of meat, two servings of fruits and vegetables, and only five servings of starch. Those teens weren't meeting their own nutritional needs, much less their baby's.[55]

What can you do?

First, make sure you are eating three meals a day, with a few in-between snacks. Then, look at what you are eating. Take the food test on page 61. Then compare it to the values in the Teen-Mom Diet.

Your diet should have AT LEAST the number of servings below:

Teen-Mom Diet

10 servings of starch/bread
1 serving is 1 piece of any type of bread, 1 medium potato (or ½ cup), ⅓ cup rice, ½ cup pasta, 6 crackers, 1 ounce snack food, 10 French fries.

6 to 7 servings of fruits and vegetables
1 serving is 1 fresh fruit, ½ cup canned fruit, ½ cup fruit or vegetable juice, ½ cup cooked or raw vegetables.

3 servings of protein food
1 serving is 3 ounces of beef, chicken, fish, or cheese, 2 large eggs, ¾ cup of cottage cheese, 1 cup dried beans or peas.

5 servings of dairy product or high-calcium equivalent
1 serving is 1 cup of milk or yogurt, 1 ounce of cheese, 1½ cups soft-serve ice cream or frozen yogurt, 1 cup of pudding, 2 cups of soup made with milk. (See page 59 for other sources of calcium.)

5 servings of fat
1 serving is 1 teaspoon of margarine, oil, or mayonnaise, 1 tablespoon salad dressing, 20 peanuts, ⅛ of an avocado.

Ten Eating Tips for the Teen Mom-to-Be

1. Eat three meals a day. Begin taking a multivitamin or prenatal vitamin as soon as you suspect you are pregnant. Take it daily. It cannot take the place of a good diet, but it can fill in the gaps!

2. If you eat fast food, have a salad and milk or milkshake with it. Drink juice instead of soda. (See page 207 for healthy fast-food menus.)

3. You must gain enough weight to have a healthy baby–thirty to thirty-five pounds if you were normal weight before pregnancy.

4. If you have trouble gaining weight, snack on ice cream, milk shakes made with instant breakfast mix, and cheese.

5. Calcium in your diet is very important. If you can't tolerate milk, try to eat as much yogurt and cheese as possible. (If you don't like milk, see page 58 for "Twelve Ways to Sneak Calcium into Your Diet" and page 34 for information on calcium supplements.)

6. Snack on fresh or dried fruits, vegetable sticks with dip, or a sandwich instead of eating chips or candy.

7. If you don't have time for breakfast, try these meals on the go: tortilla with cheese rolled inside; peanut butter and honey sandwich with banana; granola bars and yogurt; or cold pizza. Breakfast doesn't have to be boring! Or participate in a breakfast program at your school if it has one.

8. Easy snacks to take with you to school are cheese or peanut butter crackers, boxes of raisins, fresh fruit, granola bars, string cheese, pretzels, or a sandwich.

9. If it is hard for your family to buy food, you may qualify for the WIC Program (Women, Infants, and Children Program), a supplemental food program and nutrition education program for pregnant and nursing women and their children. Contact your local or state health department or your school nurse for more information.

10. If you are having a hard time coping with the fact that you are pregnant, this can affect your appetite. Find help through programs for pregnant teens, or ask your school nurse for help. Talking with someone can help you deal with the many challenges of teen parenthood.

What Can You Expect?

Teen moms can give birth to healthy, normal babies. The health of your baby depends on you. The amount of weight you gain can directly affect how much your baby weighs and the risk of premature birth. So, don't worry about gaining weight. I've seen some teens return to their prepregnant weight almost immediately.

How Much Weight Should You Gain?

The Subcommittee on Nutritional Status and Weight Gain During Pregnancy recommends that you gain thirty-five pounds if you are considered normal weight for your height. If you were underweight before pregnancy, you should gain about forty pounds. If you were overweight, you should aim for closer to twenty-five pounds.[56] Though this may seem like a lot, remember, you have only one chance to make a healthy baby!

Almost as important as how *much* you gain is *when* the weight is gained. Teens who gained little weight in the first six months (less than ten pounds by the twenty-fourth week) had a higher risk of having small babies, even if their weight gain caught up at the end of the pregnancy. Inadequate weight gain also seems to be a factor in preterm birth (birth of a baby who is less than thirty-seven weeks old.) Girls who gained less than a pound a week at the end of the pregnancy had more premature deliveries.[57]

The problem with "premies" is that the babies usually aren't quite ready for our world yet. Their lungs may not be devel-oped and they can have many other problems. Premies are often kept in the special care unit or intensive care unit for infants and won't be able to go home for a while. This is no fun for a baby– he may have to be be fed intravenously, and have his blood taken frequently. Intensive care, if necessary, could cost you and your family a lot of money–tens of thousands of dollars.

Other Nutrient Needs

Concern for calcium in the diet is shared by all women. A low intake of calcium, especially before the age of thirty, increases your risk of osteoporosis, or brittle bones. You've perhaps seen older women slumped over– their curved back is probably due to osteoporosis. Or maybe you know a relative who fell and broke a hip. This is probably also due to the brittle-bone disease. How does that affect you now?

Your diet now actually affects how thick your bones will be when you become forty years old. The thicker and stronger your bones are, the lower your risk for osteoporosis.

The Zip of Zinc

Zinc is a nutrient important for cell growth, division, and brain development. In one study, researchers gave zinc supplements to teens who didn't have enough zinc in their diets. The zinc apparently reduced the rate of prematurity and caused the pregnancies to last longer than they did in average teens. The babies of teens who took zinc supplements needed less help in breathing. What zinc may have done was to help the underweight women gain weight, which is vital in preventing premature babies.

What Does This Mean to You?

You should never take any supplement not prescribed by your doctor since some supplements can be poisonous to your baby.

However, you can make sure your diet has plenty of zinc. (See page 31 for good food sources of zinc.) Also, you should be taking your prenatal vitamin every day.

Look back to the "Essential Guide to Vitamins and Minerals" on page 27 to learn more about the nutrients most important to you and your baby.

Considering Breastfeeding

My Experiences with Breastfeeding

When my first son, Nicolas, was born, I never questioned which feeding method I would use. In fact, this decision had been made long before I even met my husband! As a health professional who knew all the physical benefits of breastfeeding and also as a registered dietitian who had recommended breastfeeding to thousands of women, I had to breast-feed.

The pressure was on! The most difficult week of my life was that first week after Nicolas was born. I had a long labor and a difficult delivery. Nicolas and I didn't catch on to the fine art of breastfeeding right away. When Nicolas did not breast-feed for twenty-four hours, I felt guilty and gave permission for him to have a bottle–big mistake!

Nicolas continued to receive bottles in the hospital. At home, our breastfeeding attempts got worse: during a feeding, he latched on and pulled away more times than I could count (or bear). As a last resort, I called our pediatrician, who referred me to a lactation consultant. She was our savior.

We had two problems, Nicolas and I. He had "nipple confusion" (sounds like the making of a good joke) and that explained his frequent latching on and pulling away. He had gotten used to a plastic nipple in the hospital, and so he couldn't get the "hang" of mine. And I wasn't positioning him correctly. A week or two after having seen the lactation consultant, we started to learn how this special process worked.

If I hadn't known about the benefits of breastfeeding, and if I hadn't recommended it to so many women, and if there hadn't been that financial pressure (I had quit my job and the formula cost about forty dollars a month), I would surely have quit breastfeeding that first week. That's why I feel compassion for all the women who want to breast-feed, but who also may have difficulty.

Looking back, I'm so glad that I nursed Nicolas. The time we spent together was wonderful. And Nicolas was never sick while I was nursing him. One of my most memorable nursing sessions took place at an outdoor jazz concert that Frank, Nicolas, and I attended when Nicolas was three months old. I felt very comfortable feeding him under the privacy of a blanket. Actually, I felt proud, because we were enjoying our own little routine. I didn't feel embarrassed about breast-feeding in public as I had done at first, and I liked feeling so self-sufficient; no packing up the bottles, trying to keep them cold, or looking for a place to warm them.

When my second son, Robert, was born, we had a totally different experience. Very soon after the delivery, I nursed Robert and he caught on immediately! During this time I made it a point that Robert was not to have any plastic nipples while in the nursery—so he never had "nipple confusion." At home, Robert continued to eat very well. Because I felt like a pro at this, I felt comfortable breast-feeding him anywhere (with or without a blanket). This was especially convenient when we traveled overseas to visit our relatives— we didn't have to worry about

packing formula.

I would never trade the experiences of nursing both my children–both were special. Now that even more studies are citing the benefits of breastfeeding, you must give it a try!

The Feeding Decision: It's Up to You

You may have been thinking about this since the day your pregnancy was confirmed. Or because of personal observations, you may have decided long ago about how you'll feed your baby. In any case, try to base your decision on what is best for your baby, you, and your family.

Undoubtedly, breastfeeding offers the most benefits for baby and mom. However, whatever method you decide to use, make a decision YOU feel good about.

Keep in mind that you can both breast-feed and formula feed. Many women find the combination option convenient, especially if they must go back to work. Even if you breast-feed for a short time, your baby will still benefit. If you do decide to combine breast- and bottlefeeding, be sure to introduce the bottle only after breastfeeding is

well established, to avoid nipple confusion.

Since this is a nutrition book for moms, this chapter will be primarily devoted to breastfeeding. However, if you decide to combine breastfeeding and formula feeding, I have listed some hints for formula feeding on page 132.

Why You Should Consider Breastfeeding

Breastfeeding has been shown to greatly improve a newborn's short-term and long-term health. Following are just some of the benefits of breastfeeding.

Benefits to Baby

- Breast milk provides superior nutrition that is matched to your baby's needs. Colostrum, or first milk, is sometimes called "first immunization" because it contains important antibodies. As a result, breast-fed babies have fewer allergies, less diarrhea, a lower risk of serious bowel disorder, and fewer ear infections and respiratory illnesses.
- Research shows that essential fats found in breast milk

(but not found in formula) are important to brain development. Studies show that breast-fed children have a higher IQ than nonbreast-fed children—supposedly related to critical brain development during the time of breastfeeding.[1]

- Breast-fed babies have a lower risk of sudden infant death syndrome (SIDS).[2]
- Breast milk may exert life-long protective effects against insulin-dependent diabetes, cancer (including breast cancer), and Crohn's disease.[3,4]
- Breastfeeding promotes good jaw and facial development.

Benefits to Mom

- A special closeness to your baby and time to get to know him or her.
- There appears to be a protective effect against breast cancer in women who breast-feed. Women who breast-fed the longest had the most protection.[5]
- Breastfeeding uses more calories and helps mom lose "Mommy stores" of fat gained during pregnancy. By the way, Mother Nature designed us to gain a certain amount of fat during pregnancy, which is used during breastfeeding.

- Breastfeeding helps your uterus return more quickly to its normal size and can also prevent hemorrhage if you start breast-feeding right after delivery.[6]
- The time you spend breastfeeding gives you a chance to rest, recuperate, and relax, not to mention time to catch up on your reading! Life is fast-paced—perhaps breastfeeding was intended to slow us down so that we could spend more time with our new little one!
- It's easy. You always have food for your baby with you and its always at the right temperature—no running to the store at night to buy formula, no messy mixing, and no worrying about proper refrigeration when you're out!
- Your family can do their part to help with the continuation of breastfeeding—being in charge of bath time, helping around the house, giving expressed milk via a bottle, bringing baby to mom while she is in bed, and so on.

Benefits to the Family

- Saves money. Formula costs for the first year can be up to one thousand dollars! Who couldn't use a little extra cash?

- May give the family a chance to have "quiet time" together. If you have other children, you can use some of your nursing sessions as a time to read stories to older children.
- Because of the recent research indicating that breastfeeding might change the genetic predisposition to chronic disease, breastfeeding may improve the health of your family in generations to come!

Breastfeeding for the Nation

Because breastfeeding has so many health benefits, even the U.S. government recommends it. One goal of Healthy People 2000; National Health Promotion and Disease Prevention Objectives for the Nation, is to have 75 percent of infants breast-fed at the time they're discharged from the hospital and to have 50 percent of infants breastfeeding at six months of age.[7] As a nation, we're not quite there. In 1994, 57 percent of infants were breast-fed after birth and 20 percent were breast-fed at six months of age. However, individual areas are making more progress: in the western U.S., over 73 percent of newborns are being breast-fed at the time of their discharge, and

31 percent are being nursed at six months of age.[11]

Tips for Formula Feeding

If you decide to feed your baby formula, or to combine breastfeeding and formula feeding, the following information may be useful:

• If you use formula, the American Acadamy of Pediatrics recommends you choose one that is iron-fortified.[8] If formula is your baby's sole source of nutrition for the first four to six months, it has to be fortified with iron to prevent iron deficiency anemia. (Breast milk naturally provides everything your baby needs.)

• If you use powdered or concentrated formula that needs to be mixed with water, make sure your water containes adequate fluoride. You can call your local water department to find out. If your water does not contain enough fluoride, your baby's health care provider will need to prescribe a supplement.

• Whether you feed your baby breast milk, infant formula, or a combination of the two, you should not give your baby cow's milk, or products containing cow's milk, until your baby is one year old. The American Academy of Pediatrics recommends this because, among other things, the protein in cow's milk may be a triggering factor in the development of insulin-dependent diabetes.[9]

• If you use formula that has to be mixed with water, make sure that your water doesn't contain too much lead. Three common preparation practices that can increase lead in formula are:

   –Using water that is drawn from the faucet first thing in the morning. If your pipes contain lead, water that has been sitting in the pipes for several hours has the highest concentration of lead.

   –Excessive boiling. This concentrates threefold the amount of lead in just five minutes of boiling.

   –Using a lead-based kettle for boiling.[10]

(See page 36 for more information on lead.)

About Bonding

Bonding is a term often used when describing breastfeeding. However, bonding refers to touching, cuddling, and holding and can be done regardless of the feeding method. The long-term effects of bonding are very positive and are thought to affect a child's self-esteem, as well as the mother's attitude towards the child.

Unlike a formula-feeding mom, a breast-feeding mom must remain with the baby, unless she expresses milk into a bottle. Bottle-fed babies can also bond with their mom, dad, or whoever is giving them the bottle. However, some parents learn that the bottle can be propped by a blanket, which allows them to go about doing other things. This "hands-off" feeding is not recommended because of a danger of the baby's choking, and also because this practice does not promote bonding or a close relationship with the baby. Also, milk sitting on a baby's teeth (which happens if he falls asleep with bottle in his mouth) can cause decay.

Whatever method of feeding you choose, feeding your baby will be enjoyable but it can also be stressful. Since babies can't tell you what they want, figuring out what they need is sometimes difficult. Some great advice about infant feeding can be found in: *Child of Mine, Feeding with Love and Good Sense,* by Ellyn Satter, R.D., M.S. (Bull Publishing). Ms. Satter is a dietitian and a social worker who gives advice about eating and tips on how to encourage a positive feeding relationship with your child.

▼

Possible Barriers to Breastfeeding

Breastfeeding seems to have some specific barriers, and if you plan accordingly, you can prevent possible problems and enjoy a successful nursing experience.

Betty Crase of La Leche League International has nursed three out of four of her children. She feels the biggest barrier to breastfeeding is society's attitudes. "Society is still prejudiced against breastfeeding," she says. "The breast is still viewed as a sex object instead of for nourishing babies. This attitude can deter a woman from breastfeeding. Women must feel comfortable breast-feeding wherever they are."[11]

Following are some other barriers and some suggestions on how to avoid them:

Family and Friends Who are Not Supportive of Breastfeeding.

▶ **Point out the benefits of breastfeeding that would most interest the unsupportive person.**

For example, your spouse might be interested in saving money or in learning about the scientifically proven benefits of breastfeeding. Be assertive in your beliefs.

▶ **Find friends or relatives who have breast-fed who can support you in bringing your family to your way of thinking!**

Knowing someone who can share her experience and offer support may also make learning to breast-feed easier.

▶ **Invite your partner, family member, or friend to go to a breastfeeding class or La Leche League meeting.**

Hospital Staff that Is Not Supportive of Breastfeeding.

This appears to be a major problem for women who are still undecided about breastfeeding. If you have some doubt and your nurse prefers that you bottle-feed, the battle may be lost!

If possible, find out which hospital is most supportive of breastfeeding. The most supportive hospitals will have:

- Policies that are conducive to breastfeeding, such as rooming-in for the baby. Having your baby room-in with you helps you establish breastfeeding.
- A lactation specialist or consultant on staff who can visit you right after delivery to get you started. A lactation specialist is usually a nurse who has extensive knowledge about breastfeeding– they know all the answers! Some hospitals also have a lactation specialist who can visit you in your home to see how things are going. If you receive your prenatal care at a public health department or through an HMO, these facilities often have a nurse who can visit you after delivery. Check on this while you are pregnant.
- Classes about breastfeeding for expectant moms and families. These highly informative classes may "sell" your spouse, significant other, or other family members on breastfeeding, as well as give you lots of answers.
- Breast pumps for rent. These "industrial" pumps are very efficient and can usually

empty both breasts in fifteen minutes. This comes in very handy for women who work.

- A list of community breast-feeding support groups, such as La Leche League, that you can call when you have questions. Their meetings are also open to pregnant women and you may learn quite a lot about nursing just by being around other nursing women.

Pediatrician (or Staff) Who Is Not Supportive of Breastfeeding.

Before you have your baby, find a pediatrician (or family physician) who supports breastfeeding. This person will probably be the one you will call if you have any problems or doubts about breastfeeding. Do some investigative reporting and call the prospective pediatrician's office. Ask to speak to the nurse, since he or she will probably be the person you will talk with about breastfeeding. Ask a common breastfeeding question, such as: "How do I know if I'm producing enough milk?" or, "What do I do if my baby seems hungry all the time?" or, "Do you know of any lactation consultants?" If you plan to interview the doctor ahead of time, you can ask about breastfeeding during the interview. Another good way to find a doctor who is supportive of breastfeeding is to ask other nursing moms; word usually gets around quickly about who the most supportive doctors are.

Having Enough Milk.

Once a mother is breast-feeding her child, her biggest concern may be knowing whether she is producing enough milk. You can make enough milk; it's a simple process of supply and demand. The more often you nurse your baby, the more milk your body makes. Here are some tips on what a mother can do to make sure her baby is getting enough breast milk:[12]

▶ Make sure you have positioned your baby properly: tummy to tummy.

Your baby should be comfortable and have a good grasp of the nipple so she can empty the milk glands. When the breasts are emptied, more milk is made to fill the demand.

▶ Let your baby set the pace for length and frequency of the feedings.

▶ Weigh your baby to ensure adequate weight gain.

Four to seven ounces weight gain per week or one pound per month, is fine for the breast-fed infant.

▶ Monitor wet diapers and bowel movements.

These are physical signs that baby is drinking enough milk. There should be six to eight wet diapers and three to five bowel movements per day in the early months.

▶ Make a habit of drinking a glass of water or other beverage every time you breast-feed.

Betty Crase and other promoters of breastfeeding think an early visit to the health care provider may be a real benefit to nursing moms. Betty says, "An early visit builds the mother's confidence and can answer some of her questions."[13] In fact, the Colorado Breast-Feeding Task Force is encouraging the American Academy of Pediatrics to make a five-to-seven-day postpartum visit standard procedure for breast-fed babies.[14]

Most authorities on breastfeeding agree that the first two weeks are crucial for long-term breastfeeding success. If you have trouble those first few weeks, seek help from your health care provider, a lactation specialist, or a local La Leche League leader ...fast!

You can reach La Leche League International at 1-800-LA LECHE.

A Note to Dad

– from Dr. Steven Nafziger, University Family Medical Center, Pueblo, Colorado.

Until several years ago, I fancied myself as being as much of an expert on breastfeeding as anybody else, and thought that all the advice I gave women on breastfeeding was always adequate and well taken. When my wife made the decision to breast-feed our first child, I quickly learned that simplistic advice such as "just keep trying, it will all come together" fell quite short. Every day, I faced some very common-sense, but perplexing questions concerning breastfeeding that made me realize how much I still needed to know about breastfeeding, not only professionally, but also as a father.

I'm sure that most fathers at least recognize some of the merits of breastfeeding. Breast milk is by far the best food for your baby. Breast-fed babies have fewer allergies and fewer illnesses during the breastfeeding period. Breastfeeding is also economical and convenient.

When moms breast-feed instead of bottle-feed, dads do get off the hook having to feed and to mix formula, but they can do other helpful and thoughtful things. Breastfeeding requires a lot of a woman's time, which prevents her doing other things, especially in the first few weeks. Helping with the housework, laundry, cooking, caring for other children, answering doorbells and telephone calls, and bringing baby to mom for feeding are only a few examples of what a father can do. Bathing or walking the baby or spending time playing with him or her will not only free up time for mom but can also create a bond with the child, which is the best gift any parent can give a child.

Of all the things a father can do to help mom while she's breastfeeding, support is probably the key factor. Many women will make the decision to breast-feed on the basis of how much they're feeling supported. A woman will be more likely to breast-feed if her partner has an enthusiastic, supportive, and positive attitude rather than an indifferent or negative attitude. A partner's support and a willingness to help can ease any reservations or fears a mom might have toward breastfeeding. Breastfeeding for the first time is not only a new experience for the father but also for the mother and requires a commitment from both of them. A father who realizes this has

Words of Encouragement from an Experienced Mom

Helene, the mother of five children, says: "The bond between mother and child while the child is attached and being nourished in the womb is not over when the umbilical cord is cut. The bond continues and grows as the mother breast-feeds and holds that new miracle of life in her arms. It is not just a nutritional need that is being met for the baby. It is a psychological, emotional, and physical need for both as well. No sensation compares with nursing your child. Nothing is as satisfying and fulfilling as nursing. I would tell every new mother who is considering breastfeeding to do it."

taken the first and most crucial step toward the mom's successful breastfeeding experience.[15]

▼

Preparing for Breastfeeding: Before and during Hosptial Stay

Checklist: What Moms Should Do before They Deliver

▶ **Attend a breast-feeding information class or a La Leche League meeting.**

Look in the phone book to find a local chapter or call the toll-free number on page 135.

▶ **Find someone who has breast-fed whom you can call when you have questions or concerns.**

This person could be a La Leche League leader or member.

▶ **Find a hospital and a pediatrician who is supportive of breastfeeding.**

▶ **If returning to work, find out if your company and boss will be supportive of your decision to breast-feed.**

Do whatever you can now to prepare them.

▶ **Prepare yourself for breastfeeding.**

Though some nipple soreness during nursing is usually a result of incorrect positioning, some soreness may be due to sensitive skin around the nipple. Alleviating the soreness can be as simple as going braless or topless around the house or not washing your nipples with soap. Nipple and breast preparation techniques are no longer recommended because they can cause premature labor. Ask your health care provider for more details.

▶ **Have these things on hand:**

Nursing pads (washable cloth pads and disposable cotton pads are available) and breast pump, or access to one (a breast pump will be useful if you have trouble with engorgement). I found that a battery-operated pump worked much better than a hand pump. Some women prefer to rent an electric pump.

Source: Modified from the Colorado Breast-Feeding Task Force.

Checklist: What Moms Should Do and Ask For in the Hospital

▶ **In addition to telling the doctors and nurses you plan to breast-feed, write a note ahead of time that states you plan to breast-feed and give the note to the nurse upon your arrival.**

▶ **Ask to "room-in" twenty-four hours a day with your baby.**

This enables you to feed your baby "on demand" more easily. However, some moms would rather rest, knowing that their babies are well taken care of, and to have them brought in frequently to nurse. Ask that your baby doesn't receive any bottles when he is not with you.

▶ **Tell them to keep anesthesia and other labor medications to a minimum so you and your baby will be alert during breastfeeding.**

▶ **Tell staff you want to breast-feed as soon as possible after delivery– on the delivery table or recovery room.**

▶ **Tell staff not to give your baby supplemental water, sugar water, or formula unless medically necessary.**

According to Dr. Nancy Krebs, a Denver Pediatrician, "Full-term babies don't have to drink very much in the first twenty-four hours or so because most are born relatively well-hydrated. Urine (colorless, dilute urine) and stools should be watched because they are indicators of adequate nutrition. Babies who are very small at birth or who may have had a stressful delivery are more vulnerable to dehydration or low blood sugar levels"[16]

If your baby doesn't breast-feed much at first, check with your pediatrician or lactation specialist.

▶ **Ask a lactation specialist or nurse to help you get started.**

Contrary to popular belief, breastfeeding doesn't necessarily come naturally. Most of us need to learn, and some of us need help.

▶ **Nurse your baby as often as the baby wants for as long as the baby wants.**

Nurse as often as every one to three hours. You may need to wake the baby.

Source: Colorado Breast-Feeding Task Force.

Things that Might Happen in the Hospital, and What You Can Do

▶ **The nurses or doctors may tell you that you need your rest.**

Tell them you will not sleep well without your baby and that you need all the nursing practice you can get before you go home and are on your own.

▶ **The baby may only nuzzle at the first feeding.**

This is okay! It is important for you to get to know each other.

▶ **The early milk is called colostrum, or "first milk."**

Colostrum is thick and yellowish. Even though mature milk will not be in during the first few days, feeding your baby as much colo-strum as possible will help protect your baby from illness, including jaundice. It also starts you and your baby on breastfeeding, helps your baby get enough nutrition and water to begin growing, and may help your milk come in sooner.

▶ **Remember, breastfeeding can be uncomfortable at first, and all of us have different tolerances for discomfort.**

Breastfeeding however, should not *hurt*. If it does, ask a nurse to help you get your baby properly positioned and latched on.

▶ **The hospital will probably give you formula or coupons for formula in the discharge packet.**

Hospitals do this because formula companies provide the samples free of charge. This does not mean that your baby will *need* the formula. Your body can make all the milk your baby needs.

▶ **Before you leave the hospital, be sure to ask for a list of names and phone numbers of people in your area whom you can call if you have breast-feeding questions or problems.**

Source: Modified from the Colorado Breast-Feeding Task Force.

Nutrition during Breastfeeding

The Best-for-Baby Breast-feeding Diet

While breastfeeding, you actually need to eat more than you ate during your pregnancy. And you should continue to "make every bite count"! Below is a meal plan that will allow you to meet your nutrition needs during nursing. Your diet should contain at least some of the following foods, which add up to about 2,400 calories. Remember that you may need more or less than these:

12 servings of starches/grains (try to make at least 3 of the servings whole grain)
1 serving is 1 slice of any type bread, 1 flour tortilla, ½ cup pasta, ⅓ cup rice or legumes, 6 crackers, or ½ cup of potato.

4 servings of fruit
1 serving is 1 medium piece of fresh fruit, ½ banana, ½ cup canned fruit in its own juice, 1 cup melon or berries, 2 plums, or 2 nectarines.

4 servings of vegetables
1 serving is ½ cup any cooked, nonstarchy vegetable or 1 cup lettuce. (Be sure to include at least 1 fruit or vegetable that is a good source of vitamin A and 2 servings high in vitamin C.)

7 ounces of protein or equivalent
(Increase your protein intake 1 ounce for each serving of milk that you don't drink.) An equivalent to 1 ounce of protein is 1 ounce cheese, ¼ cup cottage cheese, ½ cup tofu, 2 tablespoons peanut butter, ½ cup cooked dried beans, or 1 egg.

Note: Try to eat fish twice a week while nursing.

4 to 5 servings of dairy product or high-calcium equivalents
1 serving is 1 cup any type milk or yogurt, preferably skim or low-fat. (See page 59 for vegetarian equivalents.)

5 servings of fat
1 serving is 1 teaspoon margarine, oil or butter or 2 teaspoons reduced-fat margarine, 1 teaspoon mayonnaise or 2 teaspoons reduced-fat mayonnaise, 1 slice bacon, ½ ounce cream cheese, 1 tablespoon sour cream, ⅛ avocado, 10 peanuts, or 5 olives.

Here Is an Example of a "Real" Meal Plan:

Breakfast
Corn Bran with blueberries
Whole-wheat bagel with light cream cheese
Milk

Snack
Vegetable juice
Crackers
Carrot sticks
Turkey

Lunch
Grilled cheese sandwich
Sliced tomato
Peach
Sugar cookies
Milk

Snack
Fresh fruit salad

Dinner
Grilled chicken
Grilled vegetables
Spinach salad with red pepper and mushrooms
Whole-wheat roll
Fresh orange
Milk

Snack
Peanut butter and graham crackers
Yogurt with dried fruit

Calorie Needs

Your diet should be similar to your pregnancy diet, except now you need about two hundred more calories over your pregnancy needs (or five hundred calories over the amount you ate before you were pregnant). A good way to get the extra calories is to eat an additional snack or higher-calorie snacks. (See Chapter Fourteen for snack ideas.)

The suggested calorie intake for lactation takes into consideration the hundred to hundred-and-fifty calories a day that come from fat stored during pregnancy. For this reason, breastfeeding can help you lose weight; what a wonderful way to do it! The average weight loss for breastfeeding women is one to two pounds per month, after the first-month postpartum. If you breastfeed longer than that, you will probably continue to lose weight, but at a slower rate.[17]

Some research shows that the calorie needs for breastfeeding have been overestimated. Therefore, after breastfeeding has been well established, you should evaluate your energy needs based on weight gain during pregnancy, weight loss per week during breastfeeding, and your activity level. You may need more or less than two hundred calories above pregnant needs, but it's a good place to start![18,19] To ensure you have a nutritious and adequate milk supply, make sure that your calorie intake does not go below 1,800 calories.

If you breast-feed longer than six months, if you didn't gain much during pregnancy, or if you drop below your usual weight, you may need up to 650 calories per day (or even more) over your nonpregnant calorie needs. Also, if you are very active, you will need more calories

than the average woman. If you find that you are losing weight too quickly or are having trouble eating the recommended amount of food, you should visit with a registered dietitian for some individualized advice.

Protein Needs

Your protein needs also increase during breastfeeding. You'll need sixty-five grams of protein a day (or five grams more than during pregnancy) during the first six months of breastfeeding. If you nurse longer than six months, you will need about sixty-two grams of protein per day: baby will start eating solids and so will drink less milk.[20]

If you can drink or eat the recommended four servings of dairy products, you can meet your protein needs by eating just two-and-a-half ounces of protein a day (including the amount of protein in six servings of grain products.) This is because each cup of milk contains the same amount of protein as one ounce of meat. The Best for Baby breast-feeding diet is boosted in protein to ensure that you have more of the important nutrients such as zinc, iron, and vitamin B_6, which are found in some protein foods.

If you prefer not to eat much meat, you will need to choose the rest of your diet wisely. (See

pages 61, 62, and 72 for good food sources of iron and zinc.)

Nutrient Needs

Most of your nutrient needs stay the same during lactation; some decrease and some increase. You will need slightly more thiamin, riboflavin, vitamin B_{12}, and magnesium. You will need significantly more vitamin C, vitamin E, niacin, zinc, and selenium. You will need less folate and iron than during pregnancy. However, many physicians will recommend that you continue to take an iron supplement to help replace iron deficits from pregnancy or blood loss during delivery.

Be sure to continue getting plenty of fiber in your diet. (See page 47 for "Focus on Fiber.") When I experienced some constipation during the first few weeks of breastfeeding, my doctor explained that the hormones associated with breastfeeding can slow down the digestive process.

Don't forget fluids! Although in the past it was thought that women needed to drink a lot of extra fluid to produce breast milk, it now appears that drinking to your thirst will provide you with adequate fluid. The exception is the woman who lives in a dry climate or exercises in hot weather; then thirst may lag behind actual fluid needs.

If you were to eat very poorly while breastfeeding, your body would draw from stored pools of nutrients. If you breast-fed for six months and depended entirely on stored nutrients to feed your baby, you would deplete 19 percent of protein stores, 4 percent of calcium stored, 14 percent of iron stores, 46 percent of vitamin A stores, and close to 100 percent of folate stores. Protein is not a problem since most of us get more than enough. But, if your diet does not include adequate amounts of calcium, iron, vitamin A, and especially folate, your own nutritional status could be in danger. Since pregnancy and breastfeeding are such physically demanding jobs, make sure that your own diet is as good as it can be, so that you will have all the vitality and energy you possibly can![21]

Calcium Needs

During pregnancy, women are often reminded about their need for calcium. After delivery, calcium in the diet may not seem that important; it is. The lack of calcium in the diet of a breastfeeding woman promotes loss of calcium from the bone. Osteoporosis is a real threat to American women because of their dietary habits and possibly because of inadequate amounts of calcium in their diets during pregnancy and breastfeeding. The RDA for calcium during breastfeeding is 1,200 milligrams; the same as during pregnancy.[22] (See page 61 for calcium contents of your favorite foods.) If you cannot obtain the recommended amount of calcium through your diet, consult your health care provider about a calcium supplement.

▼

Nutrients of Special Concern

When we compare average vitamin and mineral intakes of women in the U.S. to the needs of breastfeeding women, we find that several nutrients are below the RDAs, or Recommended Daily Allowances. When a woman eats 2,700 calories per day, only zinc and calcium may fall in amounts below the RDA. However, if the diet is less than 2,700 calories (and the average nursing woman's probably is), intakes of calcium, magnesium, zinc, vitamin B_6, and folate will likely fall well below the RDA.

Improved food choices are better than taking a nutrient supplement for several reasons. Most nutrients are absorbed better from foods than from supplements and there may be unidentified nutrients found in foods not included in supplements. Also, taking a supplement can give you a false sense of security; you may be tempted to make poorer food choices, thinking that your vitamin will make up the difference.

On the other hand, if you do choose to take a supplement, take one that has a broad spectrum of vitamins and minerals and contains no more than 100 percent of the RDA. Some doctors recommend that you continue taking prenatal vitamins. This is fine except that their high iron content may worsen constipation. Remember that after pregnancy, a woman's need for iron generally decreases—unless she has lost a lot of blood during delivery or is anemic. Ask your physician.

Best Sources of Food for At-Risk Nutrients

Calcium

Milk, cheese, yogurt, canned or small fish with edible bones, (salmon, mackerel, sardines), tofu processed with calcium, bok choy, broccoli, kale, collard, mustard and turnip greens, and molasses.

Zinc

Oysters, pork and beef liver, seafood, lean red meats, poultry, eggs, wheat germ, nuts, dried beans and peas, yogurt, and whole grains.

Magnesium

Bran cereal, wheat germ, Swiss chard, spinach, nuts, seeds, beans and peas, whole grains, dried fruit, shrimp, and scallops.

Vitamin B₆

Mustard greens, bananas, poultry, meat, fish, potatoes, sweet potatoes, spinach, prunes, watermelon, some legumes, soybeans, lentils, chick peas, pinto beans, fortified cereals, and nuts.

Folate

Spinach, leafy green vegetables, asparagus, liver, black-eyed peas, lentils, kidney beans, fortified cereals, legumes, broccoli, Brussels sprouts, and orange and grapefruit juices.

▼

Drugs and Breastfeeding

If you must take a medication during breastfeeding, you don't necessarily have to stop nursing. The safety of the medication depends on the drug and its dosage. For example, if you are taking an antibiotic for a breast infection, you are actually encouraged to breast-feed. However, some drugs pose a risk for your baby, including antiprotozoal compounds, antineoplastic drugs, some antithyroid drugs, and synthetic anticoagulants. Make sure your physician knows you are breast-feeding before prescribing a medication.

If you must take one of the above drugs, pump your milk temporarily to keep your milk supply up. Discard the pumped milk and resume breast-feeding several days after you stop the medication. Ask your health care provider or pharmacist when the medication will leave your system so you can start breast-feeding again. If you take a lactation-suppression drug to stop breast-feeding, don't give your baby any of your milk while your milk supply is dwindling.

Some over-the-counter drugs should not be taken while you are breast-feeding. For example, acetaminophen (such as Tylenol) is usually recommended for pain instead of aspirin. Consult your health care provider about which over-the-counter medications he or she recommends—before the need arises.

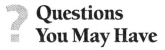

Questions You May Have

Q: I've heard that if I eat gassy foods such as broccoli, onions, and even milk and chocolate, my baby can get gas. Do I have to stop eating all my favorite foods?

A: No. Although strongly flavored vegetables and spices may give your milk a different flavor or may cause your baby gas, to stop eating such foods is not necessary for everyone. After talking to many women, I have learned that baby's reaction to mom's diet seems to be a very individual matter. One friend of mine continued eating plenty of garlic while nursing and her baby had no problem with it. Another friend loved to eat hot peppers, and baby apparently liked them too.

Keep in mind that a lot of "gas" can simply be a result of the baby's immature digestive system. Both my children had a problem with gas pains. I altered my diet in every way possible but nothing seemed to help. I chalked it up to their own digestive system and used a lot of infant over-the-counter gas medicine. They finally outgrew it.

If your baby has gas, you

might try changing your diet for several days to see if the change makes a difference. A baby's sensitivity to flavors and gas-causing foods seems to vary from baby to baby. If your baby has no problem with gas, I wouldn't worry about eating any foods, in moderate amounts.

Q: We have a lot of food allergies in my family. Can breastfeeding help prevent them in my baby?

A: It's possible, but it's not been proven conclusively. Some studies suggest that components of food eaten by the mother can pass into the breast milk and cause allergic reactions in the baby. There has been some success in controlling food and other allergies by eliminating common allergy-causing foods from the mother's diet during nursing and during pregnancy. However, the relationship between breast-feeding and allergies has not been studied enough to recommend this regimen for everyone.

Evidence does show, though, that the occurrence of atopic dermatitis, a type of eczema that is sometimes a reaction to a specific food, can be decreased through breastfeeding. As reported in *Annals of Allergy,* "Among infants at high risk of developing atopic disease because of positive family history,

exclusive breastfeeding is associated with a lower incidence and thus a delay in the occurrence of allergic disorders."[23]

Probably the best advice for women who have allergies or a family history of allergies is to breast-feed as long as possible and to eat a large variety of foods so that no one food will be passed in large amounts to the baby through the milk.[24]

Q: Can I start drinking my coffee again?

A: Your baby will receive about 1 percent of the caffeine kick that you get in your coffee or other caffeinated beverage. The equivalent of one or two cups of coffee per day is not likely to have a negative effect on baby.[25] However, caffeine can accumulate and cause your baby to be irritable and to have trouble falling asleep. So again, go easy on the coffee!

Q: I have gone into premature labor. Though I am now on bed rest and medication to stop the labor, I am concerned that I won't be able to breast-feed if my baby arrives prematurely. Any advice?

A: Breastfeeding a premature infant can be even more rewarding than nursing a full-term infant. One study shows that feeding an infection-prone prema-

ture infant with colostrum (first milk) may have even more significant anti-infective factors than in full-term infants.[26] Another study reports that pre-term infants who were tube-fed breast milk in their early weeks of life had significantly higher IQs at seven-and-a-half to eight years of age than those who did not. This difference was still significant after allowing for the mother's education and social class.[27]

If your baby comes very early, he or she may have to stay in a special area of the nursery to be monitored and to have the environment kept at a precise temperature. You may have to express milk so that it can then be fed to your baby through a special bottle or tube. In this case, you will need to pump your breasts.

The fact that you are thinking ahead is wonderful; you can arrange to rent a good-quality breast pump (Medela is one brand of electric pump), or find out whether you can get one while you're at the hospital. Taking pictures of your baby and keeping them near you while pumping may help you to be more successful in expressing milk. Not being able to breast-feed "in person" may be disappointing, but think of the benefits you are still able to provide for your baby.

Q: My mother says I should drink a beer before I breast-feed to increase my milk supply. Will it? And is it safe for my baby?

A: This old wives' tale has not been scientifically proven. On the other hand, alcohol is released in the milk, and excessive drinking has caused problems with let-down, high alcohol level in breast milk, and lethargic babies. There has been one report of lowered psychomotor development scores in babies with increased alcohol exposure.[28] Since fetal brain development continues to occur during the first year of life, your avoiding alcohol or drinking in limited amounts makes sense.

A recent study showed that the smell of alcohol could be detected immediately in the breast milk of moms who had drunk the equivalent of the amount of alcohol in one can of beer. The smell was strongest at thirty to sixty minutes after the mom imbibed. The babies drank less milk during the feeding, possibly due to the change in taste and smell of the milk. Another theory is that alcohol could decrease the mom's milk supply.[29]

If you'd really like to go "out on the town" and have more than one or two drinks, just pump your breast milk afterward and discard it. You can give your baby some previously pumped milk. Or, if you'd just like an occasional drink, use common sense. Don't drink on an empty stomach, as this will speed the flow of alcohol into your bloodstream and to your breast milk. Ask your health care provider for more information.

Q: I still smoke. Can this somehow affect my milk?

A: Nicotine and cotinine (another component of cigarette smoke) have been found in breast milk. No symptoms of exposure to the chemicals have been seen in infants, though nicotine can affect how much milk you are able to produce. Some researchers advise that if you do smoke (it would be best to quit!), you should not smoke for two-and-a-half hours before nursing and avoid smoking while near your baby.[30]

For information on kicking the habit of smoking call 1-800-4CANCER.

Q: Can the HIV virus be transmitted through breast milk?

A: There have been reported cases of breast milk infected with the HIV virus (the virus that leads to AIDS). In 1985, the Center for Disease Control advised mothers who test positive for HIV-1 not to breast-feed.[31] On the other hand, Dr. Frank Oski, professor of pediatrics at John Hopkins School of Medicine, reports that breast milk contains a substance that can block attachment of the AIDS virus and that may protect a breast-fed infant from HIV infection.[32] If you are concerned about HIV infection, discuss it with your health care provider.

Q: If I breast-feed, will my baby have a smaller risk of being overweight when he gets older?

A: Early studies indicated that breast-fed babies were much leaner than formula-fed babies; later studies show a weaker link. This discrepancy may be due to different compositions of formulas, which are now closer to breast milk in nutrient and calorie content. Currently, the specific role of breastfeeding in obesity remains unclear, though breastfeeding is thought to give long-term protection against such diseases as diabetes and cancer.[33]

Q: Should I try to lose weight while breastfeeding?

A: You will probably lose weight without even trying. Your priority is to eat all the nutrients you need to supply good-quality breast milk for your baby. A diet containing less than 1,800 calories usually provides inadequate amounts of some nutrients.[34]

However, some research shows that the current energy needs for nursing women are overestimated. Since individuals burn calories at different rates, effects of weight loss are also individual. Healthy women can lose up to a pound a week while breast-feeding without it affecting their milk.[35] Any more than that may be a sign that your milk may not contain enough energy. Of course, monitoring the growth and general health of your baby is also a good checkpoint for the quality of your milk.

Q: I want to have another baby right away. Should I still breast-feed if I get pregnant?

A: In undeveloped countries, mothers commonly continue to breast-feed well into the second trimester of another pregnancy. However, breastfeeding during pregnancy can take its toll on you. Pregnancy and lactation are nutritionally and physically demanding. One study showed that moms who breast-fed while pregnant had babies that weighed slightly less than the babies of mothers who did not.

Much depends on your nutritional status. Not only must you meet the nutritional demands of your growing fetus, but also the nutrition and calorie requirements of your growing baby. These demands can add up to as much as nine hundred extra calories a day, depending on the age of your baby! In addition, you need more calories, protein, vitamins, and minerals because the nutrient requirements can leave you nutritionally depleted.

Although breast-feeding while pregnant is possible, you may want to wait at least a few months after weaning your baby before conceiving again.[36]

Q: I've heard that women who breast-feed several children for longer than ten months have a greater risk of developing osteoporosis later in life. Is that true?

A: Although earlier studies suggested that may be true, it was later hypothesized that women regain bone mineral content after they stop breast-feeding.[38] Another study looked at women who had breast-fed from one to four children for a long period of time. Their bone mineral mass of the wrist, spine, or hip was not significantly different than those of women who did not breast-feed. It's important to note here that all of those women consumed the RDA for calcium before and during pregnancy and while breast-feeding.

Other researchers found that the bone mass of women's wrists who breast-fed was actually higher than of those who didn't. A similar study looking at bone mass in the spine found that breastfeeding actually increased bone mass 1.5 percent for every child that was breast-fed.[39,40]

Another study showed that increasing the calcium content of nursing adolescents' diets to 1,600 milligrams prevented a 10 percent calcium loss from the wrist, as compared with teens who consumed only 900 milligrams of calcium.[41]

Of course many other factors are involved in osteoporosis. The factors that you can control are calcium intake, regular weight-bearing exercising (such as walking, aerobics, etc.), moderate intake of protein, and regular exposure to sunshine.

Q: Does my diet really affect my breast milk?

A: Yes. In one study, the fat content of the woman's diet directly affected that of her milk. In another study, a very high-carbohydrate diet also increased the fat content of the milk. Women on a higher-protein diet tended to have higher-calorie milk than those on a lower-protein diet. In addition, your dietary intake of many vitamins and minerals directly affects your breast milk. Every dietary component can affect breast milk, so your best bet is to continue sticking to a basic, balanced diet that contains a variety of foods.[37]

Q: I've heard stories about PCBs being found in breast milk. How can this affect breastfeeding?

A: Environmental chemicals such as PCBs (a family of industrial chemicals) and DDT (a colorless insecticide banned in the U.S. in 1972) have been found in breast milk of mothers who have consumed minute amounts of these substances over their lifetime. The levels of PCB and DDT in their milk vary according to the number of children a woman has breast-fed, the length of time she breast-feeds, where she lives, and her occupation.

In addition, alcohol drinkers, smokers, and women who eat recreationally caught fish have significantly higher DDE (another pesticide) levels in their breast milk. Also, as women get older, the levels of both PCB and DDE passed on in their milk increases because these chemicals are consumed and stored in a person's body fat over a lifetime.

In the rare event that you have had direct exposure to a hazardous chemical some time in your life, share this information with your health care provider during your pregnancy and discuss the implications. In one study, only about 25 percent of the women who had had direct exposure to hazardous chemicals had higher levels of the chemicals in their milk compared to women who had had only a "normal" exposure.[42]

Betty Crase, Director of Scientific Information at La Leche League International says, "Unfortunately, we live in a contaminated world. However, the known and documented benefits of breastfeeding still outweigh the risks of contaminants that may be found in breast milk. What many people don't realize is that artificial infant formula can also contain environmental contaminants, especially if the water used to prepare it contains lead or other chemicals."[43]

The common sense approach is to limit your present and future exposure to chemicals in the environment:

▶ **Avoid recreationally caught fish not caught by you–fish that is caught by friends or sold at a roadside stand.**

These fish are more likely to come from contaminated water or from water with specific state health department consumption recommendations for breastfeeding women. Friends who give you leftovers from their fishing trip may not know you are breast-feeding or may not have paid attention to the sign at the reservoir that says "pregnant and breast-feeding women should avoid fish A," etc. If you

or your family catch fish, be sure to read any posted signs regarding recommended consumption levels, or call your local health department. (See page 193 for more information on food safety.) However, you should still eat fish–the omega-3 fatty acids found in fish are important to your baby's brain development, which still occurs during the first year of life.

▶ **Avoid quick weight loss while breastfeeding.**

Undesirable toxins in the environment are stored in body fat. If you go on an extreme weight loss diet, some of these accumulated chemicals can enter the milk in larger amounts as your body fat is released from storage.[44]

▶ **Avoid use of pesticides, herbicides and insecticides in your home–even those that claim to be nontoxic.**

▶ **Avoid eating the skin and fat of poultry, meats, and fish.**

Q: I just had a case of food poisoning. Can the bacteria that caused my illness be passed to my baby in breast milk?

A: According to Dr. Steven Nafziger of the University Family Medical Center in Pueblo, Colorado, "The bacteria that cause most common types of food poisoning do not pass through the breast milk. However, some rarer forms of food poisoning involve bacteria that make toxins. These toxins can directly affect the baby through the mother's breast milk. I encourage a breast-feeding mom who is experiencing flu-like symptoms to come into the office so I can evaluate her condition and make a specific recommendation."[45]

Q: I'd like to start a vigorous exercise program. Can I still successfully breast-feed?

A: Yes. In one study, women who exercised about one-and-a-half hours per day were found to produce the same amount of milk containing about the same number of calories as sedentary breast-feeding moms. Though these women burned many calories exercising, they also consumed more. These women were

very devoted to their exercise; one had previously completed an Iron Man Triathlon and another was a gold medalist in swimming! And their devotion to fitness (in addition to their devotion to their babies) may have also motivated them to eat all the right foods.[47]

Q: I am a total vegetarian. Is there anything that my milk will be missing?

A: People who eat no animal protein or dairy products sometimes need another source of vitamin B_{12}, since it is naturally found only in animal products. You need to consume foods fortified with vitamin B_{12} or take a B_{12} daily supplement of 2.6 micrograms.[46] (See page 79 for more information about vitamin B_{12}.)

The calcium requirement for vegetarians is thought to be less than for meat-eaters because their diets are lower in protein than the diets of meat-eaters.

If you consume no dairy products, you may need to carefully plan your diet to include high-calcium foods, or take a calcium supplement. Zinc and iron are other nutrients that may require you to "work" at getting sufficient amounts. (See page 72 for vegetarian sources of zinc; pages 58 and 59 for calcium; and pages 61 and 62 for iron.) If you have concerns about your diet, discuss them further with your baby's health care provider or seek a registered dietitian to help you analyze your diet.

Q: Can breastfeeding lower my breast cancer risk?

A: Yes. Several studies indicate that breastfeeding has a protective effect against breast cancer.[48,49] Breastfeeding can also cut your child's breast cancer risk when the child becomes older.[50] What a special gift!

CHAPTER NINE

Now That You Can See Your Feet Again or …

The First Weeks With Baby

This chapter answers such questions as:

• *When will I be able to eat if I have anesthesia during delivery?*
• *How can I possibly eat balanced meals if I'm too tired to cook?*
• *What is the difference between breast- and bottle-feeding?*
• *What's a good weight loss diet?*
• *How can I tell a good weight loss program from a bad one?*
• *How long should I wait before I get pregnant again?*

What to Expect after Delivery

The first few days of postpartum life will likely be spent "oohing" and "ahhing" over your new arrival as well as recovering from a very tiring event. You'll need to eat especially well those first few days at the hospital so that you have all the strength possible when you go home.

You may be too tired after delivery to eat a meal–that's normal for some women. You may just feel like drinking some juice or a decaffeinated soda for quick energy. For example, Mary never drank sugared sodas, but after eighteen hours in labor, she drank eighteen ounces of 7-Up in just five minutes! And some women are so hungry after delivery that they call out for a pizza!

High-carbohydrate snacks that might be available at the hospital include toasted English muffin, bagel, toast, bran muffins, raisin toast, canned or fresh fruit, graham crackers, milk, yogurt, milkshake, sherbet, angel food cake with fruit, fruit juices, and sodas.

When you do feel like eating, these tips will help you get back on your feet:

▶ **If you select from a menu in the hospital, pick as many high-fiber foods as possible to get your digestive track moving normally.**

Labor, as well as anesthesia, slows down your digestion immensely. Some women have hemorrhoids from pregnancy or from the "pushing" stage of labor. Eating high-fiber foods will make your bowel movements softer and easier.

Some high-fiber foods you are likely to see on your menu are Raisin Bran cereal, All Bran, 100% Bran Flakes, wheat bread, wheat rolls, fresh apple, orange, banana, strawberries, prunes, raw vegetables, salad, baked potato, legumes, peas, corn, and sliced tomatoes. Also, drink plenty of liquids when eating high-fiber foods.

▶ **Those first few days, eat as much as you want, and especially drink plenty of fluids.**

If you had a long labor, you probably didn't drink much and you'll need to rehydrate. If you are planning to breast-feed, you will need to continue drinking eight to ten cups of fluids per day.

▶ **Concentrate on getting your strength back and taking care of the baby those first few weeks.**

Hopefully, you cooked some meals ahead of time and froze them. Now is the time to start using them! If not, let Dad, or other family members cook. Or, send them out for fast or convenience foods. (See Chapter Thirteen for healthy, fast, and convenient food menus.)

▼

Menus for the First Week with Baby

Those first few days will most likely be too hectic to plan menus. Here are a week's worth of quick meals—some from take-out, and some made quickly at home. You can find the recipes for some of these dishes by looking at the page indicated in the parenthesis following the dish.

Day 1
Chinese take-out night!
Chicken and Snow Peas,
    Moo-Shoo Shrimp
Steamed rice
Fresh fruit
Milk

Day 2
Canadian bacon pizza
    on whole-wheat crust
Tossed salad
Raspberry sorbet

Day 3
Grilled chicken breast
Grilled zucchini and grilled
    carrot kebobs
Bulgur or brown rice
Wheat rolls
Frozen yogurt

Day 4
Minute steaks
Mixed vegetables

Easy Microwave Potatoes
    (page 305)
Cantaloupe or canned peaches

Day 5
Broccoli Quiche (page 296)
Sourdough rolls
Sliced tomatoes with basil
Tropical Pudding (page 237)

Day 6
Bean tostadas
Mexican rice
Avocado and tomato salad
Frozen bananas

Day 7
Pasta with Quick Alfredo
    Sauce (page 229)
Garlic bread
Mixed green salad
Fig bars

▼

Going Back to Work

Whether because of economic necessity or for personal fulfillment, most women go back to work when their babies are six weeks old. Going back to work can affect your feeding decision. In the previous chapter you have read about both bottlefeeding and breastfeeding. You may even have decided that the many important benefits of breast-feeding make it worthwhile to breast-feed. However, many women view going back to work as an insurmountable obstacle to breastfeeding.

During my counseling sessions with pregnant women, I often found that if a woman knew she was going back to work, she threw the idea of breastfeeding right out the window. However, more and more companies are being supportive of breastfeeding. In fact, one study showed that infant illnesses were reduced by 36 percent and women who breast-fed missed 27 percent fewer days due to their sick children.[1] You can continue to nurse and to return to work. Here are three examples of how working women handled their feeding decisions:

• Barb was determined to breast-feed Joshua. Her company was supportive of breastfeeding. She rented a breast pump from the hospital and used it at work. She used the Medela pump attachment that emptied both breasts at the same time, which allowed her to use her hands to read, eat a snack, etc. During her lunch break, she came home and fed Josh. Barb found that breast-feeding Josh was just the contact she needed after being away most of the day. I admired Barb for her determination. She carried on this routine for nine months, until she started

daycare in her home, where she continued to nurse.

• Sarah had a high-stress job. Her boss and company policies were not too supportive of motherhood. Yet Sarah wanted to breast-feed. She learned that breastfeeding didn't have to be done "full-time." She established a good milk supply while she was home with Erin, then she gradually worked out the routine that best worked for her family. She nursed Erin in the morning, Erin's daycare fed Erin two bottles of formula in the early afternoon, and Sarah nursed Erin in the late afternoon while her husband was preparing dinner, and again before she went to bed. Sarah's milk supply adjusted according to Erin's feeding schedule. On the weekend, Erin's dad helped out with the midday bottles, giving Sarah a break.

• Nicole didn't want to have to pump at work, but she wanted to breast-feed. By planning ahead, she and her husband saved some money so that she could work part-time after Sean was born. While at home for ten weeks after her delivery, she built up her milk supply and arranged her schedule to be away four hours each morning. By working part-

time, Nicole had the best of both worlds.

If you will be returning to work, your environment at work will influence your feeding decision. Try to look ahead to arrange the following things:

Parental leave time. If your company allows an extended maternity leave, this will give you more time to be with your baby. And if you decide to breast-feed, additional time off will allow you time to increase your milk supply. Even if you decide to breast-feed for just a month, your baby will still receive the colostrum, which contains important disease-fighting agents.

Required travel. If your job requires you to frequently be out of town, you might want to cut down your travel time to a minimum, whether you breast-feed or not. However, nursing is not impossible, but it will require diligent planning to make it work. Kristen arranged daycare with a national franchise when she traveled, so she could take Katie with her. Not many people can make such a commitment, but Kristen's example shows how creative a person can be if needed!

Flex-hours. Many companies offer flexible hours. A flexible schedule is useful for the two-career couple. For example, some people work four ten-hour days and have the fifth day off. If both partners can arrange this type of schedule, daycare would only be required three days a week, giving both parents extra time with baby. Flex-hours can also help a breast-feeding mom. For example, if you can take a long lunch and work later, you might be able to be with your child and feed him lunch. (On-site daycare makes this even easier!)

Supportive boss and coworkers. Going back to work with an infant at home may be emotionally hard. Seek out supportive coworkers; perhaps those who also have children. A supportive boss will understand if you need to take breaks to pump your breasts or take a little extra time off to feed your baby

▼

Your Body Is Changing!

The "fourth trimester" refers to the twelve weeks after you have your baby. This often-neglected period is important to understand. You are now adjusting from having been pregnant to being a mother. Life is different in many ways and you will face many new experiences and emotions. It is important that you take care of yourself physi- cally and mentally. Proper diet and a gradual return to exercise can help you feel much better. Listed below are the different changes that will be occurring in different parts of your body.

Uterus

Immediately after birth your uterus weighs about two pounds and is the size of a grapefruit. In the next six weeks, it will shrink down to normal—around three inches long and two ounces in weight. Nursing your baby will help your uterus contract and reduce in size. You may feel these contractions for two or three days, especially if this is your second or third baby.

Lochia

Lochia is the vaginal discharge that occurs the first few weeks after delivery. It is the body's way of getting rid of leftover debris from pregnancy and is a combination of blood cells, skin cells, mucus, white blood cells, bacteria, and occasionally some of your baby's stool or hair.

Your blood flow will be red and plentiful for the first few days following delivery. Remember that your body generated a greater volume of blood during your pregnancy and now much of that excess is being reduced. Amount of blood flow is individual, yet within two to three weeks, many women return to having a whitish discharge.

If you revert to bright-red bleeding, you are being too active—slow down and enjoy these simple days of newborn life. If your flow remains bright red or has a foul odor, please contact your physician. Remember that ovulation can occur within weeks after delivery, even if you are breast-feeding. However, ovulation may not occur in the breast-feeding mom until after weaning. The first periods may be heavy and irregular for several months. Discuss contraception with your doctor if you want to resume having sex within three to four weeks after delivery.

Perineum and Vagina

The area between your vagina and rectum is called the perineum. This area will feel sore due to the tremendous stretching it has undergone, even if you did not have an episiotomy. Ice will be applied in the first twelve hours after your delivery to reduce swelling. After this time, heat will promote healing. Many women take sitz baths (sitting for a short time in warm water).

Kegel exercises will help to tone muscles in the perineum area. You should have learned how to do kegels in your childbirth education class or prenatal exercise class. If not, ask your health care provider.

If you had an episiotomy, your stitches will dissolve by themselves. Your vagina will have decreased mucus until ovulation returns to normal, and intercourse might need additional lubrication. Please note that if you are nursing, ovulation may be delayed for a while, so you may continue to have reduced mucus.

Abdomen

After the birth of a baby, your abdomen will still look very much "pregnant," yet flabby. This may be one of your biggest disappointments after delivery, unless you are prepared for it. You can start doing exercises to help tighten your abdominal muscles again. Remember that good muscle tone will take time and discipline; diet, good posture, and exercise are important. If you have no energy or time to think about exercise in the first few months, tighten your perineum (do a kegel) and abdomen every time you turn on a water faucet!

▼

Losing That Baby Fat–Sensibly!

Are you ready to get rid of the extra pounds you gained during pregnancy? Not so fast! Remember that it took nine months to gain the weight; it's not going to come off in a week or two! The key to long-term weight loss is a balanced, reduced-calorie diet combined with exercise.

However, you'd better not exercise vigorously the first six weeks due to hormonal changes. (Personally, I didn't have to worry about doing anything vigorous the first six weeks; I was too tired!) Remember those hormones that were discussed in the third trimester chapter–the ones that cause your joints and pelvis to become more elastic? Well, they haven't quite returned to normal yet, so take it easy for a while or you could damage some joints or ligaments. A simple walking regimen should be fine. It's a great way to show off your new baby to the neighbors or to meet other new moms at the mall.

Chances are, if you were at your ideal weight before your pregnancy, you won't need any "diet" at all. If you are nursing, you shouldn't reduce your calorie intake below 1,800 calories. You may just need to consciously cut back on the "extras" and the fat that you eat, and increase your activity level. The weight will come off gradually.

However, many women want a "program" to follow, even if they have just ten pounds to lose. Some women were over-weight when they became pregnant; they may want something more structured. Later, we will review steps to help you evaluate a weight-loss program.

Regardless of your situation, my advice is to lose as much of your excess weight as possible before you become pregnant again (that is, if you are planning to have another child). Many of the women I see for weight loss are in their fifties and explain that they never lost all their weight between pregnancies or after their last baby. By the time they see me, they are often forced to lose weight because of a medical reason: diabetes, high blood pressure, or heart disease. Avoid any of those problems now by doing something sensible about losing weight.

I believe many people's weight "yo-yos" because they are in a hurry to lose weight. I've seen this situation in my weight-loss classes. For example, "Mary" has been overweight for fifteen years, but now she has a class reunion to attend, and all of a sudden she wants to lose her weight NOW. It's human nature.

Something motivates us to move, and we'll do anything to reach our goal. The problem in applying this mindset to weight loss is that most people quickly become discouraged and their weight loss battle is lost before it really begins.

According to some experts, people need almost six months to truly change their habits. Yet, Mary expects to do a major overhaul on her diet and lifestyle in two weeks or less!

When people change their diet drastically, they may at first lose weight quickly because much of it is water. Then, when their weight loss tapers to a pound or less a week, they feel they're unsuccessful and give up. What they have forgotten is that a pound a week adds up to fifty-two pounds a year! That's a lot of pounds!

The key to losing weight is to determine which diet or lifestyle habits need changing, and then gradually altering eating habits, setting realistic goals and adopting an exercise program that you can stick with for life. Remember—any temporary changes may result in temporary weight loss.

Following are some of the characteristics I've observed in people who are the most successful in losing weight. People who lose weight successfully . . .

- exercise regularly.[2]
- set realistic goals. When they don't meet their goals, they learn from the experience instead of considering themselves failures and giving up.
- have social support from either family, friends, co-workers, or support groups.[3]
- work on liking themselves (or they already do).
- are motivated to lose weight for internal reasons rather than external reasons.[4] For example, Judy used to lose weight to fit into her old size-six jeans. Now she loses weight to improve her health.
- concentrate not on the bathroom scale, but on some positive outcome, such as lowered cholesterol or being able to walk further without becoming tired.
- have conquered emotional eating (eating when bored, angry, depressed, or stressed), or are working on it.[5]
- have learned to eat sensibly at restaurants, at parties, while traveling, etc.
- work at self-monitoring. This may mean keeping a food diary, keeping track of the amount of fat they eat in a day, or keeping a log of how many hours per week they exercise.
- control their diet; they don't let their diet control them! This means they make educated and conscious choices about the food they eat. If they want to splurge for a special occasion, they do. They are honest with themselves about the reasons they eat.

▼

Weight Loss Programs

Many diet programs and diet books are available, but beware! Many diet programs promote quick weight loss, which is unhealthy. Others may recommend unbalanced diets, which leave out one or more foods or food groups. Some can be downright dangerous. Virtually all diets work—for the short term. However, many diets fail over the long term. Continued dieting and regaining weight, often called "weight cycling" or "yo-yo" dieting, can be harmful to the body and devastating to a dieter's self-esteem.

Evaluating Weight-Loss Programs

The steps below should help you evaluate a weight-loss program.

1. *Does the program promote a balanced diet, allowing all foods in moderation? Does it omit certain foods or food groups?*
A balanced program should allow all foods, even the so-called "bad" ones, at some point in the program.

2. *Does the program include an exercise plan or regimen?*
Since exercise is so important for long-term success, avoid any

program that doesn't address exercise or recommend a specific activity program.

3. *Does the program include behavior modification (looking at changing current behaviors)?*
For long-term weight loss, you must learn what your problem behaviors are so you can work to change them. Some tools used for behavior modification might include self-monitoring (keeping a diet record), or exercises that promote an awareness of eating patterns.

4. *Does the program use trained professionals as their "counselors" or do they use people whose only qualifications are that they have lost weight?*
Many programs use people who have lost weight, or people who are good salespeople, as their counselors. Though these people may be very helpful and motivating, they may unintentionally give out inaccurate information.

A number of "quacks," professional and otherwise, are also out there–trying to make a quick dollar! Beware of anything that sounds too good to be true (it probably is). Look for counselors who are licensed, registered, or have a degree from an accredited university.

5. *Does the program involve buying special foods or supplements?*
Personally, I feel that learning how to eat "real" food is better

for long-term weight loss. However, some people just want the convenience of buying packaged foods.

6. *Does the program provide a foundation for future good-eating habits?*
Hopefully, the program teaches you how to cook more healthfully, plan menus, and learn to eat sensibly in social situations.

The Moderate Approach

The recommended postpregnant weight loss is about one pound or less a week. You're probably thinking, "One pound a week! I'll never lose this weight!" Consider the importance of long-term success, which means keeping the weight off. People who lose weight slowly seem to keep it off the longest.

To lose a pound a week, you can either cut your food intake by five hundred calories a day, use more calories by exercising, or combine eating less and exercising more. For example, Colleen walks about two miles every evening, which uses approximately two hundred calories. She has also cut three-hundred-calories-worth of extras out of her diet. The diet/exercise approach that Colleen uses works best for long-term weight maintenance. Besides being good for muscle tone, cardiovascular

health, and endurance, exercise is also good for your mental health! Following is an example of a good fitness program. As you can see, fitness doesn't have to be boring!

Suggested Activity Program for Colleen
Height: 5'4"
Weight: 160 pounds
Goal Weight: 120 pounds
Exercise-Activity Goal: 1 hour 6 times a week

Monday: 1 hour of light aerobics burns 217 calories

Tuesday: 1 hour of walking (26-minute mile) burns 217 calories

Wednesday: ½ hour of bicycling at 10 mph burns 200 calories

Thursday: 1 hour of walking (26-minute mile) burns 217 calories

Friday: Day off!

Saturday: 1 hour of lawn mowing burns 261 calories or 1 hour of hiking burns 399 calories

Sunday: 1 hour of gardening burns 232 calories

Source: Fit III Analysis Program.

By following this activity program, Colleen burns over 1,700 calories! To lose one pound per week, she also needs to reduce her diet by 1,800 calories per week or about 250 calories per day. (Please note that the numbers of calories burned are calculated specifically for Colleen.)

The chart below lists a few of the extras Colleen eats that she can easily cut from her diet.

These changes add up to a reduction of over seven hundred calories per day! Colleen will only need to follow half the proposed changes to lose one pound per week!

Depending on your weight, height, and activity level, you will probably want to eat between 1,200 to 1,800 calories per day to lose one pound a week. Eating below 1,200 calories is usually not advised unless you have a petite build.

Lose Weight by Leaning toward Vegetarianism

Cutting down on animal protein is often a way to cut calories and fat, which can lead to weight loss! Leaning toward vegetarianism, or even becoming vegetarian, might be your goal. While testing meatless recipes for the book *Make the Change for a Healthy Heart,* I was losing weight without trying and I had to consciously eat extra snacks to avoid losing weight! (See Chapter Six for more on vegetarian eating.) In addition, here is a good source to help with weight loss for vegetarians: *Simple, Low-Fat, and Vegetarian,* by Suzanne Havala, M.S., R.D., Vegetarian Resource Group, 1994, and *Vegetarian*

Weight Loss Guide, by Suzanne Havala, M.S., R.D., published in *Vegetarian Journal Reports,* Vegetarian Resource Group, 1990.

Fifteen-Hundred-Calorie Meal Plan

This meal plan is meant to be a guideline of a healthy weight-loss program—it's not meant to take the place of individual counseling with a health professional. If you are breast-feeding, this meal plan does not contain enough calories or nutrients for your current needs.

7 servings of starches/grains

1 serving is 1 slice of any type bread, 1 flour tortilla, ½ cup pasta, ⅓ cup rice or legumes, 6 crackers, or ½ cup of potato.

3 servings of fruits

1 serving is 1 medium piece of fresh fruit, ½ banana, ½ cup canned fruit in its own juice, 1 cup melon or berries, 2 plums, or 2 nectarines.

3 or more servings of vegetables

1 serving is ½ cup of any non-starchy vegetable or 1 cup lettuce.

5 ounces of protein or equivalent

1 serving is 1 ounce of lean meat, 1 ounce reduced-fat cheese, ¼ cup cottage cheese, ½ cup of tofu, 2 tablespoons peanut butter, ½ cup cooked dried beans, or 1 egg.

Low-Fat Food Substitutions			
Food	Calories	Action	Calories Saved
1 tablespoon margarine	100	Substitute Butter Buds or Molly McButter	100
1 cola drink	150	Substitute diet soda	148
2 chocolate chip cookies	140	Substitute 1 peach	100
1 cinnamon roll	230	Substitute 1 Quaker Caramel Corn Cake	180
3 cups whole milk	450	Substitute 2% milk	90
3 tablespoons blue cheese dressing	180	Substitute Wish Bone Healthy Sensation Chunky Blue Cheese	120

**2 to 3 servings
of dairy products**

1 serving is 1 cup of skim or 1% milk or low-fat yogurt.

3 servings of fat

1 serving is 1 teaspoon margarine or butter or 2 teaspoons reduced-fat margarine, 1 teaspoon mayonnaise or 2 teaspoons reduced-fat mayonnaise, 1 slice bacon, ½ ounce cream cheese, 1 tablespoon sour cream, ⅛ avocado, 10 peanuts, or 5 olives.

For more information about weight loss or healthy eating, see the reference section in the back of this book for recommended weight-loss books and low-calorie cookbooks.

? Questions You May Have

Q: I've never been much of a breakfast eater, but I've heard that it's good for you. Is it?

A: You may have heard that "breakfast is the most important meal of the day." In many respects, that's true. A recent study showed that people who skipped breakfast had trouble working on tasks that required concentration. According to Diane Odland, nutritionist at the U.S. Department of Agriculture Human Nutrition Information Service, "When you consider it's been eight or nine hours since you've had a meal, it's obvious that refueling at breakfast will make you feel and perform better during the day."[6]

Eating breakfast can also help you lose weight. People who skip the first meal of the day often make up for it later by eating larger meals or snacking on high-fat, high-sugar foods. Whether you stay home with a child or work outside the home, eating breakfast will definitely improve your energy level.

Q: Will I lose all my pregnancy weight without really trying?

A: It depends on how much you gained. In one study, women who gained more than twenty pounds retained from five to ten pounds between pregnancies. Those who gained over forty pounds were an average of seventeen pounds heavier at the start of their next pregnancy. Since the current recommendation for weight gain is over twenty-five pounds, you will probably have to make an active effort to lose the weight.[7]

Q: How long will it take me to lose my "baby" fat?

A: Again, it depends on how much you gained, how much you eat, and your activity level. A lucky few fit into their "un-pregnant" clothes right after delivery (though that wasn't the case for me or any of my friends).

The amount of time needed to lose the weight and get your "old body" back is probably a big surprise to every mother. Much to my dissapointment, I needed almost nine months to return to my normal weight. I thought I'd be back to my old self within a few months. Doing aerobics three times a week made the biggest change in the way my body looked. I was also able to lose those stubborn last five pounds.

When I surveyed other dietitians about this book, several suggested that I include some realistic expectations for weight loss and body size after pregnancy. Here are some things you should expect:

- Very few people go back to wearing their "skinny" clothes right after delivery. Expect to wear your maternity clothes for a few more months (even though you probably feel like burning them!).
- You may need to buy a few outfits in "the next size" until you get your shape back.
- Your body may have reproportioned itself. For example, Kate weighs the same as she did before pregnancy, but her hips are a few inches wider. Most of us continue

to have a little "tummy" unless we diligently practice abdominal exercises. Some find their ribcages permanently expanded and need to wear a larger bra size. Believe it or not, some women even wear a larger shoe size after pregnancy.

- If you are breast-feeding, you may feel as though you are "busting" out of your blouses. Judy was exasperated because for the first few months of breastfeeding, the only shirts she could wear were her husband's t-shirts and her old maternity shirts. However, Sandy was glad to have an excuse to buy new clothes!
- Many women lose the last few pounds after they stop breast-feeding.
- Exercise can't be emphasized enough. It will help you lose baby fat and tone up some of the muscles you haven't used lately.
- Overall, be patient. I clearly remember asking my aerobics teacher how fast I could

get into shape after the baby came, if I worked out regularly. I wanted *real* numbers. She said it could be done in six to eight weeks, but I might need time for recovery. Not me, I thought. I was going to be supermom! Well, after a tough labor and delivery, and a long adjustment to motherhood, months passed before I had the time and energy to restart my exercise program. After my second son was born, I didn't have a problem losing the weight. I breast-fed him longer and I was much more active chasing two kids around!

Preparing for Your Next Pregnancy

Sometime between your labor anesthesia wearing off and sending out birth announcements,

someone will ask, "So, when are you going to have another baby?" You may not be ready to answer that question for a long time. However, you may want another baby right away or in the next year. Waiting at least nine months between pregnancies is a good idea to shape-up your body and to build up your nutrient stores. When you are ready to think about getting pregnant again, turn to Chapter One, Contemplating Pregnancy, to learn what you can do for a healthy pregnancy *before* you conceive.

No matter when you decide to have another baby, or even if you decide not to, don't lose the good habits you established during pregnancy. A healthy diet is one of the most important things you can do to ensure good health for you and your children, and teaching your children good eating habits is one of the most precious gifts you can give them.

Fitting Fitness In

Benefits of Exercise

Throughout the book, I've mentioned exercise many times. I'm hoping repetition will bring home the message. Exercise is one of the most important things you can do for your health—now and later. Regular exercise can bring you numerous benefits, with just a little of your time invested.

While you are pregnant, exercise offers even more benefits:

- Exercise helps battle the fatigue many women feel during pregnancy.
- Exercise makes you physically fit and helps your body get ready for labor.
- Exercise helps you feel better about your expanding body size.
- Once you've established a fitness routine, resuming exercising after you have the baby (when you're trying to lose weight) will be easier.
- Regular exercise will help you sleep better; and you may need all the sleep you can get during those last few weeks of pregnancy!
- You will probably feel better all over—you'll have a better emotional outlook and you may have improved immunity.

A former "couch potato" says: "I was never interested in exercising, but when I became pregnant, my doctor suggested I get involved in an exercise program for pregnant women at the YWCA. I went to an aerobics class, mostly for my baby, and much to my surprise, I began to really enjoy it. I shared labor and delivery stories with other Moms-to-be and began a "Mommy Network." Toward the end of my pregnancy, I think the exercise really helped me sleep better. Also, I felt much less tired than I did with my first pregnancy. I had more energy and felt vivacious."

If you didn't exercise before you were pregnant, you should ask your health care provider about exercising. He or she may have some special guidelines for you, depending on your current situation. If you had exercised routinely before pregnancy, you can probably continue your exercise program with some modifications.

What Every Pregnant Woman Should Know about Exercise

Note: For the most part, these guidelines also apply to the postpartum period.[1]

▶ Don't do too much at first.

Have you ever watched the Olympics and gotten so inspired that you jumped up and decided that you were going to run two miles? Don't! Start out slowly and run maybe as little as five minutes a day; and don't forget to warm up and cool down.

▶ Be kind to your joints.

The hormones of pregnancy make joints very elastic, which prepares them for childbirth. Exercise that involves lots of bouncing, jerky movements, jumping, or quick changes in direction could cause joint pain or injury. Also, avoid deep flexing or extending of your muscles. Use gentle stretches (instead of stretching to the limit) to cool down.

▶ Avoid "Iron Man Marathons" and other rigorous events (unless you are already an athlete and you have your health care provider's permission).

Stay away from competitive sports. Stick to walking, swimming, or low-impact aerobics (preferably classes developed just for pregnant women).

▶ Do kinder, gentler exercise.

With the extra weight gain in pregnancy, which changes your body's center of gravity, you should avoid sports that have the potential for falling, which include downhill skiing, skating, skateboarding, etc. Exercise on a wooden floor or a tightly carpeted surface to reduce shock and provide sure footing.

▶ Be consistent.

Regular exercise is best, even if only for a few minutes. Thousands of people are "would be" exercisers and have good intentions. Their homes are full of treadmills, stationery bikes, rowing machines, and weight sets. Unfortunately, this collection of exercise paraphernalia serves mostly as dust collectors and clothes racks. Those people would be much better off if they set aside fifteen minutes a day to simply go for a walk.

▶ Warm up and cool down.

Always begin with a five-minute warm-up period of less-intense exercise (such as slow walking, cycling, or water walking for swimmers) to warm up muscles. Strenuous exercise should last no longer than fifteen minutes. Follow a period of intense exercise with five to ten minutes of "cool down"—a gradual slowing down of your workout that ends with gentle stretching.

▶ Exercise at least three times a week.

Exercising just twenty minutes a day, three times a week, is much better for you than being a "weekend athlete."

▶ Measure your heart rate during exercise.

Exercising too intensely can increase your body's internal temperature, which can harm the fetus. Measure your pulse at the peak of your activity and also before cool down. To measure your pulse, place your index finger at your carotid artery on your neck. Keep moving. Count your heart rate for either six or ten seconds. Pregnant women's heart rates should not exceed 140 beats per minute. This is fourteen beats in six seconds or twenty-three beats in ten seconds. Check with your health care provider for alternate guidelines.

▶ Take your time.

Get up from the floor slowly and gradually to avoid dizziness or fainting caused from a drop in your blood pressure.

▶ Drink, drink, drink!

Drink water before, during, and after exercise to prevent dehydration. Drinking will also help cool you off. Take a squirt bottle filled with water on your walk or to aerobics.

▶ Stay out of the heat.

Don't do any vigorous exercise in hot, humid weather, or during an illness when you have a fever.

▶ Watch out for danger signs.

Stop your activity immediately and call your doctor if any of these symptoms occur: pain, bleeding, dizziness, shortness of breath, rapid heartbeat, back pain, pubic pain, and/or difficulty walking.

▶ Be kind to YOU!

Think of exercise as a special time for YOU. You may not always agree, but exercise is a way to pamper yourself!

▶ Eat enough food.

During pregnancy, blood sugar levels are usually lower than nonpregnant levels and your body uses carbohydrates at a greater rate. So, you might have low blood sugar during strenuous exercise. Make sure you don't exercise on an empty stomach. You may want to eat a piece of fruit, some crackers, dried fruit, or drink some juice before your workout for more energy.

If you worked out regularly before pregnancy, and continue to have a vigorous workout schedule, keep in mind that you will need to increase your calories accordingly. Your weight gain will let you know if you're eating enough.

Some reasons why exercise should be "toned down" or done differently during pregnancy are:

- Your heart rate at rest is higher than a nonpregnant woman's and rises more quickly during exercise. So, watch the intensity of your exercise.
- Your body temperature may rise more rapidly than a nonpregnant woman's. And since your baby's body temperature is always one degree warmer than yours, an elevated body temperature could mean trouble for your baby. Be careful of how hard and how long you exercise.
- After your fourth month, your uterus may compress the vena cava, a major vein. This could interfere with blood flow to the fetus. (After your fourth month, don't do any exercise while laying flat on your back.)
- Some hormones make joints and connective tissue relax (to get ready for delivery) and can make joints susceptible to injury. Treat your joints gently by doing slow stretches daily and don't forget to warm up and cool down!
- Some studies have shown that vigorous activity can cause contractions, which may lead to premature labor. One study done with women who had gestational diabetes showed that the safest exercises were those that used mostly the upper body or those that applied little stress below the waist.

The researchers found that walking on a treadmill was fine, but jogging was likely to cause contractions. Exercising on a stationary bike caused contractions in half of the women, though exercising on a recumbent bicycle (one in which you sit back with your legs in front of you, not under you) caused no contractions. The upper arm ergometer proved to be the safest form of exercise. This is a machine similar to a stationery bicycle except that the arms do all the pedaling.[2]

For more specific information about exercise, ask your health care provider or childbirth educator. Always check with your health care provider before starting an exercise program, especially if you haven't recently exercised.

When You Shouldn't Exercise

According to the American College of Obstetricians and Gynecologists, several conditions totally restrict you from exercising vigorously. If any of these conditions apply to you, ask your health care provider before exercising.

- History of three or more miscarriages
- Ruptured membranes
- Premature labor
- Diagnosed multiple gestation (twins, triplets, or more)
- Incompetent cervix
- Bleeding or a diagnosis of placenta previa
- Diagnosed cardiac disease

Some conditions may require you to limit strenuous exercise. If any of these conditions apply to you, be sure to talk with your health care provider before starting an exercise program.

- High blood pressure
- Anemia or other blood disorder
- Thyroid disease
- Diabetes
- Cardiac arrhythmia or palpitations
- History of premature labor
- History of intrauterine growth retardation (slowed growth of fetus)
- History of bleeding during current pregnancy
- Breech position of baby in last trimester
- Excessive obesity
- Extreme underweight
- History of extremely sedentary lifestyle

Source: American College of Obstetricians and Gynecologists. *"Exercise During Pregnancy and the Postnatal Period."* ACOG Home Exercise Programs. Washington, D.C.: ©1985. Reprinted with permission.

▼

Fitting Fitness into Your Busy Lifestyle

Here is where the "fitting fitness in" comes in. Some people don't exercise regularly because they don't have time. It's true, we live in a very fast-paced society. Yet, most of us have fifteen minutes a day that we probably waste. Here are a few ideas for fitting fitness into your lifestyle:

▶ **Take a walk every morning before work.**

If you happen to have a treadmill, you can walk while watching the morning news.

▶ **Make more trips up and down the stairs.**

One suggestion is to unplug the downstairs phone so that every time the phone rings, you need to go up and down the stairs once. However, although these kinds of "tricks" will give you more activity, such activity uses only short bursts of energy and won't improve your overall fitness much.

▶ **Use half your lunch hour to take a walk.**

I did this on the days I didn't go to aerobics. The funny part of it was that I had to turn down many rides. Everyone must have felt sorry for this big pregnant woman walking down the street!

▶ **Write your exercise "date" on your calendar and keep it!**

▶ **Exercise with your spouse or a friend.**

▶ **Walk the dog; she'll love you for it!**

▶ **Sign up for an exercise class just for pregnant women.**

Sometimes if you pay for a class, you are more motivated to go.

▶ **On the weekend, take a drive to the country where you can walk while admiring scenic views.**

▶ **Get the whole family into exercising!**

Take walks or hikes together.

▶ **Rent or purchase an exercise video just for pregnant women.**

The American College of Obstetricians and Gynecologists have approved a series of exercise videos: *Pregnancy Exercise Video* and *Postnatal Exercise Video* ($19.95 each). You can order them by calling 1-800-424-3463.

Your Personal Exercise Schedule

Take just a moment to write your plan for exercising.

My goal is to exercise _____ times per week, for _____ minutes each time.

My Exercise Schedule:

Monday (at)_____
(time)

Tuesday _____

Wednesday _____

Thursday _____

Friday _____

Saturday _____

Sunday _____

Ten Ways to Exercise without Exercising

Not everyone truly enjoys exercising! If you fit into that category, you'll like the following list that will increase your physical activity level without a planned exercise routine.

▶ **Walk the dog.**

▶ **"Shop 'til you drop."**

Or you can go once around the mall and window-shop.

▶ **Go dancing–ballroom, country and western, even square-dancing will do.**

Or put on your favorite music at home and dance!

▶ **Take a stroll around a scenic place, a lake, down a tree-lined avenue, or along a forest trail.**

▶ **Go canoeing or paddle-boating.**

▶ **Do arm exercises using one-pound weights or cans of soup while watching your favorite show.**

▶ **Go to the pool and just walk from side to side.**

Bring a friend. Chatting away, you won't notice the time passing.

▶ **Aerobic lawn mowing!**

Supposedly, the latest trend is to cut your grass with a push mower. Start a fad in your neighborhood!

▶ **Plant a garden.**

Gardening is a fun activity and you get to enjoy the fruits of your labor! Or clean house more often–vacuuming *can* be aerobic.

► **Set a walking date with a neighbor or coworker.**

Once you get to talking, you'll hardly notice the time (or the exercise).

Exercise after Pregnancy

Women often face weight problems, especially after having had children. Those last five pounds just don't seem to come off. Then you add another five pounds from your next pregnancy, and before you know it, you're fifteen or twenty pounds overweight. So what does exercise have to do with weight?

Research has shown that people who exercise regularly lose more weight and have the best odds of (and here's the hard part) keeping it off! Other benefits of exercising include improved cardiovascular fitness, lowered heart rate, lowered blood pressure, decreased blood lipids, decreased blood sugar, toned muscles, less body fat, improved immunity, and more!

After you have your baby, you may need some time to feel motivated to exercise. That's okay. You have just gone through one of life's biggest events. You may need some time to get used to a new baby in the house and to set up a new routine. (I needed four months to adjust!) Remember those hormones that made your joints more elastic so that your pelvis could stretch for birth? Weeks will pass before those hormones drop to their normal levels. Most physicians will approve an exercise program after the six-week check-up. Until then, walking is generally fine.

A new mom says: "I was one of those people who thought I would be out of the house and back to exercising within days after delivery. Surprise, surprise! After a week, I still had trouble walking! My neighbor had a C-section and she was taking her baby on a walk in the stroller when he was just four days old! I was jealous!"

Women have very individual labor experiences. Some breeze through their labor in a few hours. Others may last a day and a half. If you had a long labor, it may have taken a lot out of you. If you had stitches, hemorrhoids, or a combination of the two, it may seem even longer before you'll feel okay walking and sitting. Be prepared for the best or worst situation, but remember that this too shall pass.

You Don't Have to Be a Race Walker to Lose Weight!

One study compared the effects of low-intensity and high-intensity exercise. Women who walked four days a week for twelve weeks lost five pounds of body fat, whether they exercised slowly or vigorously. Both groups burned three hundred calories during each workout. However, low-intensity walkers lost more body fat in the abdomen and buttocks area. If those areas are a problem for you, you may want to exerciese at a slower rate.[3]

Tips for Starting a Postpartum Exercise Program

► **Start at your own pace, no matter how slow it seems!**

► **Stretching will be important, even if you don't feel like exercising.**

► **Find activities you enjoy and, if possible, include other family members.**

▶ **Join a fitness class for moms and babies.**

You won't feel as though you are the only one out of shape; you can meet other moms; and you can take along your baby! (Call your YMCA.)

▶ **While you are at home the first six weeks, the days seem to drift by.**

Make a schedule for yourself that includes some activity. The schedule will give you a sense of purpose.

▶ **When you have time between baby's naps, pop in an exercise video.**

American Health magazine rates the following as the Ten Best Exercise Videos. The first three are beginner/intermediate level, and may be best if you weren't very active during your pregnancy. Videos four through eight are intermediate/advanced level and may be appropriate for those who kept up a regular fitness routine during pregnancy. Videos nine and ten are advanced level and may be appropriate for those whose fitness levels have increased.

1. *Richard Simmons: Sweatin' to the Oldies*

2. *Basic Stepping with Walk Aerobics*

3. *Jane Fonda's Complete Workout*

4. *Victoria's Power-Shaping Workout*

5. *Kathy Smith's Instant Workout*

6. *Kathy Smith's Weight Loss Workout*

7. *Jody Watley: Dance to Fitness*

8. *The Firm; Aerobic Workout with Weights, Volume I*

9. *The Firm; Aerobic Workout with Weights, Volume II*

10. *Technifunk 2000*

Source: *American Health Magazine*, March 1992.

Possibly the most important fact about exercising is that you're doing it. Do what you have to do to get started, but as that sports-shoe commercial says, JUST DO IT! (See the resource section in the back of this book for references on fitness.)

❓ **Questions You May Have**

Q: Doesn't exercise make you more tired?

A: At first you may feel a little more tired after exercising while pregnant. This tiredness is a result of the extra weight you are carrying and the extra blood that must be pumped through your heart. (During the first trimester, hormonal changes can cause fatigue.) However, since exercise increases endurance, you will gradually feel less tired once your body gets accustomed to exercise. Of course, if you are already exercising, you shouldn't feel as tired. If you do, you may not be eating enough foods or the right foods.

Q: How will I know if I'm eating enough while exercising during pregnancy?

A: The rule of thumb here is to eat when you're hungry and to watch your weight gain. If you're not gaining enough, you need to eat more. If you have a vigorous schedule and just can't seem to eat enough, you may need to slow down. (See page 218 for "Snack Ideas for High-Energy Moms.")

Q: I'm on bed rest. How can I prevent my body from turning into flab?

A: Pregnancy often causes us to make changes in our lifestyle and habits. Bed rest takes this to the extreme. You *will* lose your level of fitness while on bed rest. However, by stretching and doing isometric exercises (if approved by your health care provider), you can retain some of your muscle tone. Ask your health care provider for a list of suggested exercises to keep yourself limber and for permission to do arm exercises. Also, remember that after you have the baby, your endurance for exercise will be very low. You'll need to start out slowly! I thought I would need practically *forever* to get back into shape after I was off bed rest. In just a few weeks, my endurance felt normal. Your body *will* bounce back and you *can* become fit again, so think of your situation as a temporary one.

Q: My back hurts all the time lately. What can I do?

A: I can sympathize with you. During the last two months of my pregnancy, I couldn't sweep and mop the kitchen floor in the same afternoon, because my back hurt so much. I finally gave that job to my husband (one of the unexpected benefits of pregnancy!).

Your back undergoes a great deal of stress during pregnancy.

Most traditional back-strengthening exercises are not recommended during pregnancy because they are performed lying on your back. One that is recommended is the pelvic tilt. If you are attending an exercise class for pregnant women, you probably already know this exercise.

How to Do a Pelvic Tilt

1. Stand with feet shoulder-width apart and knees slightly bent.

2. Contract the muscles of the buttocks and abdomen and gently thrust your pelvis forward, rotating your pubic bone upward. Hold this position for ten seconds and release.

3. The pelvic tilt can be done while lying or while squatting on your hands and knees.

Source: American College of Obstetricians and Gynecologists. *ACOG Guide to Planning for Pregnancy, Birth, and Beyond.* Washington, D.C.: ACOG ©1990. Reprinted with permission.

You should try to do the pelvic tilt as often as possible during the day. Keep in mind that after your delivery, lifting and carrying can still be painful. Continue the pelvic tilts and other back-strengthening exercises to improve your back health. Keeping your stomach muscles strong will support the back muscles and will prevent back strain. Stomach crunches (or half sit-ups)—lifting your shoulders off the ground while keeping your knees bent—is a great tummy exercise for the postpartum period.

For more information on exercise, I recommend *Essential Exercises for the Child-Bearing Year*, an excellent book by Elizabeth Noble.

Section II

Shopping, Cooking, and Eating Out

CHAPTER ELEVEN

Stocking the Pregnant Kitchen

So, now you're motivated to eat well! If your diet is already good, you may not need much help. But, if you're "turning over a new leaf" nutritionally, you may be thinking "where do I begin?"

The best place to start improving your diet is, not surprisingly, your own kitchen. First, you need to find out what your shopping and eating patterns are so you can change them if you need to.

Look inside Your Pantry

1. What takes up the bulk of room in your freezer? Frozen vegetables? Ice cream? Frozen juice? Fish, chicken, meat? Fish sticks? Frozen dinners? Frozen pies or cheesecakes? Pizza?

2. Does the top shelf of your fridge hold milk or soda?

3. Are your produce drawers bulging with fresh fruits and veggies or are a few lonely, shriveled carrots all they contain?

4. Does your pantry hold many convenience and ready-to-make foods? Canned vegetables? Canned fruits? Potato chips? Candy?

5. Do you have a mix of grains, such as brown rice, pasta, bulgur, quinoa, whole-wheat flour, wheat germ, oats, and barley or just white flour, rice, and pasta?

6. Do you keep a variety of vegetables in the house, or do you regularly eat your favorite two vegetables and fruits?

A Peek inside My Pantry

As a registered dietitian, people are always curious about how I eat at home. Sometimes I think they envision me and my family eating "perfectly" all the time. What they don't realize is that we are just like any other family; we have our habits, our likes, and our dislikes. But to show you how my family eats and shops, I'll let you take a look into my kitchen.

This Is What You'll Usually Find in My Pantry:

Various canned tomatoes, tomato sauce, and tomato paste

Jarred spaghetti sauce without meat

Corn, peas, sweet potatoes, pumpkin

Canned black beans, vegetarian refried beans, kidney beans

Fantastic Foods Soup-in-a-Cup (usually Jumpin' Black Bean or Leapin' Lentils)

Dried lentils, split peas, twelve-bean mix

Canned tuna, salmon

White and whole-wheat flour, skim evaporated milk,

Yeast, sugar, brown sugar, molasses, honey

White rice, brown rice, bulgur, barley, pasta, pasta, and more pasta!

Sun-dried tomatoes

Raisin Bran, All Bran, old-fashioned oatmeal (super-economy size!), grits, Product 19, Multibran Chex, low-fat granola

Raisins, mixed dried fruit

Canola oil, olive oil, soy sauce, many miscellaneous spices

Apple cider vinegar, red wine vinegar, tarragon wine vinegar

Boboli bread

Graham crackers, popcorn cakes, pretzels, Fig Newtons, Le Petite Beurre

Tobler or Cadbury Chocolate (My motto: buy the best but eat one square at a time!)

Lay's Baked BBQ Potato Chips, Tostitos Baked Tortilla Chips, or Guiltless Gourmet Oil-Free Tortilla Chips

Freezer:

Miscellaneous frozen juices

Nutri-Grain waffles

Healthy Treasures Fish Sticks/regular fish sticks

Trout, salmon, sole, and/or shrimp

Chicken, turkey breast

Top/bottom round, ground buffalo

Mashed bananas (to use later for banana bread or pancakes)

Chopped spinach/broccoli, mixed vegetables, peas

Miscellaneous combination vegetables

Budget Gourmet Light & Lean Pockets, and/or Michelina's Frozen Entrees

Refrigerator:

1% milk, eggs, Kraft Free cheese, regular American cheese, part-skim mozzarella or farmer's cheese, reduced-fat or fat-free Cheddar, fresh Parmesan cheese, light Velveeta

Juice, Diet Coke, decaffeinated iced tea

Miscellaneous meat, fish, or chicken, thawing

Yoplait flavored low-fat yogurt, Land O' Lakes fat-free sour cream

Ham/turkey breast deli meat

Brummel & Brown Yogurt Spread/I Can't Believe It's Not Butter!, light

Natural-style peanut butter

Mayonnaise, fat-free mayonnaise, homemade vinaigrette dressing, homemade Hidden Valley Ranch dip or dressing (almost fat-free), Good Seasons fat-free Zesty Herb dressing, barbecue sauce, teriyaki marinade, ketchup, hoisin sauce, grated ginger, chopped garlic in a jar, Dijon mustard, capers, horseradish, lemon juice, wheat germ and wheat bran (to prevent rancidity)

Various leftovers

Produce Drawers:

Summer: all kinds of berries, cantaloupe, watermelon, apricots, nectarines, peaches, mangos, pine-apple, lemons, tomatoes, carrots, romaine, leaf or Boston lettuce, cucumber, zucchini, eggplant, red and green peppers, alfalfa sprouts, ready-to-eat European salad mix

Winter: apples, bananas, pears, grapes, oranges, grapefruit, dates, figs, egg-plant, acorn squash, butter-nut squash, carrots, leeks, cabbage, broccoli, cauli-flower, tomato, lettuce, cucumber

▼

What's on a Food Label

Chances are, you are more concerned than you were just a few months ago about what you (and your baby) are eating. Your favorite new pasttime may be studying food labels. Why should you read labels? It's the perfect way to put nutrition knowledge into practice by helping you make informed food-buying choices.

What Can Be Learned from a Label?

Introducing The New and Improved Food Label—in 1990, Congress passed the Nutrition Labeling and Education Act, and in 1991, the Food and Drug Administration proposed label revisions in accordance with the new law. According to Dr. David Kessler, Commissioner of the Food and Drug Administration, "This game of 'food label roulette' is a costly game and places the consumer at a disadvantage. It is time to take the guesswork–and the element of chance–out of food labeling."

The label contains a virtual gold mine of information. For example, by looking on my box of Raisin Bran, I can see how many calories, how many grams of fiber, and how much sugar or sodium a serving contains. I can also find how much protein and fat it has and see how all these numbers compare to a standard based on the 2,000-calorie diet called Daily Value. The standard is pretty close to the number of calories you may be eating, so this is a good comparison.

I can also check out how vitamin A, vitamin C, calcium, and iron stack up to the Daily Value (formerly the U.S. RDAs on the label). Suppose I'm allergic to milk protein. I can look for it on the list of ingredients.

Following is a list of everything that is required on the food label:[1]

- Total calories
- Calories from fat
- Total fat
- Saturated fat

- Cholesterol
- Sodium
- Total carbohydrate
- Dietary fiber
- Sugars
- Protein
- Vitamins A and C, calcium, and iron (listed as "Percent of Daily Value")
- Nutrient information (listed in customary serving sizes and in household measures)

You'll also find that terms that were "loosely" defined in the past will have standard meanings:[2]

Fat-free: Less than ½ gram of fat per serving and no added fat.

Low-fat: Contains 3 grams of fat or less per 3½-ounce serving.

Light: Has at least ⅓ fewer calories or ½ the fat than a comparable product. Can also mean that a low-calorie, low-fat food has had its sodium reduced by 50 percent. It can still mean light texture or color.

Reduced: A nutritionally altered product that has at least 25 percent less of a nutrient or calories than the regular product.

Low in saturated fat: 1 gram or less per serving.

Lean: Less than 10 grams of fat, 4½ grams of saturated fat, and less than 95 milligrams of cholesterol per serving.

169

Extra lean: Less than 5 grams of fat, less than 2 grams of saturated fat, and less than 95 milligrams of cholesterol per serving.

Cholesterol-free: Less than 2 milligrams of cholesterol per serving and 2 grams or less of saturated fat per serving.

Low in cholesterol: 20 milligrams or less per 3½-ounce serving and 2 grams or less of saturated fat per serving.

Percent fat-free: Can only be used on products that meet low-fat or fat-free definition.

Low sodium: less than 140 milligrams per 3½-ounce serving.

Very low sodium: Less than 35 milligrams per 3½-ounce serving.

Calorie-free: Fewer than 5 calories per serving.

Sugar-free: Less than ½ gram per serving.

High: Contains 20 percent or more of the Daily Value for a particular nutrient.

Good Source: Contains 10 to 19 percent for a particular nutrient.

Nutrition and Health Claims

For the first time, health claims describing the relationship between a food or nutrient and the risk of a disease or health-related condition are allowed on a label. The health claim must meet certain requirements and must be phrased so that consumers can understand the food-disease relationship. Some of such pairs are:

- Folic acid and neural tube defects
- Calcium and osteoporosis
- Sodium and hypertension
- Saturated fat and cholesterol and coronary heart disease
- Fruits, vegetables, and grain products that contain fiber and risk of coronary heart disease
- Fat and cancer
- Fruits and vegetables and cancer
- Fiber-containing grain products, fruits, and vegetables and cancer

The Ingredient List

Products contain a list of ingredients—by weight, in descending order. The new labeling law requires that even standardized foods, such as mayonnaise and ice cream, have a list of ingredients. In addition, all FDA-certified color additives will be listed by name. Another helpful requirement is that beverages that claim to contain juice must declare the total percentage of juices present. For example, "Juice blend—2 to 7 percent juice."

Sugar is Sugar by Many Other Names

Some ingredients have many names, which makes deciphering the food label even trickier. For example, corn syrup, high-fructose corn syrup, dextrose, glucose, corn sweetener, sucrose, sugar, brown sugar, fructose, maltose, sorbitol, mannitol, honey, and fruit-juice concentrate are all types of sweeteners.

Additional sweeteners are "artificial" sweeteners, which are sometimes called nonnutritive or noncaloric sweeteners, widely found in diet products: Nutra-Sweet (the sweetener in Equal), Saccharin (found in Sweet'n Low, Sugar Twin, etc.), and Acesulfame K (found in Sweet One). Several other nonnutritive sweeteners are currently awaiting FDA approval. (See page 110 for information on using these products during pregnancy.)

Let's find out how looking at a food label can help you make a healthier food choice. To most people, jam is jam. You may look at the price per ounce and pick up the cheapest. Or you may be partial to a particular brand and don't look twice at the others. After all, jam is jam...right? Let's see.

Jam # 1

Ingredients: High-fructose corn syrup, strawberries, pectin, natural flavoring.

Jam #2

Ingredients: Strawberries, high-fructose corn syrup, pectin, natural flavoring.

The better choice would be Jam #2 that, ounce per ounce, contains more strawberries than sugar.

Other Ingredients to Look For

Hey, what are all those funny words on the food label? You may have noticed there are many more things on the ingredient list besides food; these other ingredients are called food additives. An additive is a substance other than a basic foodstuff that is in food as a result of production, processing, storage, or packaging.

The media has been giving a lot of attention to food additives; so much so that the word "additive" may bring to mind something negative. In truth, additives often protect our food from spoilage (and therefore keep us from getting sick) and bring clear benefits. For example, many foods are fortified with vitamins and minerals; these are considered additives. Many new fat-free products contain plant gums or seaweed derivatives that have

been safely used for centuries. Those are also considered additives.

Listed below are the main categories of additives and what they do:

Preservatives: Help give food a longer shelf life by retarding spoilage.

Antimicrobials: Prevent food spoilage from bacteria, mold, or fungus. For example, calcium propionate is used to keep bread from molding.

Antioxidants: Prevent oil-containing foods from going rancid and also delay browning. Vitamin C (ascorbic acid) is commonly used in meats as an antioxidant.

Curing agents: Prevent spoilage in meats. Sodium nitrate is often found in smoked meats.

Flavoring agents: Directly or indirectly add flavor to a product.

Sweeteners (including natural and artificial): Many new artificial sweeteners are awaiting FDA approval.

Flavor enhancers: Enhance flavor without leaving a flavor of its own. Monosodium glutamate (MSG) occurs naturally in food and is also added to food to bring out the natural flavors.

Artificial flavoring: Adds flavor lost in processing or increases natural flavor.

Coloring agents (natural, nature-identical, and synthetic FD & C colorings): Most foods we eat have some added coloring, even Cheddar cheese! Color is often added to a product because consumers expect food to be a certain color.

Texturizing Agents

Emulsifiers: Help to evenly distribute tiny particles of liquid: keep oil and water mixed, as in creamy salad dressings.

Stabilizers or thickeners: Give body or texture. Gums and other thickeners are used in fat-free salad dressings to give them the consistency of regular dressing.

Fat replacers or fat substitutes: Replace the properties of fat. They may be added to give a product moisture, or the taste or texture of fat. Fat-replacers include natural plant substances, such as guar gum, xanthan gum, and carageenan, or they may be products developed specifically for replacing fat, such as Simplesse (found in Simple Pleasures ice cream) or Olestra (a new fat substitute to be used for frying snack foods) recently approved by the FDA. Olestra should be avoided during preganacy.

Nutrients: Vitamins, minerals, and fibers are often added to replace nutrients lost in processing or to fortify a food to improve its nutritional value.

Miscellaneous: Other types of additives include leavening agents, propellants, pH control agents, humectants, dough conditioners, and anticaking agents.

Are Food Additives Safe?

Yes; the vast majority of food additives are safe. Some are beneficial; others may cause reactions in sensitive individuals. Questionable additives continue to undergo evaluation. Keep in mind that overconsumption of any one food or food component can have consequences. Lack of variety in the diet causes an excess of some dietary elements and a deficit of others.

For example, sodium nitrate, which is found in cured meats, can be converted to nitrosamines, which may be cancer causing. Vitamin C is often added with nitrates to prevent their conversion to nitrosamine. Sulfites, used as antibrowning agents, are another type of additive. They are most often found in dried fruits and in some beer and wine. Up to 10 percent of the population is sensitive to sulfites; particularly people with asthma. If a food contains sulfite, it is listed on the nutrition label.

If You Are Concerned about Food Additives

▶ **Make sure to eat a wide variety of foods.**

▶ **Eat as many "whole foods" as possible, limiting mixes and convenience foods.**

▶ **Use fresh meat more often than cured or smoked meats.**

▶ **Eat fresh fruits, vegetables, milk, and whole grains for snacks instead of packaged snack foods.**

▼

Eating on a Budget

Let's face it, raising children is expensive. If you are pregnant with your first child, you may have already found that just furnishing the nursery can cost a bundle! You may be looking for ways to cut costs on food. You can eat a nutritious diet and limit your food costs. But eating on a budget, yet nutritiously, does take some advanced planning and, in some cases, thinking about saving for the long term.

Saving for the Long Term

Invest in a Deep Freezer.
Though this represents a great investment, owning a deep freezer can allow you to buy in bulk and stock up on sale items. A grocer in my city often has "buy-one, get-one-free" sales, with no limit on the number that you buy. Take chicken for example. If you could buy enough chicken for six months and get it for half price, that would be quite a bargain. If you live near a cattle ranch, you can invest in a side of beef (or split with a friend) and you'll have tremendous savings as well as very lean cuts of meat.

Try making a double pot of beans or lentil soup and freeze half. This ready-made meal will be wonderful on a cold winter's night. You can also freeze leftovers instead of eventually throwing them away or feeding them to the dog when everyone is tired of them. Consider freezing in microwaveable containers for your own "frozen dinners" for lunch or dinner.

Buy in Bulk—Store or Share with a Friend.
This only works if you will actually use the food. If half of it spoils before you use it, this strategy is not a bargain anymore! A friend of mine makes

homemade granola and lots of other homemade goods. She buys fifty pounds of oatmeal at a time from a health-food store and saves lots of money!

Plant a Garden with Enough to Can or Freeze.

Fresh produce is sometimes the most expensive food. Having your own garden and canning or freezing what's left for the next winter can save you a "bushel."

Plant Fruit Trees that Will Yield Fruit in a Few Years.

Can you imagine stepping out in your back yard and picking a fresh grapefruit? My cousin in Florida does. Or how about some fresh apples to make a fresh apple pie? Check with local agricultural specialists to find out which fruit trees grow well in your area.

While Shopping:

▶ **Clip coupons and shop the sales.**

Many stores offer double and triple coupons. One Saturday I took this advice a bit too far. I went to three stores, buying up all the great bargains. This store-hopping was tiring, but I saved at least 30 percent on my groceries that week!

▶ **If you have other children, make sure they are not hungry or tired when you shop. If they are, try to leave them at home.**

You will not only have time to concentrate on reading labels and comparison shop, but you'll not be temptd to buy extra treats to keep the kids happy.

▶ **Don't go shopping when you are tired or hungry.**

▶ **Always shop with a list.**

▶ **When using coupons, make sure to first compare the price of the food with its coupon; then compare it to the store or generic brand.**

Often I find that the couponed item is more expensive, even with the coupon.

▶ **Go to farmers' markets.**

In the summer, farmers' market prices are often cheaper. Again, if you can arrange to buy in bulk, you can save. For example, we bought a large box of tomatoes for just five dollars and made homemade tomato sauce, which we then froze for future soups and sauces.

▶ **Buy your bread at a thrift store.**

I prefer a brand of bread that is probably the most expensive on the market! However, by buying the bread at a thrift store, I can also buy fat-free cakes, cookies, and ready-to-make pizza crusts, all at reduced prices. To top it off, if you spend five dollars or more, you get one free item!

▶ **If you buy staples such as beans, cereals, dried fruit, and oats from bulk containers, you not only save money but you reduce packaging to help the environment.**

Ditto for buying a large size of snack food instead of individual packages.

▶ **Get the best per-pound value.**

Fruit is often cheaper when in five-pound bags, but produce is not always cheaper when packaged. Mushrooms and tomatoes are good examples of this. Packaged ready-to-eat produce such as salads are more expensive than the individual ingredients. However, if you don't have the time to put together a salad and the ingredients end up spoiling in your fridge, then buying the packaged food is a much better value for your money and your body!

The Cost of Convenience

We Americans want our food fast and easy, and we pay for it. When you compare the costs of homemade to various levels of convenience foods, you may be shocked!

- Frozen pancakes are 18 cents each; pancakes from a mix are 4 cents each or close to one-fourth the price of the frozen.
- A popular Italian salad dressing costs $1.65 for an eight-ounce bottle. A mix plus oil and vinegar costs $1.52. By being creative and adding your own herbs and spices, you save the cost of the mix; eight ounces cost only 55 cents, plus pennies for spices.
- Instant packets of oatmeal cost 36 cents each. Old-fashioned oatmeal, which offers the best nutrition value, costs only 8 cents per serving–and that's for Quaker, a name brand.
- Ready-to-eat muffins from the bakery cost 69 cents each. A Jiffy Banana Muffin Mix muffin, including added ingredients, costs only 9 cents! For the cost of one ready-to-eat muffin, you could feed the whole family with muffins from the easy-to-make mix!

When Menu Planning

- Plan your menus with budget in mind. Make less-expensive foods such as grains, beans, and vegetables the main course, with more expensive meats as "the topping." Not only is a meatless or almost-meatless diet good for your food budget, it can save you the pain, anguish, and cost of having a diet-related chronic disease such as heart disease or cancer many years down the road. (See page 282 for ideas on vegetarian meals.)
- Plan your menus around what's on sale at the store.
- When cooking, use powdered milk. You can double your calcium by using canned evaporated milk (which saves money on fresh milk).
- Fresh fruit may seem more expensive than dessert, but it's usually not!
- Plan your menus with leftovers in mind. Think of different menus you can do with one dish (beef fajitas the first night; fiesta salad with beans and beef strips the second night; or freeze some in individual containers for future lunches or quick dinners. Most people end up throwing part of their food away because

they forget about it, get tired of eating the same thing night after night, or just don't like leftovers! (See page 278 for leftover menus.)
- Are you eating out because of lack of time? Frozen waffles or pancakes, even though expensive, are still cheaper than a meal at a drive-through. A frozen sandwich such as Lean Pockets is still cheaper than a burger meal (though close!). But, if you can plan ahead a bit and arrange for creative leftovers for lunch, you'll probably see the greatest savings on your food budget. The same is true for vending machine snacks, which can "eat" away at your food budget!

▼

Stocking the Kitchen Tool Box

To make great, nutritious meals, you need to have the tools of the trade! I consider the following "tools" essential for a cook who wants to eat well but doesn't have lots of time to waste in the kitchen:

Essential Items

Blender or food processor. One or both are essential for making quick soups, low-fat cheese dips, stuffings, and "meal-on-the-go" drinks.

Meat thermometer. To really know whether your meat is cooked to the right temperature, a meat thermometer is the most reliable method. If you like your meat rare, invest in a thermometer to make sure you have cooked your food to the temperature that kills bacteria.

Microwave. I didn't realize how much I used mine until I started writing down the recipes for this cookbook. Though most people use them just for warming leftovers or heating water, using them for cooking can be a real timesaver. Microwave-cooking can also preserve nutrients.

Nonstick pans. You don't have to add fat when using nonstick cookware. I also like the fact that clean-up is a breeze.

Plastic cutting board. For food-safety reasons, use a plastic or acrylic cutting board instead of a wooden one (at least for raw meats). Wooden boards are harder to sterilize and can harbor bacteria from uncooked meats.

Microwave-safe cookware. Many people use leftover margarine containers for cooking in the microwave. This is not recommended because some of the chemicals in the plastic (also from plastic wrap) have been shown to migrate into the food. Until further research is done on this, use either pyrex-type cookware or containers made especially for the microwave.

Miscellaneous gadgets. A few good-quality knives, nylon spatulas and spoons for nonstick cookware, measuring cups and spoons, and a wire whisk should be part of every kitchen. These few tools will make life easier for the cook!

Nice-to-Have Items

Minichopper. These mini food processors hold only about a cup and are great for chopping onion, garlic, or other vegetables to a fine consistency—a great gadget for women who are sensitive to the smells of cooking in the first trimester. Another nice-to-have item is a hand-held slicer/ chopper that uses different blades. You can chop an onion in about thirty seconds! Or slice a potato into paper-thin slices in a minute.

Rotating platter for microwave. This item ensures that your food is cooked evenly to the correct temperature and also saves you from having to stop the microwave every few minutes to rotate half a turn!

Salad spinner. I love salad, but I hate washing and drying all those lettuce leaves. We received a salad spinner for a wedding gift, and now the salad-making process is much easier.

Really Nice-to-Have Items

(In other words, your wish list for Christmas after you have a nice college fund going!)

Ice-cream maker. Great for making frozen yogurt and sorbets that can satisfy your sweet tooth without a lot of fat.

Breadmaker. Imagine waking up to fresh bread every morning! Making your own whole-grain bread may help you increase the fiber in your diet.

Hand-held blender. These are the type you see advertised on TV. Some of my clients have told me they really *do* whip skim milk and they really *can* grind meat, crush ice, and make milkshakes.

▼

Cooking and Storing to Keep the Vitamins

Which is better—frozen, canned, or fresh vegetables? Nothing beats freshly picked foods straight from your garden. However, in some cases, frozen vegetables can actually have a higher nutrient content than fresh.

Fresh vegetables may not be so fresh by the time you buy them, and especially if they stay several days (or weeks!) in your refrigerator. The way you cook them can also affect nutrient content. Recently, a University of Illinois researcher found that "fresh" beans from the store, which had left the farm seven days earlier, had lost 50 percent of their vitamin C. After three days in a home refrigerator, they had lost 10 percent more. However, frozen beans had lost only 30 percent of their vitamin C after four months in the freezer. In this case, frozen vegetables were a better choice.[3]

Canned vegetables don't hold a candle, nutrient-wise, to fresh or frozen. However, some people like the taste of certain canned vegetables, such as corn. And you may want to keep some canned veggies in the house for those times when there's "nothing to eat."

Caring for Vegetables Once They're Home

▶ **Store veggies in the crisper in their bags.**

Ziploc now has special vegetable bags that have air vents that let the right amount of moisture out to keep your veggies fresh.

▶ **To keep lettuce and other greens fresh, wrap in paper towels, then store in their bags.**

▶ **Don't cut, peel, or wash vegetables until you are ready to cook or eat them.**

The only exception to this might be if you like to keep carrot and celery sticks cleaned, cut, and ready to eat. Having them ready to eat will increase their chances of being eaten. Eating any vegetables, even with reduced nutrient content, is better than eating none at all!

▶ **If possible, avoid soaking vegetables to wash them–soaking will deplete water-soluble vitamins.**

Healthiest Cooking Methods

1. Not cooked
2. Steaming/Microwave cooking
3. Stir-frying
4. Baking
5. Boiling

When foods are "cooked to death," they don't taste good, they have the consistency of baby food, and they've also lost much of their water-soluble vitamins such as B vitamins and vitamin C.

Tips to Cook Your Vegetables more Healthfully:

- To cook vegetables in the microwave, add one or two tablespoons of water and cover tightly. After the microwave cycle is finished, let the vegetables stand a few minutes while covered, to continue cooking. This method is wonderful for cooking cubed potatoes, which are so moist they're great without added fat. (See page 305 for variations of this recipe.)
- When stir-frying, put the more dense vegetables in the pan first. For example, start with onion, garlic, and spices for flavor, then add carrots, celery, cabbage, broccoli; at the end, add softer vegetables such as peas, mushrooms, and greens.
- Steaming over a rack in a pressure cooker is almost too fast! Watch the time carefully to avoid overcooking.
- When boiling, use just enough water to prevent

Even if you don't read the rest of this chapter make sure to read the summary on page 193.

Low-fat, High-Fiber Cookies

Those with a sweet tooth will be happy to know that some cookies are now a bit more nutritious. The following cookies are low in fat and are made with whole grain or are high in fiber.[4]

- Health Valley Fat-Free Fruit Centers
- Health Valley Fat-Free
- Fat-Free Frookies
- Archway Old-Fashioned Molasses
- Barbara's Bakery Oatmeal
- Frookies Animal Crackers
- Health Valley Honey Jumbo Peanut Butter
- Frookies Fruitins

Since new food products come on the market every day, be sure to check your store for new products that are low in sugar and fat and high in fiber.

scorching. Some vegetables (such as potatoes) need to be covered with water. Cut the larger vegetables in pieces to shorten cooking time.

The Essential Guide to Food Safety

Most of us are so busy cooking all the right foods, exercising, and taking other measures for our baby, that we don't stop to think about how we can make our kitchens "safe." By safe, I don't mean just making sure the pot handle is not facing out. Many other dangers are lurking in the kitchen, and many are related to how you handle your food before, during, and after cooking, and even how you make your food selections.

Specifically, the dangers in your kitchen usually can't be seen, smelled, or tasted. They are hidden in the form of bacteria, fungus, and molds. According to one estimate, 6.5 million to 33 million cases of food-borne illness occur in the United States each year. About 9,000 people die of them. Pregnant women have more to risk; fetuses can be severely harmed by some bacteria. A bout of food poisoning reduces mom's nutrition intake, which could also slow baby's growth.

Even if you don't read the rest of this chapter make sure to read the summary on page 193.

Making Your Kitchen Safe

When You're Preparing Food:

▶ **Wash your hands.**

Wash hands in hot, soapy water before preparing food and after using the bathroom, blowing your nose, petting the dog, changing a diaper, and so on. This advice is common sense of course, but these are the most common ways in which bacteria are passed through food.

▶ **Keep raw meats and produce away from each other.**

Use a separate cutting board for raw meats and uncooked foods. Wash the "meat" board in the dishwasher after use. Use a plastic cutting board instead of a wooden one—the wood can't be cleaned as well and may harbor bacteria. Use paper towels instead of a reusable sponge or rag to wipe away blood from meat, fish, or poultry. Wash hands well with soap after handling meat and before handling other foods, especially raw produce.

▶ **Wash sponges, towels, and kitchen rags often; bacteria can survive quite well in them.**

Replace sponges every few weeks. Between replacing them, try washing them in the washing machine with bleach or in your dishwasher on a daily basis.

▶ **Thaw food in the microwave or refrigerator— NOT ON THE KITCHEN COUNTER.**

When Eating Out— At Restaurants, Picnics, and Friends' Homes:

▶ **Don't eat anything that has been sitting out for hours without proper refrigeration or heat.**

Recently, cantaloupe caused an outbreak of salmonella. The person who cut the cantaloupe did not wash the outside, and bacteria got onto the edible portion. After the cantaloupe was out of the refrigerator for a while, the bacteria had a chance to grow to the point that it caused illness.

▶ **If meat, fish, or chicken doesn't look as though it is cooked well enough, ask to have it be cooked more thoroughly.**

Be assertive. (Smoked foods will still look pink, even when done.)

▶ **If food that should be cold, isn't, don't eat it.**

Recently, my husband and I ordered a piece of cream pie to share. After having eaten almost

half of it, I realized that the pie wasn't cold at all and alerted the waitress. She found out that the refrigerator was broken, but no one had noticed it!

▶ **Avoid restaurants that don't practice good sanitation.**

For example, people who handle food should have a hair covering and should have clean hands. If someone takes your

Eggs, Meat, and Poultry Storage Guide

Cooked Food (General)

Food	Suggested Storage Times Refrigerator at 40° F	Freezer at 0° F
Corned beef (in pouch with pickling juice)	5–7 days	Drained, wrapped, 1 month
Egg, chicken, tuna, ham, or macaroni salad (deli or homemade)	3–5 days	These products don't freeze well
Ham, canned, unopened package	6–9 months	Don't freeze
Gravy and meat broth	1–2 days	2–3 months
Ham, cooked, half	3–5 days	1–2 months
Ham, cooked, slices	3–4 days	1–2 months
Ham, cooked, whole	7 days	1–2 months
Hard sausage (pepperoni, etc.)	2–3 weeks	1–2 months
Lunch meats, opened package	3–5 days	In freezer wrap, 1–2 months
Lunch meats, unopened package	2 weeks	In freezer wrap, 1–2 months
Meat and meat dishes, cooked	3–4 days	2–3 months
Pork and lamb chops, prestuffed, or chicken breast, stuffed	1 day	These products don't freeze well
Smoked sausage	1 week	1–2 months
Soups and stews (vegetable- or meat-based)	3–4 days	2–3 months
Store-cooked convenience foods (ready-to-eat)	1–2 days	These products don't freeze well
TV dinners, frozen casseroles		3–4 months

Fresh Meats

Bacon	1 week	1 month
Beef roast	3–5 days	6–12 months
Beef steaks	3–5 days	6–12 months

money and then directly touches your food, your food is not very clean! Also, people who work with food must wash their hands after using the restroom, blowing their nose, smoking, or eating before they handle food again. Workers who don't follow these rules should be reported to your local health department.

Is It Still Good?

Do you find yourself asking this question often? Here is a guide from the U. S. Department of Agriculture (USDA) about how long you can safely refrigerate and freeze various foods.

According to Dee Ann Whitmire, a registered dietitian and communication specialist with the Western Dairy Council, "A good rule of thumb is that you can keep a dairy product one week after the date printed on the package–the "pull" date. Also, when in doubt, throw it out, since how you handle a product can affect its freshness."[5]

When Is It Done?

Don't be impatient when you cook meats; cooking them thoroughly takes time, and thorough cooking is necessary to kill harmful bacteria.

When checked visually, red meat is done when it's brown or gray inside; poultry is done when juices run clear; and fish is done when it becomes opaque and flakes with a fork.

Cook eggs until the white is firm and yolk is no longer runny. This lessens the chances that the egg is harboring *Salmonella*.

Cook beef, pork and lamb to an internal temperature of 160° F; whole chicken or turkey to 180° F; and fin fish to 145° F for at least five minutes. In general, fin fish should be cooked ten minutes per inch of thickness.

Eggs, Meat, and Poultry Storage Guide (continued)

Fresh Meats

Food	Suggested Storage Times Refrigerator at 40° F	Freezer at 0° F
Ground turkey, veal, pork, or lamb	1–2 days	3–4 months
Hamburger and stew meats	1–2 days	3–4 months
Hot dogs, opened package	1 week	In freezer wrap, 1–2 months
Hot dogs, unopened package	2 weeks	In freezer wrap, 1–2 months
Lamb chops	3–5 days	6–9 months
Lamb roast	3–5 days	6–9 months
Pork chops	3–5 days	4–6 months
Pork and veal roast	3–5 days	4–6 months
Sausage, raw	1–2 days	1–2 months
Variety meats (tongue, brain, kidney, liver, heart)	1–2 days	3–4 months

Fresh Poultry

Food	Refrigerator at 40° F	Freezer at 0° F
Chicken or turkey, pieces	1–2 days	9 months
Chicken or turkey, whole	1–2 days	1 year
Giblets	1–2 days	3–4 months

Cooked Poultry

Food	Refrigerator at 40° F	Freezer at 0° F
Chicken nuggets, patties	1–2 days	1–3 months
Cooked poultry dishes	3–4 days	4–6 months
Fried chicken	3–4 days	4 months
Pieces with broth or gravy	1–2 days	6 months
Pieces of chicken, plain	3–4 days	4 months

Other

Food	Refrigerator at 40° F	Freezer at 0° F
Eggs, in shell	3 weeks	Don't freeze
Mayonnaise, commercial, refrigerate after opening	2 months	Don't freeze

Seafood Storage Guide

Fish Fillets/Steaks

Product	Purchased Commercially Frozen for Freezer Storage	Purchased Fresh and Home-Frozen	Thawed; Never Frozen; or Previously Frozen and Home-Refrigerated
Lean:			
Cod, flounder, haddock, halibut	10–12 months	6–8 months	36 hours
Pollock, ocean perch, sea trout, rockfish, Pacific Ocean trout	8–9 months	4 months	36 hours
Fat:			
Mullet, smelt	6–8 months	N/A	36 hours
Salmon (cleaned)	7–9 months	N/A	36 hours
Shellfish			
Blue crabmeat, fresh	N/A	4 months	5–7 days
Blue crabmeat, pasteurized	N/A	N/A	6 months
Clams, shucked	N/A	N/A	5 days
Cocktail claws	N/A	4 months	5 days
Dungeness crab	6 months	6 months	5 days
King crab	12 months	9 months	7 days
Lobster, live	N/A	N/A	1–2 days
Lobster, tail meat	8 months	6 months	4–5 days
Oysters, shucked	N/A	N/A	4–7 days
Shrimp	9 months	5 months	4 days
Snow crab	6 months	6 months	5 days
Surimi seafoods	10–12 months	9 months	2 weeks
Breaded Seafoods			
Fish sticks	18 months	N/A	N/A
Portions	18 months	N/A	N/A
Scallops	16 months	10 months	N/A
Shrimp	12 months	8 months	N/A
Smoked Fish			
Herring	N/A	2 months	3–4 days
Salmon, whitefish	N/A	2 months	5–8 days

Footnotes:

- *N/A–not applicable*
- *These storage guidelines indicate optimal shelf life for seafood products held under proper refrigeration or freezing conditions. Temperature fluctuations in home refrigerators will affect optimal shelf life, as will frequent opening and closing of refrigerator and freezer doors.*
- *Although the above storage times ensure a fresh product for maximum refrigeration storage life at 32° F, the consumer should plan on using seafood within 36 hours for optimal quality and freshness of the product.*
- *To determine approximate storage time for those species not listed, ask your retailer which category (lean, fat, shellfish, breaded, or smoked) they fall within and refer to the guide.*
National Fisheries Institute, 2000 M Street, NW, Suite 580, Washington, D.C. 20036

A Few Tips for Microwave Cooking

▶ **Choose only microwave-safe containers.**

Chemicals from packaging and from containers not deemed microwave-safe can be absorbed into food at high temperatures.

▶ **Cover the dish with a lid or heavy-duty plastic wrap turned back at one corner.**

Plastic wrap shouldn't touch food. The trapped steam will help regulate the food's temperature throughout.

▶ **Rotate the dish half way through cooking time.**

Even if the dish is on a turntable, repositioning it is still a good idea; turn over large food items. These practices help the food cook more evenly and safely.

▶ **Make sure to let food stand for an additional third of the cooking time.**

Food continues cooking after having been removed from the microwave. This helps equalize its temperature throughout.

Source: *Food Safety and the Microwave; A consumer guide to food quality and safe handling*, Food Marketing Institute.

Other Hidden Risks in Your Food Supply

Okay, you decide you're going to avoid all those preservatives by simply eating fresh fruits and vegetables, homemade grains, and fresh fish, chicken, and beef. Now you're totally safe from the undesirable compounds in food, right? Wrong!

Unfortunately, to avoid all food risks is difficult. Remember, keep food safety in perspective. Pesticide use is still common, though reduced use is becoming possible through crop rotation and biotechnology. Organic farming is also gaining popularity. Although growth hormones are being used, they are assumed safe.

Polluted waters can cause fish to be contaminated with such heavy metals as mercury and other chemicals. Improper handling of any raw fish, poultry, beef, or dairy product can cause bacterial growth. However, despite the potential dangers in our food, our food supply is one of the safest in the world. According to Dr. Martha Stone, Professor of Food Science at Colorado State University, "Our food supply is the safest, most wholesome, most abundant in the world. Aren't we fortunate?"[6]

You should be "picky" about what you eat and how you pre-

Dairy Products Storage Guide		
	Suggested Storage Times*	
Food	**Refrigerator at 40° F**	**Freezer at 0° F**
Milk	8-20 days	Not recommended due to reduced quality of product after thawing
Buttermilk	2-3 weeks	
Eggnog	1-2 weeks	
Parmesan cheese	Almost indefinitely	
Sour cream	3-4 weeks	
Ultra-pasteurized cream	6-8 weeks	
Yogurt	3-6 weeks	
Grated cheese in moisture-proof packaging, unopened	12 months	6-8 weeks
Processed cheese food in jars, unopened	12 months	Not recommended
Swiss and Cheddar cheese	1 month	6-8 weeks

Refers to the amount of time after processing, not after purchasing.

Sources: *Newer Knowledge of Milk*, National Dairy Council, 1988, and *Newer Knowledge of Cheese*, National Dairy Council, 1986.

pare foods when you're pregnant. While exposure to some contaminants may be harmless for you, it might be harmful to your baby. It's also important to eat a variety of different foods to decrease your exposure to various contaminants, and to increase your intake of a variety of nutrients.

What's Organic?

Organic simply means grown without synthetic pesticides and herbicides. Farmers use non-chemical, biological methods of pest control, such as compost and beneficial insects. A national standard for "organic" does not yet exist, although such states as California, Oregon, Minnesota, Texas, Washington, and Colorado have certification programs. However, national standards are being developed and should be in effect in a year or two. Check with your State Department of Agriculture or Department of Health for more information.

The word "organic" may not necessarily mean "free of pesticide residues." Some growers take over plots of land that contain enough pesticide residue in the soil to grow perfect-looking produce. However, they can still claim "no pesticides used."[7] The only sure way to know you are getting true pesticide-free produce is to buy "certified organ-

ic." Fortunately, organic farming is becoming more popular and we should be seeing more organic products in the next few years. According to Helen Davis of the Colorado Department of Agriculture, "Organic farming methods do not change the nutritional quality of produce. However, organically grown produce is often fresher and less processed, which slightly improves its nutrient value."[8]

▼

How to Lower Your Risk

The following section will give you tips on selecting and handling foods so that you can eat the safest food possible.

Fruits, Vegetables, Grains, and Nuts

The biggest risk regarding fruits and vegetables is not consuming enough! The slight risk of illness due to pesticide exposure is minimal compared to the risk of illness from not eating enough produce.

Safety Tips:

▶ **Grow your own.**

▶ **Buy locally grown produce.**

Such produce is fresher, picked closer to its peak ripeness, and probably isn't coated with wax or sprayed with post-harvest pesticides. Usually, a local farmers' market or roadside stand is a great source. However, last summer when I asked where the produce came from at my local farmers' market, some of it had been shipped from four states away!

▶ **Wash off pesticide residues.**

If you'd like a little help in removing pesticide residues, use a few drops of dish soap or Fit Fruit and Vegetable Rinse, a product made by Procter and Gamble. It's usually found close to or in the produce department.

▶ **Buy domestically grown produce (this is also good for local farmers).**

Questions about Using Pesticides or Their Safety?

Call the National Pesticide Telecommunications Network, funded by the Office of Pesticide Programs of the EPA at Oregon State University: 1-800-858-PEST.
Hours:
6:30 A.M. to 4:30 P.M.
Pacific Time
Monday through Friday

Ironically, pesticides that are banned in the U.S. are still produced for export. Some of those pesticides find their way back into our country on imported foods.

▶ **Buy fruits and vegetables "in season".**

If you buy a cantaloupe in the dead of winter, you can be sure it was grown pretty far south. That means it had to be picked early, and was most likely sprayed with post-harvest pesticides and wax to make sure it arrived at your store looking "just picked"!

▶ **The large national brands of peanut butter probably have the highest quality standards in terms of aflatoxins, a naturally occurring carcinogen.**

Throw away any moldy, discolored, or shriveled peanuts, pecans, walnuts, almonds, Brazil nuts, and pistachios—they can also have aflatoxins.

▶ **Store potatoes in a cool, dark place.**

Trim away any green or damaged marks—they contain a toxin (glycoalkaloids) that can affect the nervous system.[9]

▶ **Consider buying certified organic produce.**

(In Colorado, this means that no pesticides were used on the land for three years, though pesticide residues may still be present.) However, since the cost of organic produce is sometimes prohibitive, following the other tips in this chapter may work best for you. If you do buy organic products, they won't always look perfect. One reason pesticide use is so popular is that Americans demand perfect looking oranges or flawless lettuce!

Putting Pesticides into Perspective

According to Dr. Bruce Ames, Chairman of the Biochemistry Department, University of California, Berkeley, "The man-made pesticide residues in the American diet are present in trivial amounts and are not a credible risk factor for causing cancer. The danger has been widely exaggerated by piling up worst case assumptions—none of these assumptions are turning out to be true. The FDA and EPA are doing an adequate job of protecting our food supply from carcinogenic contaminants."

Instead of worrying about risks that have very little real danger, we should look at the whole picture of food safety. According to Dr. Sanford Miller of the University of Texas Health Sciences Center in San Antonio, "There

simply is no public health problem with pesticide residues. The real risks in the food supply are microbiological hazards;...risk for illness from microbes is 1 in 100, while risk of illness from pesticides is 1 in 1,000,000."[10]

Although less than 1 percent of food samples analyzed for pesticides in 1989 exceeded tolerances set by the EPA, the amounts were often just a fraction of EPA tolerances. Nevertheless, washing produce to remove any tiny amount of residue that may be present is always a good idea.

Guide to Peeling and Washing Produce

To peel or not to peel? It's a toss-up: peeling does completely remove all surface pesticides (whereas washing might not), but peeling can also mean losing valuable fiber and nutrients. As a general rule, peel produce if your diet is otherwise rich in fiber—especially produce that is obviously waxed—to remove the wax and any other surface pesticides.

Always wash produce. Adding a few drops of dish soap to a pint of water is more effective than plain water in removing many pesticides. Choose a soap brand that doesn't contain dyes and perfumes. Don't use salt water or vinegar—these won't help. Salt is something we get more than enough of in our diets. No evidence shows that specially formulated pesticide and wax-removing washes are more effective than regular dish detergent–and they can cost up to eight times as much! Use a vegetable brush, and be sure to rinse food completely.

Here are some tips for cleaning specific types of produce (instead of buying organic):

▶ **For leafy vegetables such as lettuce and cabbage, discard outer leaves and wash the inner leaves.**

▶ **Wash celery after trimming off the leaves and tops.**

▶ **For recipes that need grated peel, buy organic fruit, if possible.**

▶ **Peel carrots (you won't be losing fiber, since carrots have fiber throughout).**

▶ **Peel cucumbers if they're waxed.**

▶ **Wash eggplants, peppers, tomatoes, potatoes, green beans, cherries, grapes, and strawberries.**

▶ **Peel apples, peaches, and pears if you get plenty of fiber from other sources, since the peels of these fruit likely contain risky residues.**

▶ **Cut up cauliflower, broccoli, and spinach before you wash them, since pesticides may otherwise be hard to wash off.**

Source: Reprinted from *Safe Food*, which is available from CSPI, 1875 Connecticut Avenue NW, #300, Washington, D.C., 20009 for $9.95. Copyright 1991.

Dairy Products

The biggest potential risk from eating dairy products comes from drinking raw or unpasteurized milk and from bacterial contamination due to improper handling.

Like all perishable foods, dairy products are very safe foods, if handled properly. One issue that has gotten recent media attention is the use of BST on dairy cows.

You may have heard of cows being given a hormone called Bovine Somatotropine (BST). Dairy cows produce this naturally occurring hormone. Scientists have found a way to produce the hormone synthetically, and when given to cows, this hormone can increase the cows' milk production by 10 to 30 percent.

The National Institute of Health (NIH) has concluded that milk from BST-treated cows is safe for humans.[11] The medical community generally regards the use of supplemental BST as safe.[12]

So what's all the fuss? Actually, much of the controversy surrounding this issue is based on social or economic grounds. Some people feel that an increased milk supply may take jobs away from dairy farmers and some people are concerned that injections of BST may adversely affect dairy cows. Others are just opposed to biotechnology in general.

Safety Tips:

▶ **Buy only pasteurized milk and milk products. Avoid any raw milk, including goat's milk.**

▶ **Avoid cheeses that have been known to have been contaminated with the dangerous *Listeria* bacteria.**

These include Brie, Camembert, feta, blue cheese and Mexican-style soft cheeses (Queso Blanco and Queso Fresco).

▶ **Keep your refrigerator at or below 40° F and keep milk refrigerated.**

If you like to put milk on the table for meals, don't keep it out long. Milk left out at room temperature, even briefly, can allow bacteria to grow and will quicken spoilage.

▶ Never return unused milk to its original container after it has been sitting out for a while.

▶ See chart on page 181 for storage times for dairy products.

Eggs

The number-one food safety problem with eggs is *Salmonella* bacteria, which are often passed from the hen to humans before the egg is formed. Though rare, salmonella poisoning can be fatal, especially if it affects someone with an already weakened immune system. Unfortunately, salmonella poisoning is on the rise, especially in the northeastern states. However, you don't have to entirely avoid eggs, which is fortunate since the protein in eggs is of very high quality. Following are some tips for keeping your eggs safe.

Safety Tips: Buying and Storing

▶ Buy only eggs that have been refrigerated.

▶ Store eggs in their own container to keep them from cracking.

▶ Don't wash eggs; they are usually washed, sanitized, and coated

with mineral oil to keep out bacteria.

▶ Buy eggs that aren't cracked–bacteria can seep through the cracks.

Buy "AA" or "A" eggs, which are required by law to be clean and uncracked.

Eating

▶ Avoid any food containing raw egg or egg white.

According to Dr. Pat Kendall, Food Science Specialist with Colorado State University, most of the *Salmonella* bacteria are found in the egg yolk.[13] When you eat out, you may want to avoid "health shakes," caesar-salad dressing, and cold mousse desserts or soufflés, which may contain raw eggs. Also avoid unpasteurized eggnog and eggnog made with raw eggs, homemade ice cream, and lightly cooked egg products such as meringue and French toast.

▶ Cook your eggs until yolk and white are firm or at least yolk is beginning to thicken.

If you prefer your eggs runny, you might choose instead an egg substitute, which contains pasteurized eggs. Avoid the temptation to lick the spoon of cake batter or cookie dough that may contain raw eggs.

Beef and Pork

The potential food-safety risk from eating beef or pork is due to bacterial contamination from improper handling by processors or, more often, by the consumer. Eating raw or undercooked beef can increase your chances of getting toxoplasmosis (an illness caused by a parasite), which can be harmful to the fetus.

The danger in contracting trichinosis–another parasitic disease from pork–is much reduced as compared to past generations. Trichinosis is an illness caused by eating raw or undercooked pork that is infected with a type of worm. It is completely destroyed at 138°F.[14]

The Facts about Drugs and Hormones

Drugs

One of the main concerns regarding consumption of animal meat is that of drug residues. About forty years ago we discovered that small, preventive doses of certain antibiotics improved livestock growth. The National Cattlemen's Association recommends against routine use of antibiotics in cattle feed and most beef producers are following their recommendation. When antibiotics are used to treat illness in cows, the cow goes to the market only after a specified quarantine period.

Hormones

"Growth hormones have been used safely and successfully for almost thirty years to increase lean production and feed efficiency," says Lowell L. Wilson, Animal Science Department, Pennsylvania State University.[15]

Hormones improve animal growth. Beef cattle given a small amount of growth hormone grow faster, go to market sooner, and are leaner. According to the Beef Industry, if hormone implants were not used, the supply of beef would shrink and prices consumers pay would rise.

A Texas A & M report concluded that the scientific community now agrees that the proper use of certain hormones is harmless to the consumer and may enhance animal growth performance by as much as 20 percent.[16] The University of California *Wellness Letter,* March 1989,

reported: "At the prescribed dosages used in feed lots, these hormones have been certified safe by numerous scientific studies."

Surprisingly, hormones are present in nearly all the plant and animal foods we eat. In fact, many common foods exceed the level of estrogen found in beef that have been given a supplemental dose of the hormone.

Men, women, and children also produce estrogen in their bodies at levels thousands and millions of times greater than the levels found in beef. In the third trimester of pregnancy, your body will produce 37 million times the amount of estrogen found in a three-ounce serving of beef.

Poultry

The two greatest potential risks from eating poultry are illnesses from two food-borne bacteria,

Salmonella and *Campylobacter jejuni,* both of which can be reduced or destroyed by proper cooking and handling.

Chicken is the most popular meat among my clients. It can be prepared as a quick low-fat dish. However, it can also have two undesirable traveling companions that will make you sick; *Salmonella* and *Campylobacter jejuni.* Salmonella is a bacteria of the genus *Salmonella* found in chicken feces, and it spreads to other parts of the chicken during processing. Improper handling of raw chicken in your own kitchen adds to the risk of food poisoning from *Salmonella.*

Sanitary kitchen procedures are the best defense against coming into contact with the *Salmonella* bacteria. *Salmonella* bacteria multiply at room temperature—a good reason to thaw poultry in the refrigerator or in the microwave instead of on the countertop. You should also keep poultry foods in a cooler or on ice when having a picnic or buffet dinner. Keeping hot foods hot (above 140° F) and cold foods cold (below 40° F) keeps *Salmonella* at bay.

Chicken is often contaminated with another bacteria, *Campylobacter.* Campylobacterosis is thought to be a very common, but under-reported illness that affects 2 to 6 million people in the U.S. a year. Since the symp-

Estrogen Levels in Food		
Food	Serving Size	Estrogen, in nanograms*
Beef, from a cow implanted with estrogen	3 ounces	1.85
Beef, from a cow not given estrogen	3 ounces	1.01
Egg	1	1,750
Cabbage	3 ounces	2,016

*One nanogram is one billionth of a gram; compared to a gram, a nanogram is equal to one blade of grass on a football field.

Source: Inter-American Institute for Cooperation of Agriculture, *Report on Use of Hormonal Substances in Animals,* December 1986.

toms (cramps, diarrhea, and fever) are flu-like and can occur up to five days after eating the affected food, only one in a hundred cases is thought to be reported.

Like *Salmonella, Campylobacter* is also a "bug" that is passed between chickens during processing. Luckily, you can control its growth with sanitary kitchen procedures.

Safety Tips:

- *Campylobacter* can live in your refrigerator for weeks! Make sure to clean any juices that spill from a defrosting chicken. If juice falls on food that will be eaten raw (such as lettuce, fruit, or cheese), throw that food away.
- Because microwave ovens cook unevenly, they may not completely kill *Campylobacter* (or *Salmonella*), so traditional methods such as baking, broiling, or boiling are preferred.
- Research shows that most of the reported cases of *Campylobacter* occur during barbecue season–a hint that perhaps people are undercooking their grilled chicken! A combination of microwaving and grilling would ensure thorough and quick cooking. (An internal temperature of 180°F ensures

it's thoroughly cooked.)
- Since *Campylobacter* does not survive freezing, buy frozen chickens, or freeze for a few days before using.

For more information about poultry, call the toll-free USDA Meat and Poultry Hotline: 1-800-535-4555

Fish

Ben Franklin said "Fish and house guests begin to smell after three days." He should have said "two days," at least for fish, because it's unwise to keep fresh fish longer than that!

The greatest potential risks from eating fish are bacterial food poisoning and consumption of chemicals that fish have ingested from polluted waters. Proper handling and cooking can reduce or kill bacteria. If you are considering becoming pregnant, are already pregnant, or are breastfeeding, you should limit your tuna consumption to one or two times a week and your shark and swordfish intake to once a month.

Americans are eating more fish, up 25 percent in the last ten years. The healthfulness of fish is probably the main reason for its growing popularity. It's low in fat and calories and high in protein, and provides essential omega-3 fatty acid–a type of fat that can have very beneficial effects on your health.

However, a recent study done by *Consumer Reports Magazine* uncovered a bit of bad news about fish. They reportedly found that 30 percent of the fish they sampled were of poor quality, half the fish were contaminated by bacteria, and some species were contaminated by polychlorinated biphenyls (PCBs) and mercury. The researchers blamed polluted waters and handling of the fish (from the fishing boat, to the processor, and even in your local store) for the presence of the contaminates.[17]

Critics of the *Consumer Reports'* study thought that the study collected too few samples and used poor research methods. However, the study does give us food for thought and reminds us to not take the quality of our food for granted.

Dr. Michael Bolger, a toxicologist with the Center for Food Safety and Applied Nutrition of the Food and Drug Administration, disagreed with some findings of the study:

"The data on PCBs and mercury are uncertain. They didn't do a good job of presenting that fact. They didn't give the benefits of eating fish, making the report unbalanced. Their sample size was inadequate and there was no distinction made within salmon samples–they weren't from the Pacific Ocean but the Great Lakes, where only a small amount of commercial fishing is done.

"There is no question that in certain areas PCBs continue to be a problem, such as Boston Harbor and the Great Lakes. The problem is seen in inland waters such as rivers and lakes. In marine species, there is no evidence that it is a concern except with several in-shore species like bluefish and striped bass.

"The two main sources of salmon from the Great Lakes are from sports fishing and from Native Americans who have exclusive fishing rights. Those who fish in the Great Lakes should check with their local health department for fish advisories."[18]

In a 1991 report on Seafood Safety, the National Academy of Sciences (NAS) said that "Fish and shellfish are nutritious foods that constitute desirable components of a healthy diet. Most seafoods available to the U.S. public are wholesome and unlikely to cause illness in the consumer." The FDA agrees with the NAS conclusions and reminds consumers that fish and shellfish are highly perishable products that can spoil or lose quality between harvesting and consumption.[19]

Janis Harsila, a registered dietitian from the National Seafood Educators, says:

"The *Consumer Reports* article tells us not to eat any salmon, but that study looked at a very

small sample. When Alaska analyzed their fish they found virtually no PCBs or other pollutants, so Alaskan salmon is actually one of the safest fish to eat. Some of the purest waters are in Alaska and any fish caught there are usually safe."[20]

Did You Have Your Omega-3 Today?

In recent years a type of oil found primarily in fish–omega-3 fatty acid–shows great promise in controlling blood pressure, reducing heart disease, and improving the symptoms of rheumatoid arthritis. Now we know that developing babies need DHA (one kind of the omega-3 acids) for building brain tissue, nerve growth, and for development of the eye retina.

Before birth, your baby gets its DHA from you (especially if you eat your share of fat-rich fish), and after birth, from breast milk. Omega-3 fatty acids are so important that some scientists think that lack of the fat could result in delays or deficiencies in nervous tissue development and possibly in impaired vision.[21]

Good sources of omega-3 include anchovy, Atlantic salmon, coho salmon, herring, mackerel, pilchards, pink salmon, sablefish, sardines, sockeye salmon, spiny dogfish, and whitefish.

Moderately good sources include chum salmon, pompano, rainbow trout, shark, smelt, spot, striped bass, swordfish, Pacific oysters, and squid.

Source: National Fisheries Institute.

The Facts on Fish

Fish are among the most perishable of foods. They have a shelf life of seven to twelve days once they're out of the water. Some fish stay on the fishing boat for several days, so once they arrive at the store they may have little "life" left! If fish get warmer than 32°F, their shelf life decreases but it can be cut in half if kept at 42°F. Fattier fish and cold-water fish spoil even faster.

Poor sanitation practices, such as using unwashed knives and cutting boards, can increase bacterial growth. So can some store display procedures. For example, if a fish is kept under a hot light, the fish gets warm and bacteria can multiply quickly. If raw fish is displayed next to cooked fish, the cooked fish can be contaminated. (Fortunately, the bacteria in fish can be killed with proper cooking.)

Other contaminants found in fish include PCBs and methylmercury, neither of which pose an immediate threat to most people, but which can be harmful to the fetus. PCBs (chemicals previously used in transformer fluids) were banned in the 1970s, though some of its residues remain and will be around for years to come. They accumulate in fatty body tissue, so they can be passed up the food chain and back down again as fish eat other fish and when some fish is turned into fish feed.

Too much accumulated PCB in the body is thought to affect neurological behavior and cognitive development in the growing fetus. Methylmercury is thought to have the same effect. Not much data is available to support how the fetus reacts to these chemicals. One example of methylmercury poisoning was a tragic accident in Japan when, during a certain period, fish sold in stores were highly contaminated with methylmercury. The infants born during this time had severe problems similar to cerebral palsy.

Dr. Bolger of the FDA sees the subject of mercury contamination as a "gray" area: "What we know about lead and mercury is like night and day." When comparing our fish eating habits with the those of the Japanese, he says, "The Japanese eat five times more seafood than we do. If mercury has the effect that we think it has (on neurological development) you would expect to see the effects in academic achievement and economic success. Why is it then that the Jap-

anese are doing as well as they are?[18] Good questions, Dr. Bolger.

Surely Someone Inspects Fish?

Most of us assume that all fish is inspected, but up until now inspection procedures have been "hit or miss." The National Marine Fisheries Institute has had a voluntary inspection service for years. Fish processors can pay to have their store or plant sanitation conditions and procedures observed and be issued a seal of approval. According to the *Consumer Reports* study, about 18 percent of the fish eaten in the U.S. is currently inspected under this program. Local and state health departments also do some inspection of seafood, mostly through control of shellfish harvesting.

However, there's good news for fish lovers. A newly created Office of Seafood under the Food and Drug Administration will play an increasing role in sea-

Buyer Beware

Labels that say "USDA Inspected," or "U.S. Govt. Inspected" are sometimes incorrectly found on fish labels. USDA inspects beef, pork, and chicken, but not fish.

food's safety. Already the office has inspected over three-quarters of all seafood-processing facilities in the U.S. during its first year in existence.

Are All Fish Safe for Pregnant and Breast-feeding Women to Eat? Should any Fish be Limited or Avoided?

Among the controversy over safe levels of consumption of fish that could contain PCBs, mercury, and other environmental contaminants, those questions frequently have many answers. After consulting with toxicologists and organizations across the country, my advice is to try to eat fish several times a week, but eat tuna not more than once or twice a week, and shark and swordfish just once a month. Avoid fish from the Great Lakes area. Variety and moderation are the keys.

Remember, you should not entirely avoid eating fish during pregnancy or while breast-feeding. Fish contain important nutrients for your baby. Just limit the high-risk fish intake and eat a variety of others.

What You Can Do

You can eat fish without worry by taking a few precautions.

Safety Tips: Buying Seafood

▶ **From a health-risk standpoint, frozen fish is often the best choice.**

Fish is usually quick-frozen or frozen right on the boat where it was caught, resulting in fish that is actually fresher than "fresh." Look for and avoid freezer burn, ice crystals, and broken wrappers. Avoid buying fresh salmon, bluefish, and catfish and freezing it when you get home. According to Clare Vanderbeek of the National Fisheries Institute, "Fish with a higher fat content will deteriorate more quickly than low-fat fish. Consumers should buy those fish already commercially frozen, which will ensure a higher-quality product."[22]

▶ **If you choose to buy fresh fish, learn how to recognize "freshness."**

Fish gills should be bright red and moist, not brown and covered with mucus. Eyes should be bright, clear, and bulging. Avoid fish with cloudy or slime-covered eyes. The skin should have a translucent "varnished" look. Fish with skin that is starting to discolor, that has tears or blemishes should be left at the store.

▶ **Watch for troubling display habits.**

Do not buy fish in stores where fish is stacked in large piles (harder to keep at coldest temperatures), where raw fish is displayed next to cooked fish, where you smell a strong "fishy" odor (means more bacteria), or where fish is displayed under bright, hot lights.

▶ **Find out, if possible, where your fish came from–the further from shore, the better.**

You can also ask to see a tag for shellfish, which indicates when the fish was caught and shipped. However, both pieces of information may require some real "fishing."

▶ **The National Fisheries Institute recommends avoiding recreationally caught fish.**

Fish caught recreationally are more likely to be from contaminated waters or not handled properly. It's probably best to avoid buying shellfish at roadside stands; they can be "bootlegged"–or caught from polluted waters.

▶ **Good choices for pregnant women and women who breast-feed include flounder, cod, pollock, orange roughy, squid, clams, rockfish,**

Alaskan salmon, shellfish, and sole.[17,20,23]

Variety is important!

Storing and Handling Seafood

To keep your fish as fresh as possible:

▶ **Before refrigerating, remove fish from its package, rinse under cold water, and pat dry with paper towels.**

To keep cleaned fin fish more than twenty-four hours, place the fish on a cake rack in a pan, fill with crushed ice, and cover tightly with plastic wrap or foil. Rinse the fish daily, cleaning the rack and changing the ice.

▶ **Keep fish stored at 32 to 38°F or in the coldest part of your refrigerator and use within one day.**

Keep frozen fish at 0°F and use within six months.

▶ **Store live oysters, clams, and mussels in the refrigerator.**

Keep damp by covering with a clean, damp cloth or moist paper towel, but do not place on ice or allow fresh water to come in contact with seafood. Never store live in an airtight container because it will kill them.

► **Keep freshly shucked oysters, scallops, or clams in their shells and store in the coldest part of the refrigerator, preferably packed with ice.**

► **Keep live lobsters, crawfish, and crabs in the refrigerator in moist packages (use seaweed or damp paper strips), but not in airtight containers, fresh water, or salt water.**

Lobsters should remain alive for about twenty-four hours.

► **Be sure to discard any fish juices and marinade used for raw fish, and do not reuse sponges, utensils, or cutting boards used for raw fish.**

Don't forget to wash your hands well after handling raw seafood.

► **Throw out fish that smells "fishy" or like ammonia.**

► **Discard any shellfish that die during storage.**

For more information, see *Consumer Reports Magazine,* February 1992, pages 103-120; *FDA Consumer* 91-2246; and *Seafood A to Z,* by Janis Harsila, R.D., and Evie Hansen, National Seafood Educators.

Cooking Seafood

► **Avoid raw and undercooked fish and shellfish at all times!**

► **Don't leave raw or cooked seafood out of the refrigerator for more than two hours. (This includes preparation time and time on the table.)**

► **Cooking fish well will destroy most or all bacteria present.**

Fish is done when the flesh is opaque and begins to flake easily when tested with a fork at its thickest part. You can also check doneness with a thermometer. Fish is ready when its internal temperature reaches 145°F.

Fin Fish:

Although you don't want to undercook fish, overcooking it will make your fish less tasty. National Seafood Educators suggest the following for perfectly cooked fish every time:

► **For baking (400 to 450°F), broiling, grilling, poaching, steaming, and sautéing, measure fish at its thickest part.**

If the fish is stuffed, measure after it's stuffed. Then cook ten minutes per inch, turning half-way through cooking time. Pieces that are less than half an inch thick don't need to be turned.

► **Add five minutes to cooking time if fish is cooked in foil or sauce.**

► **Double the cooking time for frozen fish that hasn't been defrosted.**

Shellfish:

• One pound of medium shrimp in the shell needs three to five minutes to boil or steam.

• Shucked oysters, clams, and mussels become plump and opaque when done. Overcooking causes them to shrink and toughen.

• Oysters, clams, and mussels in the shell will open when cooked. Remove them one by one as they open.

• Sea scallops take three to four minutes to cook through; the smaller bay scallops may take as little as thirty to sixty seconds.

• Sautéed or deep-fried soft-shell crabs take about three minutes each. Steamed hard-shell crabs or rock crabs take about twenty-five to thirty minutes for a large pot of them.

• If you poach or steam fish, let liquid come to a boil first, then add fish and cook as described above.

Microwaving

▶ **Split-second timing is important when cooking fish in the microwave.**

Since fish will continue cooking after it has been removed from the microwave, take it out before it looks done—when the outer edges are opaque and the center is still slightly translucent. Allow the fish to stand covered for a few minutes before serving.

▶ **Use a shallow microwave-safe dish.**

▶ **Arrange fillets with the thicker parts pointing outward and the thinner parts toward the center of the dish.**

Rolled fillets cook more evenly than flat fillets.

▶ **Cover the dish with plastic wrap and lift one corner to vent.**

▶ **Cook three to six minutes per pound of boneless fish on high.**

▶ **Cook thawed, shucked shellfish two to three minutes per pound, stirring and rotating half a turn during cooking.**

Allow to stand for a third of the cooking time.

▶ **Place clams, mussels, or oysters in the shell in a single layer in a shallow dish.**

Cover with plastic wrap, venting one corner. Cook two to three minutes on high. Check and remove shellfish as they open.

The above information comes from *Seafood, a Collection of Heart-Healthy Recipes* by Janis Harsila, R.D., and Evie Hansen, National Seafood Educators. This book has everything you want to know about seafood, including how to buy, store, cook, and even how to introduce it to picky eaters. The 180 recipes give new meaning to "fast food," since recipes can be cooked and on the table in thirty minutes or less.

Food Safety Issues— Whom to Believe?

In 1989, two stories about food safety hit the headlines and people all over the country lingered at their plates, wondering whether anything was safe to eat.

First the alar scare came (alar was a pesticide banned by the EPA in 1989 because it was carcinogenic), from which Washington apple growers are just now recovering. Soon after, a story about two cyanide-infected grapes made the news. As a result, the purchase of all imported foods from Chile dropped off, causing economic hardship in that country.

Food safety issues often appeal to our emotions, since the safety of our children is often cited. However, when we react with our hearts instead of our minds, our opinions and decisions are likely to be based on feelings, not facts.

Many activist groups are involved in food safety issues and for the most part, their claims are valid. However, when scientific information is taken out of context and blown out of proportion to its real effect on our health, people are needlessly misled, confused, and frightened.

Depending on which side of the issues you are on, you can probably find a scientific study to back you up. Frankly, we don't know all the answers about nutrition and health, which is why you may hear one story today and hear a completely different story tomorrow. When an issue or scientific study hits the headlines, you should ask yourself these questions:

1. *Who is reporting the information?*
Is it a neutral group or someone with something to gain from the results? For example, someone who is selling vitamin supplements may recite this or that study. Though the points made may be valid, the person's opinions may be biased—so try to separate facts from opinion.

On the other hand, many large companies commonly fund research by well-respected universities. However, this doesn't mean the research is biased or of lower quality. Let's face it, besides the producers of the food, who would want to put up millions of dollars for research on oatmeal?

2. *If the study is scientific, was it done on animals or humans?*
Though many effects are the same in animals and humans, you can't always assume that the results can be equally compared.

3. *How large was the sample size?*
Research using a group of ten people won't be as reliable as research on a group of a thousand.

4. *How many studies have been done on the subject?*
Only after many studies can anything be proven conclusively. One study shouldn't cause you to change dietary habits drastically, unless the evidence is very strong.

▼

Food Safety in a Nutshell for Pregnant Women

DO

▶ **Do keep raw and cooked foods separate.**

Use separate cutting boards and knives for each to prevent transfer of bacteria.

▶ **Do wash hands, utensils, and preparation areas with hot soapy water after contact with raw meats.**

A weak bleach-and-water mix can help kill germs on kitchen surfaces—see label for details. Don't forget to wash hands after using the restroom, blowing your nose, or changing a diaper.

▶ **Do wash sponges in the dishwasher daily to prevent bacteria from growing.**

▶ **Do choose low-fat fish and meats (pesticides, chemicals, and metals accumulate in the fat).**

▶ **Do remove skin and inner organs of fish before making soups and stews.**

▶ **Do thoroughly reheat leftovers or ready-to-eat foods such as hot dogs until steaming hot.**

▶ **Do store fish in the coldest area of your refrigerator and cook within a day.**

▶ **Do keep your refrigerator clean and at 35 to 40°F.**

▶ **Keep hot foods over 140°F and cold foods at or below 40°F.**

If you are serving hot food that will be out for a while, use a hot plate. Refrigerate or freeze leftovers as soon as possible.

▶ **When serving, do keep hot or cold foods at room temperature as short as possible.**

▶ **Do eat a variety of foods.**

▶ **Do cook raw meat to an internal temperature of 160°F, poultry to 180°F, and fish to 145°F.**

Avoid any raw or undercooked animal protein.

▶ **Do make sure to use refrigerated ground meat and patties in one or two days after buying or defrosting.**

▶ **Do avoid raw or unpasteurized milk.**

▶ **When refrigerating large portions of food, do divide into smaller containers so the food can cool more quickly.**

DON'T

▶ **Don't eat foods with uncooked or under-cooked eggs, such as eggnog, caesar salads, uncooked soufflés, and homemade ice creams.**

Pasteurized eggnog and eggnog made with pasteurized eggs are safe.

▶ **Don't eat any raw fish or shellfish.**

▶ **If you have animals, don't allow them on food-preparation areas.**

▶ **Don't eat such soft cheeses as Mexican style cheese (Queso Fresco or Queso Blanco), feta, Brie, blue cheese, and Camembert.**

These can harbor a bacteria called *Listeria,* which is particularly harmful to fetuses.

▶ **Don't drink hot liquids such as coffee or tea in ceramic mugs that may contain leaded glaze.**

The hot acidic coffee can cause small amounts of lead to leach into your beverage.

▶ **For women of child-bearing age, the FDA recommends not eating shark or swordfish more than once a month.**

If you live in the Great Lakes and Hudson River area, eat as little as possible of swordfish, shark, bluefish, and salmon from the area. They can be contaminated with heavy metals or chemicals that can harm the fetus (more details on page 188).

▶ **Don't store fruit juice or acidic foods in ceramic containers (especially imported ones), or leaded crystal decanters, because lead can be leached into the food or drink.**

Also choose seamless cans or welded-seam cans instead of soldered-seam cans, which may contain lead.

▶ **Don't drink or use water with high levels of lead.**

The only way to know for sure if your water contains lead is to have it tested. If you have lead pipes or lead-soldered pipes, let the water run for a few minutes before using to decrease lead content. Avoid using warm tap water for drinking or cooking. (See page 36 for more information on lead exposure.)

If you are concerned about the quality of your tap water because of bacteria, lead, or other contaminants, consider getting a water purification system. According to Consumer Union, publisher of *Consumer Reports Magazine,* federal regulations for city water systems appear to be getting weaker, not stronger.

For more information on food safety or food-borne illnesses call the USDA Meat and Poultry Hotline: 1-800-535-4555 (in the D.C. area 202-720-3333) or the Seafood Hotline: 1-800-FDA-4010 (in D.C. 202-205-4314).

Sources: *Safe Food; Eating Wisely in a Risky World,* Michael Jacobson, Lisa Lefferts, and Anne Witte Garland, Center for Science in the Public Interest, 1991; Background Paper; *Preventing Food-borne Listeriosis,* USDA, U.S. Department of Health and Human Services and FDA, April 1992; FDA Consumer, 9/94; and FSIS Backgrounder "Escherichia coli Update." 5/93.

Fast Foods–Eating Out and Eating In

This chapter answers such questions as:

- *What can I add to a frozen entree to make a quick, complete meal?*
- *Are there any fast foods that are high in iron?*
- *Which fast-food restaurants serve grilled chicken?*
- *Is it possible to eat out and have a low-fat meal?*
- *What can I keep at home in the pantry to put together a quick meal?*

We live in a very fast-paced society and we often don't have time to cook. Approximately forty cents of every food dollar is spent on food prepared away from home. You may be wondering whether you can eat out or prepare convenience foods and still have a balanced diet. The answer is yes–with a little thought and planning.

Tips for Choosing Convenience Foods

Convenience foods such as frozen dinners, shelf-stable meals, and dinners-in-a box are becoming more and more popular. Some are better than others. Consider these points when looking for dinners:

- Are the dinners balanced (do they contain protein, starch, and vegetable and/or fruit)?
- How much fat do the dinners contain? A good rule of thumb is to look for no more than ten grams of fat per three hundred calories.
- How is the sodium content? More than eight hundred milligrams per serving could be excessive. However, since you need more sodium during pregnancy, excess sodium should not be a concern unless you were following a low-sodium diet before pregnancy and your physician has advised you to continue doing so. (See page 198 later in this chapter for more on sodium.)
- Are the dinners a good value? One often pays for convenience, so cost is something to consider. When considering the total price of a dinner, make sure to consider the cost of ingredients that you add, such as chicken or tuna.
- Is there a long list of additives and preservatives? If you are concerned about this, read the ingredient label.

Frozen Convenience Foods: How to Have a Complete Meal

The following frozen dinners offer convenience and good nutrition. Thousands of new foods enter the grocery store every year. The exclusion of some items on our list does not imply that those items are bad choices.

Below you can find out what to add to the different types of frozen convenience foods to create a balanced meal:

Low-Calorie Entrees

Budget Gourmet
Healthy Choice Entrees
Weight Watchers Ultimate 200 and Entrees
Lean Cuisine Entrees

Start with one of the entrees above and add:

1 cup milk or yogurt
1 fruit and/or raw veggies (consider buying a bulk bag of oranges, apples, or canned individual servings of fruit to keep at work)
1 piece of bread, bagel, bran or corn muffin, or roll

Then maybe add a dessert and you have a complete meal!

Low-Calorie Dinners

These dinners offer a complete meal, but still contain about 300 calories:

Healthy Choice Dinners
Budget Gourmet Light and Healthy Dinners
Budget Gourmet Hearty and Healthy Dinners
Lean Cuisine

To have a complete meal add:

milk or yogurt
some type of starch
fruit and/or vegetable

"Lite," or lower-calorie, meals are good choices because they are low in fat. Too much fat could give you heartburn, as well as add too many extra calories. However, the entree-type meals don't always include a fruit or vegetable and they can be too low in calories. Additional foods are necessary to make a balanced meal.

Reading the nutrition label can help you pick the healthiest meals. By looking at the label, you can pick the meal with lower fat, lower sodium, or perhaps the one with the least number of additives or the most vitamin C. Scanning the percentage of vitamins A and C at the bottom of the label can help determine the amount and healthfulness of fruits and vegetables in the meal.

Meal Starters

These offer yet another choice for a quick nutritious meal; they can be prepared in the microwave or on the stovetop. Some include meat–such as Tyson Fajita Kit. Others, such as Green Giant Create-A-Meal and Bird's Eye Meal Starter don't, so you have the option of adding chicken, shrimp, beef, or leaving the meal meatless. An added benefit to these meals is that if you cook the meal as little as possible, the vegetables will retain more vitamins. These meals are especially nutritious because they include a lot of vegetables. You just need to add another starch, fruit, and milk for a complete, healthy meal.

Chicken Pot Pies, Frozen Pizza, Fried Chicken, Chicken Nuggets, Fish Sticks

These foods get 50 percent or more of their calories from fat, and they are usually less expensive than other frozen dinners. However, many "lite" versions of those foods are now available, which are better choices (but more expensive). If you are having a hard time gaining weight or don't have an appetite, you can choose the "original" versions, in moderation. Just watch out for indigestion due to their high fat content.

Doing Your Math

Remember, the average pregnant woman needs about 2,200 calories. (Your calorie needs can range anywhere from a modest 2,000 calories to more than 3,000 calories, depending on your size and activity level.) You can count on about 400 calories for breakfast, 500 calories for lunch and dinner and two 300-calorie snacks or three 200-calorie snacks. Most low-cal dinners have 300 calories. After adding milk, fruit, and starch, you have 550 calories and a well-balanced meal for you and your baby!

Frozen Pizza, Burritos, and Pocket Sandwiches

These foods are often less expensive, but are missing the vegetables. Some are high in fat, so read the label. Make sure to add some fruit and vegetables to make a balanced meal.

Quick Extras to Add to Your Meal

Starches: Bulgur, instant brown rice, whole-wheat English muffin or bagel, bran muffin, bread sticks, canned legumes, corn, or peas

Fruit: Any fresh fruit, frozen bananas or grapes, frozen melon balls, canned pineapple, instant pudding with bananas, fruit shake, yogurt parfait, fresh fruit, or fruit juice.

Vegetables: Ready-to-make coleslaw or salad, precut vegetable sticks, shelf-stable vegetables, canned or frozen vegetables, or vegetable soup.

▼

Using Convenience Foods for the Whole Family

Frozen meals are fine for just one person, but how about when you need something quick for the whole family? Here are a few ideas for using convenience items when making a meal. Consider stocking some of these items in your freezer for those days when you have no time to cook! (See page 210 for "Fifty Quick-and-Easy-Meals or Snacks.")

Bird's Eye Meal Starter Primavera
Bird's Eye Meal Starter Teriyaki Meal Starter
Contessa Classics Shrimp Fajitas
Frozen turkey roasts

Garden Chef Garden Mexi-Burgers
Gorton's Grilled Italian Herb Fish Fillets
Gorton's Grilled Lemon Pepper Fish Fillets
Gorton's Shrimp and Seafood Stir Fry Teriyaki
Green Giant Create-A-Meal Garlic Herb
Green Giant Create-A-Meal Sweet and Sour Stir Fry
Green Giant Harvest Burger
Jennie-O Chicken Breast Fillets in Cacciatore Sauce
Morning Star Farms Veggie Burger
Mrs. T's Pierogies
Rosetto Cheese Ravioli or Tortellini
Tuna Helper Au Gratin Creamy Broccoli
Tuna Helper Garden Cheddar
Tyson Chicken Stir-Fry Kit
Tyson Chicken Fried Rice Kit
Van De Kamp Crisp and Healthy Fish Fillets

Shelf-Stable Foods

Don't have access to a refrigerator? Or are you stuck on bed rest? Shelf-stable foods are those that don't need refrigerating until you open them. The variety of shelf-stable foods are expanding quickly. Good examples are "meals in a box," stews and soups in microwaveable containers, and "Cup of Soup"-type meals.

Many canned soups also offer healthy quick meals. These foods redefine the meaning of fast food; they can be ready to eat in one-and-a-half to two minutes! To top off your shelf-stable meals, keep dried fruit or individual servings of applesauce or other fruit or pudding on hand too. These foods also work well for camping and hiking.

Read the labels on the shelf-stable products; some of the smaller products are soups or side dishes, not entrees.

Make sure to add milk or yogurt, fruit, vegetable, and a starch to the entrees so that you have adequate calories and nutrients.

Dinners:

Dinty Moore American
   Classics (a few are
   high in fat)
Top Shelf (a few are
   high in fat)

Entrees/Side Dishes:

Campbell's Microwave Soups
Chef Boyardee Main Meals
Fantastic Foods
   Bombay Curry
Fantastic Foods Jumpin'
   Black Bean Soup
Healthy Choice Garden
   Vegetable or Country
   Vegetable Soup
Hormel Micro Cup
Libby's Dinner
Nile Spice Couscous
   Lentil Curry

Progresso Lentil Soup
Knorr Black Bean Soup

Watching Your Sodium?

Most "lite" frozen meals and entrees contain seven hundred milligrams or less of sodium. Watch the label for sodium if sodium intake is a concern for you. Remember that your need for sodium during pregnancy goes up. However, your physician may ask you to moderate your salt intake if you had a prepregnancy condition such as hypertension or kidney disease. Most Healthy Choice, Lean Cuisine, Weight Watchers, and Budget Gourmet meals are reduced in sodium.

▼

Putting It All Together: Healthy Convenience-Food Menus

These menus can give you ideas on how to make a complete, balanced meal starting with a frozen dinner.

Mexican/Southwest

Top Shelf Chicken Fiesta
   (shelf-stable)
2 wheat tortillas
1 ounce reduced-fat cheese
Orange

Weight Watchers Chicken
   Enchiladas Suiza
Baked tortilla chips
   (or homemade chips)
Refried black beans
Tomato slices
Strawberries
Milk

Tyson Chicken Fajita Kit
Refried vegetarian beans
Frozen melon balls
   and bananas
Milk

Healthy Choice Chicken
   Enchilada Suprema
Three-bean salad with tomato
Yogurt with peaches
Vegetable juice

El Chico Lean Olé Enchilada
   Combination Dinner
Mixed fresh fruit salad
Milk

Weight Watchers Fiesta
   Chicken with Rice
Raw broccoli and carrots
Bran muffin
Watermelon
Milk

Italian

Weight Watchers
Ravioli Florentine
Wheat roll
Green beans in vinaigrette
Yogurt with blueberries

Weight Watchers Lasagna
with Meat Sauce
Bread sticks
Spinach salad with
artichoke hearts
Melon
Milk

Lean Cuisine Cheese
Lasagna with Chicken
Breast Scallopini
Garlic toast
Tossed salad with green
peppers
Grapefruit half

Budget Gourmet Bay Shrimp
and Clams Marinara
Dinner
Minestrone soup or Minute
Minestrone (See page 254
for recipe.)
Wheat crackers
Fresh peach
Milk

Healthy Choice Supreme
French Bread Pizza
Caesar salad
Strawberry sorbet
Milk

Americana

Weight Watchers Broccoli
and Cheese Baked Potato
Tossed salad with
kidney beans
Fresh apple
Vanilla pudding with banana
Milk

Budget Gourmet Stuffed
Turkey Breast Dinner
Spinach
Corn muffins
Fresh mango
Milk

Healthy Choice Mesquite
Beef with Barbecue Sauce
Coleslaw
Lemon yogurt with
blueberries

Continental

Budget Gourmet Special
Sirloin of Beef
in Wine Sauce
Cucumber and tomato slices
Dinner rolls
Tangerine
Milk

Budget Gourmet Fettuccine
Primavera in Herb Sauce
with Chicken
Wheat rolls
Vegetable soup
Mixed fruit salad
Yogurt

Healthy Choice Honey
Mustard Chicken Entree
Carrots
Bran muffin
Fresh strawberries
with yogurt

Healthy Choice Lemon
Pepper Fish Dinner
Tossed salad with carrot
and bell pepper strips
Fruit cocktail
Milk

Healthy Choice Garlic
Chicken Milano
Zucchini slices with dip
French bread
Milk

Budget Gourmet Beef
Stroganoff
Vegetable soup
Sourdough roll
Tropical fruit salad
Milk

Budget Gourmet Herbed
Chicken Breast with
Fettuccine
Caesar salad
French bread
Frozen yogurt with
raspberries

Oriental

Weight Watchers Sweet 'N
Sour Chicken Tenders
Budget Gourmet Spinach
Au Gratin Side Dish
Cherries
Milk

Budget Gourmet Teriyaki
Chicken Chow Mein
Red peppers and cauliflower
with dip
Wheat roll
Cinnamon applesauce
Milk

Lean Cuisine Beef Lo Mein
Pineapple chunks
Milk

Lean Cuisine Chicken
in Peanut Sauce
Tossed salad with tomato
Banana and strawberries
with yogurt

Budget Gourmet Mandarin
Chicken with Plum Sauce
and Vegetables
Cabbage with vinaigrette
dressing
Honeydew melon
Milk

Yu Sing Cashew Chicken
Raw broccoli
Wheat roll
Yogurt with raisins and
sugar cookie

Grab-and-Go Lunches

These sandwich-type meals are
great to eat at your desk while
working.

Turkey, Broccoli, and Cheese
Lean Pocket
Yogurt
Banana
Milk

Papa's Turkey and Swiss
Piroshki
Baby carrot sticks
Fresh apple
Milk

Pizza Lean Pocket
Yogurt
V-8 juice

Ruizz Beef Steak Fajita
Tomato slices
Banana
Yogurt

Healthy Choice Hearty
Handful–Turkey and
Vegetable
Baked tortilla chips
Salsa
Grapes
Milk

Economy Frozen Meals

Little Juan Bean and
Cheese Burrito
Fruit cocktail and yogurt
Milk

Fish sticks
Easy Microwave Potatoes
(See page 305 for recipe.)
Sliced tomatoes
Peach halves
Milk

Totino's Canadian Bacon
Pizza
Tossed salad
Pineapple slices
Milk

Banquet Turkey and Gravy
with Stuffing and
Mashed Potatoes
Fresh apple
Milk

Macaroni and cheese
Carrot and pineapple salad
Tomato juice
Pudding

Meatless Entrees

If you prefer meatless, here is a
selection of entrees that contain
cheese and milk, but not meat.
Some are higher in fat. To make
a complete meal, add milk
or yogurt, vegetable, fruit, and
in some cases, beans or other
sources of protein.

Budget Gourmet Macaroni
and Cheese with Cheddar
and Parmesan
Budget Gourmet Three-
Cheese Lasagna
Budget Gourmet Cheese
Ravioli Parmigiana
Healthy Choice Manicotti
with Three Cheeses
Healthy Choice Pasta
Shells Marinara
Lean Cuisine Angel Hair
Pasta
Lean Cuisine Fettuccine
Primavera
Lean Cuisine Macaroni and
Cheese with Broccoli
Michelina's Spaghetti
Marinara
Weight Watchers Kung Pao
Noodles and Vegetables

Weight Watchers Paella Rice
and Vegetables
Weight Watchers Pasta
and Spinach Romano
Weight Watchers Peking Style
Rice and Vegetables
Weight Watchers Parisian
Style White Beans
with Vegetables
Weight Watchers Pilaf
Florentine
Weight Watchers Risotto with
Cheese and Mushrooms
Weight Watchers Santa Fe
Style Rice and Beans

Sit-Down Restaurants: Making the Best Choices

Dining out offers many choices; which foods are best for the mom-to-be? If you eat out often, your diet will most likely be higher in fat and lower in other nutrients such as calcium, folacin, and vitamin C, unless you make your choices wisely! Some specific challenges for the pregnant diner are:

- Typically large servings may tempt you to overeat; take half of it home in a doggy bag! Or order a half portion or from the appetizer menu.

- Higher-fat foods and fried foods may cause heartburn. What you would think of as low-fat (such as Oriental food) can sometimes surprise you!
- Servings of vegetables and fruits are usually minimal–leaving your meal just meats and starches. Consider ordering a side salad, coleslaw, or appetizer vegetable to round out the meal.
- Milk may not be available–this could be a problem if you dine out regularly.

Salad-Bar Savvy

Most people think a salad bar means a healthy meal! It can be–but beware the high-fat foods! Here are a few tips for making your trip to the salad bar a healthy one!

▶ **Go easy on the hidden fats: sunflower seeds, Chinese noodles, coconut, salad dressing, bacon bits, olives, marinated vegetables, puddings, mousses, and salads made with mayonnaise, such as potato salad, coleslaw, and egg salad.**

Also try to stay away from the fried foods such as fried zucchini and potato skins on the "super bars."

▶ **Make sure to eat enough protein foods: ham, turkey, cottage cheese, kidney beans, garbanzo beans, and/or Cheddar cheese.**

At the Table

▶ **Try to avoid meals described with these words: butter, butter sauce, hollandaise, raw (as in seafood), au gratin, alfredo, creamed, cream, sautéed, pan fried, or fried.**

▶ **Choose wisely from the menu.**

You should be able to order a healthy entree by looking for these key words: marinara sauce, vegetarian, grilled, baked, poached, steamed, stir-fried, lean, and light.

▶ **Order foods that contain one or two servings of vegetables.**

You may want to order á la carte to get what you want. Pasta, potatoes, and brown or wild rice are good side dishes. Avoid fried potatoes.

▶ **Order all salad dressings or sauces on the side.**

▶ **Are you tempted by the chips or bread brought to your table before you order? Eat a raw fruit on the way to the restaurant or before you leave home.**

You'll then be less likely to over-indulge in before-dinner snacks. Or ask that those foods not be brought to the table and ask for a salad to snack on.

Some Typically Healthy Entrees Include:

Mexican
Chicken, beef, or shrimp
    fajitas
Chicken enchiladas
Bean tostadas or burritos

Italian
Pasta with marinara sauce
Pasta primavera
Tortellini or ravioli with
    marinara sauce
Vegetable lasagna

Bistro Style
Grilled chicken sandwich
Chef salad
Chicken caesar salad
Grilled shrimp with pasta

Steak House
Small fillet of beef
    (such as Filet Mignon)
Seafood brochette
Grilled salmon

Here are some examples of healthy menu items from national chain restaurants—mix and match to create your own healthy meal:

Au Bon Pain
Minestrone soup
Turkey breast and Swiss
    cheese on four-grain bread
Vegetarian chili with
    onion bagel

Boston Market
Chicken soup
Chicken breast
New potatoes
Home-style mashed potatoes
Zucchini marinara
Steamed vegetables
Cinnamon apples
Fruit salad

California Pizza Kitchen
Field greens salad
Moo Shu Chicken Calzone
Mixed Grill Vegetarian Pizza
    with honey-wheat crust
Sorbet

Chili's
Chicken fajitas
Southwest salad
Nonfat frozen yogurt

Cracker Barrel
Tossed Salad
Grilled Farm-Raised
    Catfish Fillets
Carrots
Country Vegetable Plate
Corn bread

Friday's
House salad
Garden Burger with house
    salad
Pacific Coast Tuna Sandwich
Thai Chicken Salad with
    dressing on the side
Sherbet

Houlihan's
Dinner salad
Vegetable lasagna
Chinese Chicken Salad
Fruit sorbet

Kenny Roger's Roasters
Side salad
BBQ Chicken Pita
Roasted Chicken Salad
Cinnamon apples

Olive Garden
Salad with bread sticks
Minestrone soup with
    bread sticks
Shrimp Primavera
Grilled Herb Chicken
    with Peppers
Raspberry sorbet

Ponderosa
Salad bar
Broiled salmon
Teriyaki steak
Baked potato
Rice pilaf
Carrots
Green beans

Quincy's Family Steakhouse

Dinner salad

Club Steak with Mushroom
Sauce

Baked potato

Broccoli spears

Red Lobster

Caesar salad

Shrimp cocktail

Seafood gumbo

Lemon sole

Baked potato

Fresh vegetables

Cheese-garlic biscuit

What's for Dessert?

Fresh fruit, sorbet, sherbet, and low-fat frozen yogurt are good choices. If you want to indulge in something heavier, split it with your dining partner.

▼

The Most Nutritious Fast Foods

Which fast foods are healthiest? A good question; and the answer depends on what you are looking for: Low-fat content? High vitamin C or A content? High fiber content? Every day the choices available at the drive-through seem to expand. You can now eat a healthy, balanced diet when you eat fast food regularly. The key is to make the best choices (many of us have good intentions!) and to round out your diet by snacking on fruits and vegetables that might not be available when you eat in the "fast lane."

Fast Foods Highest in Vitamin C	
The best sources of vitamin C are, of course, fruits and vegetables. However, you will find it hidden in some fast foods where you least expect it. Keep in mind that some of the foods listed here are high in fat and calories.	
Company/Product	**Percentage of RDA for Pregnancy**
Taco Bell Taco Salad with shell	107
Orange juice, 6 fluid ounces	102
Grapefruit juice, 6 fluid ounces	86
Carl's Jr. Fiesta Potato	86
Taco Bell Bean Burrito with red sauce	75
Wendy's Baked Potato, sour cream, and chives	64
Arby's Baked Potato, Broccoli and Cheddar	64
Taco Bell Beef Tostada with Red Sauce	64
Wendy's Cauliflower, ½ cup	60
Wendy's Baked Potato, Broccoli and Cheddar	51
Wendy's green peppers, ¼ cup	51
Burger King Garden Salad	49
Taco Bell Mexican Pizza	44
Jack in the Box Chef Salad	39
Taco Bell Combination Burrito	38
Subway Chef Salad or 6-inch sandwich (any choice)	36
KFC coleslaw	31
Long John Silver's Seafood Salad	26
Wendy's honeydew melon, 2 ounces	21
Pizza Hut Traditional Hand-Tossed Pizza, Supreme, medium, 2 slices	17
McDonald's Wheaties, fortified	17

Source: Adapted from the *Completely Revised and Updated Fast-Food Guide*, Copyright 1991, CSPI. Available from CSPI, 1875 Connecticut Avenue NW, Washington, D.C. 20009 for $7.95.

Fast Foods Highest in Calcium

Calcium is a mineral that is very important to your future bone health, and you can jeopardize that health if you don't have enough calcium in your diet while you are pregnant or breast-feeding. However, if you choose a fast food just for its calcium content, you're likely to get a lot of extra calories in the forms of fat and sugar that you probably don't need. For example, if you choose the Pizza Hut Personal Pan Pepperoni Pizza, you would get 675 calories and twenty-nine grams of fat along with your calcium. Hardee's shakes will give you 41 percent of the RDA for calcium, along with nine grams of fat and ten teaspoons of sugar or more! McDonald's offers a low-fat milkshake that provides 30 percent of the RDA for calcium, with eight-and-a-half teaspoons of sugar and just one gram of fat. Sometimes it's worth it to splurge—just not too often!

Company/Product	Percentage of RDA for Pregnancy
Pizza Hut Traditional Hand-Tossed Pizza, Cheese, large, 2 slices	83
Wendy's Taco Salad	66
Pizza Hut Thin 'n' Crispy Pizza, cheese, medium, 2 slices	55
Carl's Jr. Shake, large	41
Hardee's Shakes	41
Dairy Queen Heath Breeze, regular	41
Carl's Jr. Cheese Potato	37
Domino's Pizza Double Cheese/Pepperoni, 16 inch, 2 slices	32
Wendy's Frosty Dairy Dessert, medium (11 ounces)	32
McDonald's low-fat milk shakes	30
Carl's Jr. Breakfast Burrito	29
Baskin-Robbins low-fat frozen yogurt, large (9 ounces)	28
Taco Bell Taco Salad, with shell	27
Milk, 1%, or 2% low-fat, 8 ounces	25

Source: Adapted from the *Completely Revised and Updated Fast-Food Guide*, Copyright 1991, CSPI. Available from CSPI, 1875 Connecticut Avenue NW, Washington, D.C. 20009 for $7.95.

Tips for Making the Healthiest Fast-Food Meal

▶ **Remember that having a food high in vitamin C with your meal will increase the amount of iron your body absorbs.**

You can do this by drinking orange juice, having a salad with high-vitamin C veggies such as tomatoes, broccoli, or cauliflower, or having fresh fruit or other vegetables from the salad bar.

▶ **Cut the fat on sandwiches by asking for no mayonnaise or sauce.**

You can also ask for any sauces on the side. Cutting the cheese will also cut the fat; skip it unless cheese is your primary source of calcium.

▶ **If you eat at the salad bar, choose raw vegetables, such as tomato, broccoli, cauliflower, carrot sticks, and fresh fruits.**

Have cottage cheese, beans, ham, or chopped eggs for a protein source. Go sparingly on the puddings, olives, mayonnaise-based salads, etc. Be sure to have a source of starch, such as bread sticks or crackers.

▶ Try to bring along fresh fruit or vegetables to go with your meal or order a side salad.

▶ If you are trying to keep your weight gain down, choose lower-calorie fare such as grilled chicken, fajitas, or bean burritos.

Skip the additional toppings such as cheese, sour cream, and guacamole. Choose low-calorie or fat-free salad dressings.

▶ If you have trouble with heartburn, avoid fries, burgers, fried pies, and other fried foods, which are high in fat and will aggravate your heartburn.

▼

Healthiest Fast-Food Menus for Pregnancy

The following menus have been chosen because of their lower fat content as well as higher values for some nutrients. All foods listed have less than 50 percent of their calories from fat. The main dishes marked with an asterisk (*)

Fast Foods Highest in Zinc	
Company/Product	Percentage of RDA for Pregnancy
Arby's Beef and Cheese Sandwich	36
Taco Bell Regular Taco	26
Arby's Roast Beef Sandwich	22
KFC Fried Chicken, drumstick and thigh	21
Taco Bell Beefy Tostada	21
Taco Bell Bean Burrito	20
Taco Bell Beef Burrito	15

Source: *Nutritionist III Analysis Software.*

Fast Foods Highest in Folate	
Company/Product	Percentage of RDA for Pregnancy
Taco Bell Regular Tostada	18
Taco Bell Bean Burrito	18
Arby's Ham and Cheese Sandwich	18
McDonald's Egg McMuffin	11
Taco Bell Burrito Supreme	11
Arby's Beef and Cheese Sandwich	10
McDonald's French Fries, large	10
Arby's Roast Beef Sandwich	10
Burger King Egg-Cheese Croissant	9

Source: *Nutritionist III Analysis Software.*

Fast Foods Highest in Vitamin B_6	
Company/Product	Percentage of RDA for Pregnancy
KFC Fried Chicken, breast and wing	26
Arby's Beef and Cheese Sandwich	15
KFC Fried Chicken, leg and thigh	15
McDonald's French Fries, large	14
Taco Bell Burrito Supreme	12
Arby's Roast Beef Sandwich	12
Burger King Egg-Cheese-Ham Croissant	10

Source: *Nutritionist III Analysis Software.*

have 30 percent or fewer of their calories from fat. Most meals average five hundred calories.

Breakfast Fast-Food Menus

With a few exceptions, "fast-food" breakfast means a high-fat, low-fiber meal. The closest thing to fresh fruit is orange juice. So if you do eat fast-food breakfast regularly, try to supplement the meal with fresh fruit of your own or make healthier choices the rest of the day to balance the breakfast out.

Arby's
*Blueberry muffin
Low-fat milk

Ham biscuit
Orange juice
Low-fat milk

Burger King
Bagel with egg and cheese
Low-fat milk
Orange juice

Plain bagel with cream
  cheese
Orange juice

Carl's Jr.
*Bran muffin
Orange juice
Low-fat milk

*Hotcakes
Orange juice
Low-fat milk

Scrambled eggs
*English muffin with
  margarine
Low-fat milk

Del Taco
Breakfast burrito
Water or hot chocolate

Dunkin' Donuts
*Bran muffin with raisins
Low-fat milk
Orange juice

Apple and spice muffin
Low-fat milk
Juice

Hardee's
*Pancakes with 2
  bacon strips
Orange juice
Low-fat milk

Ham and egg biscuit
Orange juice
Low-fat milk

Jack in the Box
Scrambled egg pocket
Orange juice
Low-fat milk

*Breakfast Jack
Orange juice
Low-fat milk

McDonald's
*Apple bran muffin
  (Contains no fat.)
*Cheerios or Wheaties
Low-fat milk
Orange juice

Egg McMuffin
Low-fat milk
Grapefruit juice

*Hot cakes with margarine
  and syrup
Orange juice
Low-fat milk

Wendy's
Mushroom, green pepper,
  and onion omelet
Orange juice

Breakfast sandwich
Orange juice

Whataburger
Egg omelet ranchero
Orange juice

*Pancakes
Low-fat milk

Lunch and Dinner Fast-Food Menus

Arby's
Light Roast Beef Deluxe
  Sandwich
Lumberjack Mixed
  Vegetable Soup
Low-fat milk

*Light Roast Chicken Deluxe
   sandwich
*Plain baked potato
   Orange juice

---

*Light Roast Turkey Deluxe
   sandwich
*Side salad
   Low-fat milk

Roast chicken salad with
   light Italian dressing
Potato soup with bacon
Low-fat milk

Broccoli and Cheddar
   Baked Potato
Side salad with light
   Italian dressing
Low-fat milk

French Dip sandwich
Garden salad
Low-fat milk

Burger King

BK Broiler
Side salad
Orange juice

---

*Chunky Chicken Salad
Newman's Own reduced-
   calorie Italian dressing
Crackers
Low-fat milk

Carl's, Jr.

*Charbroiler BBQ "Lite
   Menu" Chicken Sandwich
Cream of Broccoli Soup
Low-fat milk

*California Roast Beef
   and Swiss Sandwich
*Small vanilla shake

---

*Lumber Jack Mixed
   Vegetable Soup
*Chef Salad-to-Go
   with reduced-calorie
   French dressing
Low-fat milk

Dairy Queen

*BBQ Beef sandwich
Side salad
*Yogurt cone

---

*Grilled Chicken Fillet
   sandwich
Side salad
Low-fat milk

Fish Fillet sandwich
Side salad
Low-fat milk

Domino's Pizza

*2 slices, 14-inch, cheese,
   bell pepper, and
   mushroom pizza
Tossed salad
Fresh fruit salad (from home)
Low-fat milk

El Pollo Loco

*Vegetarian burrito
Side salad
Low-fat milk

Chicken breast
Coleslaw
Corn
Low-fat milk

Chicken Fajita Meal
Orange juice

Hardee's

*Grilled Chicken Sandwich
*Mashed potatoes
Side salad
Low-fat milk

Roast beef sandwich
Side salad
Low-fat milk

---

*Grilled Chicken and Pasta
   salad with reduced-calorie
   French dressing
*Chocolate Cool Twist
Orange juice

Jack in the Box

*Chicken Fajita Pita
Guacamole
Side salad
Low-fat milk

---

*Chicken Teriyaki Bowl
Low-fat milk

Garden Chicken Salad with
   low-calorie Italian dressing
Crackers
Strawberry milkshake

KFC

Rotisserie Gold Chicken
   Breast (skip the skin)
Garden salad
Corn on the cob
Low-fat milk

Meatless Meals at KFC

*Baked beans
*Corn on the cob
*Coleslaw
Low-fat milk

Long John Silver's

Baked Fish Entree with
 sauce, coleslaw, and
 mixed vegetables
Low-fat milk

---

*Lemon Crumb Fish
Hush puppies
Rice pilaf
Green beans
Low-fat milk

---

*Seafood chowder with cod
*Shrimp salad with crackers
 and reduced-calorie Italian
 dressing
Coleslaw
Low-fat milk

McDonald's

*McGrilled Chicken Classic
Garden salad
Low-fat milk

---

*Chunky Chicken Salad
Crackers
Strawberry frozen-yogurt
 sundae
Low-fat milk

Pizza Hut

Canadian Bacon Pizza,
 2 slices
Salad bar
Lemonade

Cheese Thin n' Crispy
 Pizza, 2 slices
Salad bar
Water or low-fat milk

Rax

Salad bar
Cream of broccoli soup
Low-fat milk

Regular Roast Beef Sandwich
Lighterside Garden Salad
Low-fat milk

Skipper's

Create-A-Catch Green Salad
 with low-calorie Italian
 dressing
Create-A-Catch Fish Fillet
Baked potato
Low-fat milk

Shrimp and Seafood Salad
Create-A-Catch Cup
 Clam Chowder
½ serving fries
Low-fat milk

Subway

Following are the best choices—
choose the six-inch sandwich on
a honey-wheat roll. In addition
to one of the toppings below, add
lettuce, tomato, vinegar, peppers,
etc., but skip the oil. It doesn't
add anything but empty calories!

Ham
Roast beef
Seafood and crab
Subway Club
Tuna
Turkey

Good accompaniments include
garden salad and broccoli cheese
soup.

Taco Bell

*Light Burrito Supreme
Low-fat milk

---

*Light Soft Chicken Taco
Pintos n' Cheese
Orange juice

---

*Light Seven-Layer Burrito
Low-fat milk

---

*Light Taco Supreme
*Light Chicken Soft Taco
Low-fat milk

Wendy's

*Grilled Chicken Sandwich
Salad bar with fruit
Low-fat milk

Hot Stuffed Chili Cheese
 baked potato
Side salad
Low-fat milk

---

*Grilled Chicken Salad
Breadstick
Low-fat milk

Salad bar
Breadsticks
Low-fat milk

Luscious Snacks and Desserts

When you feel like splurging on
dessert, the following are low in
fat, but delicious:

*Arby's Chocolate Shake
*Baskin Robbin's Nonfat
Frozen Yogurt
*Dairy Queen Small
Strawberry (yogurt) Breeze
*I Can't Believe It's Not
Yogurt's Nonfat Frozen
Yogurt
*McDonald's or Dairy
Queen's Frozen Yogurt
Cone
*TCBY's Nonfat Frozen
Yogurt
Wendy's Frosty Dairy Dessert

(Also available is sugar-free yogurt at TCBY and "I Can't Believe It's Not Yogurt".)

Source of nutrient information:
Manufacturer's nutrient analysis.

▼

Last-Minute Meals from the Cupboard

The time is "ten minutes to famished." You look in the cupboard and see a can of tomato sauce, some olives, and a can of salmon. What do you do? Improvise! If you think creatively, you can make a lot of great meals from the cans in your pantry. And, by keeping a supply of staple ingredients on hand, you can avoid spending too much of your food budget on convenience foods or calling out for pizza!

Last-Minute Meals from the Cupboard

Ingredients	Meals
Pasta, Spaghetti sauce	Spaghetti with marinara sauce
Boboli pizza, English muffin, or pita bread, Canned chicken, Canned mushrooms, Pasta, Capers, Artichoke hearts, Canned biscuits	Pizza with artichoke hearts, Chicken with mushrooms and capers over pasta with Italian sauce, Quick calzone (using biscuits), Chicken Tetrazzini
Mozzarella cheese, Cottage cheese, Tuna, Salmon, Evaporated skim milk, Pasta, Parmesan cheese, Olives, Canned peas, Mushroom soup (reduced-salt and reduced-fat)	Fettuccine alfredo with tuna or with peas, Tuna casserole, Linguini, salmon, and Parmesan cheese toss, Macaroni and cheese
Refried beans, Taco shells, Pineapple tidbits, Tostada shells, Instant brown rice, Mixed vegetables, Canned tomatoes, Potatoes, Black Beans, Corn, Chicken broth, Fat-free dressing, Tostadas/corn tortillas, Black bean soup	Bean tostadas, Chicken tacos, Chicken salad with pineapple, Spanish rice with chicken, Canned chicken and vegetables, Baked potatoes with chicken topping, Black bean and chicken soup, Black bean tostadas, Black Bean and Corn Salad (see page 224 for recipe) with tortilla chips
Baked beans, Cornbread mix, Kidney beans, Rice or bulgur	Cornbread and bean bake, Hoppin' John (see page 306 for recipe)

Using the ingredients on the left side of the table on page 209, you can make all the foods on the right; some of them make great gourmet dishes!

▼

Fifty Quick-and-Easy Meals or Snacks

Some of my best meals are the kind thrown together in a hurry from what's available. I hope these give you some ideas for quick-but-healthy meals.

Pizzas

Pizza can start with different kinds of crusts:

English muffin
French bread
Pita bread
Corn bread baked
    in a round pan
Flour or corn tortilla
Boboli crust
Refrigerated pizza dough
Pizza-dough mix
Homemade crust
Frozen bread dough

And can have any number of toppings:

Italian: Pasta sauce, cheese, and your choice of meat or veggies.

Mushroom: Cream of mushroom soup, mushrooms, onions, and mozzarella and Parmesan cheeses.

Spinach: Pasta sauce, cooked chopped spinach mixed with cream cheese, and mozzarella cheese.

Ratatouille (see page 311 for recipe).

California: Sun-dried tomatoes, cheese, pizza sauce, ham, mushrooms, and chopped fresh basil.

Chile Con Queso: Refried beans with sauce of melted Velveeta cheese with salsa over baked corn tortilla or English muffin.

All-white pizza: White sauce, shrimp, crab, mushrooms, and mozzarella cheese. (My version of the sauce is flour, margarine or butter, and milk; another is olive oil and garlic; or you can just skip the tomato sauce and have a white pizza.)

Pepper and olive: Using light Creamy Italian or Creamy Garlic dressing, add a mix of red, yellow, and green peppers, and black and green olives. Top with mozzarella cheese.

Ham and crushed pineapple.

Mexican: For sauce, mix salsa and tomato sauce. For topping, use refried beans, Monterey Jack and Cheddar cheeses, chili or bell peppers, chopped tomatoes, and cilantro or parsley.

Grilled veggie: Pasta sauce with grilled eggplant, mushrooms, zucchini, and olives. Add grilled chicken pieces if desired.

Cold Pizzas (These make great appetizers and snacks.)

Seafood: Cream cheese, cocktail sauce, and boiled shrimp or crab make great appetizers.

Cream cheese mixed with Ranch dressing mix: Top with chopped broccoli, carrots, green onions, cauliflower, peppers, shredded cheese, and sliced black olives.

Layered Mexican pizza: Start with Boboli crust or other baked crust. Top with refried beans, guacamole, sour cream flavored with taco seasoning, chopped tomatoes, shredded cheese, and sliced black olives. This can be made fat-free or full-fat. Also works well as a dip without crust.

Sandwiches

Tired of the same old peanut butter and jelly on white bread? Try these ideas for a change of pace! A variety of breads help beat brown-bag boredom:

Rye
Whole-wheat pita
French bread
Flour tortilla
Graham crackers
Saltine crackers
Melba toast
Wheat bread

Sourdough bread
Oat bread
Hamburger bun

Try any of the following fillings:

Warm

Leftover stir-fry vegetables (with or without chicken, pork, beef, or tofu) in pita pocket or tortilla.

Light pastrami over sauerkraut with Swiss cheese on rye.

Grilled vegetables and cheese on crusty whole-wheat French bread.

Refried beans and cheese in flour tortilla or on baked corn tortilla. (Top with shredded lettuce and tomato.)

Vegetarian burger (found in frozen food section or with frozen chicken patties).

Salmon patties.

Cold popcorn shrimp with melted mozzarella on top of tomato slice on an English muffin.

Grilled fish-fillet burgers.

Sloppy Joes (with lean ground beef, ground turkey, or Textured Vegetable Protein–TVP).

Spiced black beans with reduced-fat cheese and bell peppers in a folded tortilla.

Delightful Spinach (see page 223 for recipe) in a whole-wheat tortilla.

Thinly sliced roast beef and microwave-steamed bell peppers on a French roll with beef broth for dipping on the side.

Cold

Chef salad stuffed in a pita pocket with light Italian dressing on the side.

Cooked and chilled asparagus spears rolled up with ham and cheese in a whole-wheat tortilla.

Chopped chicken with light mayonnaise, fat-free sour cream, curry powder, green onion, mango, and raisins stuffed in a pita pocket (or serve as a salad over torn spinach leaves).

Boursin Cheese Spread (see page 288 for recipe) or light cream cheese, chopped parsley, alfalfa sprouts, and thinly sliced cucumbers and tomatoes on thinly sliced bread.

Popcorn shrimp or imitation crab in a sauce of light mayonnaise and ketchup over English muffin topped with chopped tomato and avocado.

Peanut butter with banana on graham crackers.

Light ricotta cheese on raisin English muffin topped with fruit of choice.

Cottage cheese with chopped carrots, broccoli, green onion, and celery on wheat-berry English muffin.

Main-Dish Salad Ideas

These are great for the summer when no one feels like having a hot meal. To save time, keep chopped, cooked chicken in the freezer or use canned, chopped white chicken meat.

Tortellini with ham, shredded cheese, tomatoes, artichoke hearts, and vinaigrette dressing.

Rice or bulgur with corn, kidney beans, green beans, chopped red peppers, reduced-fat Cheddar cheese, and vinaigrette dressing.

Linguini with imitation crab, steamed carrots and broccoli, and creamy Italian dressing.

Mixed greens with grilled fish, walnuts, and cucumber dressing.

Black Bean and Corn Salad (see page 224 for recipe).

Spaghetti with stir-fried chicken, snow peas, and red peppers with peanuts and teriyaki sauce.

Oriental Salad with grilled chicken (see page 228 for recipe).

Leaf lettuce, canned tuna in water, white beans, kidney beans, cherry tomatoes, cucumbers, olives, and green onion with light Ranch dressing.

Small shell pasta, popcorn shrimp, chopped avocado, and tomato over bed of shredded romaine lettuce with fat-free vinaigrette dressing.

Chicken and Spinach Salad (see page 227 for recipe).

Chicken and pineapple chunks over shredded cabbage with Catalina dressing.

Mixed fresh fruit salad with fruit-flavored yogurt and bran muffins.

Peas with light mayonnaise and cheese chunks over mixed greens garnished with tomato slices and yellow bell pepper rings.

Fajita salad: Grilled marinated chicken, beef, or shrimp, peppers and onions over torn lettuce.

Serve with baked flour tortilla triangles or Baked Tostitos.

Rotini pasta with honey dijon dressing, ham chunks, and three-bean salad.

Taco salad with Baked Tostitos topped with shredded romaine lettuce, canned or leftover warmed chili, reduced-fat cheese, chopped tomatoes or salsa, and fat-free sour cream.

Menus and Recipes for the First Trimester

About the Eating Expectantly Menus

Many people have trouble planning menus, but when you're pregnant, planning can be even tougher due to what I call the "eating moods" of pregnancy. You know—when you're so hungry you could eat a horse, but nothing sounds good. Or when you'd rather stay in bed because you feel queasy, but you've got to get your son ready for school. Some days you just feel exhausted and would like an idea for how to get dinner on the table in fifteen minutes (or less)! In the menus that precede each chapter of recipes, I've tried to take some work out of menu-planning by giving you lots of ideas. The types of menus in each chapter are listed at the beginning of each of the recipe chapters, as well as in the end of Chapters Three, Four, and Five.

Beverages are not necessarily included in the menus, although it is assumed that milk will be your choice of beverage at least two times per day! Other good choices for drinks include vegetable and tomato juice, fruit juices, soymilk, and sparkling water mixed with fruit juice. Of course, you should also try to drink plenty of water throughout the day.

The recipes included in the menus list the page number on which they appear, in parentheses. Recipes are usually located in the same chapter, although some will be located in other sections of the book.

About the Eating Expectantly Recipes

When it comes to food, I have my likes and dislikes like anyone else, so the recipes in this book reveal my own food biases. For example, you won't find any recipes that contain mustard greens or liver since these are not among my favorites! You will also find some French recipes, since my husband is French, and a few southern recipes, since I am originally from Texas. The Eating Expectantly recipes were developed and chosen primarily for their taste, and then for nutritional value and ease of preparation. (After all, if food doesn't taste good, who would eat it even if it is nutritious?) Most recipes call for ingredients that are readily available; the majority will be found in your own pantry. Vegetarian recipes may call for a few ingredients that you may have to buy from a large health-food store.

Nutritional Analysis

All recipes were analyzed using Nutritionist III Software Version 7.2 from N-Squared Computing. All numbers are rounded off. When more than one ingredient or more than one serving amount is listed, the first number listed is the one used for analysis.

Protein is listed so that you have an idea of how a recipe compares to your total goal for protein intake. Fat is included because most people are interested in fat content these days; women who have heartburn will be interested in choosing the lowest-fat recipes. Carbohydrate is listed for the benefit of diabetics and health professionals, so they can plan special diets. The fiber listed is dietary fiber. If fiber is not listed, it is because the recipe contains less than one gram per serving.

Key Nutrients

Recipes were compared to the RDAs for pregnancy and are listed as a percentage of the RDAs. By looking at the key nutrients, you can pick foods high in a variety of nutrients; you can also learn which types of foods are most nutritious.

Diabetic Exchanges

Diabetic exchanges are included to assist in meal-planning for women who have diabetes or gestational diabetes. They are calculated according to the Exchange Lists for Meal-Planning developed by the American Diabetes Association and the American Dietetic Association. Exchanges are also rounded off as needed. Women who have diabetes should consult with a registered dietitian to receive an individualized meal plan based on their weight and activity level.

The diabetic exchanges are based on principles of good nutrition, so women who are not diabetic can also use them for keeping track of how many servings of food from the different food groups they are eating.

Diabetic Variations

A few of the recipes contain a significant amount of sugar; a sugar-free variation follows each recipe. These variations contain Equal. (See page 110 for information about the use of artificial sweeteners during pregnancy.) Use Equal only with your physician's approval. When a diabetic variation is listed, the exchanges that follow it are for the diabetic variation.

First-Trimester Menus

Keep in mind that during the first trimester, your priority is not to gain weight but to make your diet as high-quality as possible and to improve your other lifestyle habits. Don't worry if because of nausea, you don't eat much at all for a little while. Lack of appetite should only become a concern if you begin losing weight.

Don't Feel Like Eating Menus

Many women find that drinking their liquids between, instead of with, meals helps with nausea. Remember–eating what you crave may help you get past your nausea, so don't worry if your craving seems a little weird.

Cream of mushroom soup
Wheat toast
Peach slices

Chicken noodle soup
Saltine crackers
Lime sherbet

Jell-O with pears
Cottage cheese
Toast

Low-fat yogurt and
  banana shake
Graham crackers

Egg custard
Graham crackers

Granny apple slices with
  peanut butter
Pretzels

Plain pasta
Applesauce

Macaroni and cheese
Frozen grapes

Creamy Asparagus Soup
  (page 220)
Wheat crackers

Boursin Cheese Spread
  (page 288) or cream
  cheese on bagel
Pears

Don't Feel Like Cooking Menus

(Also look at Vegetarian Convenience-Food Choices in Chapter Six and at Using Leftovers with Flair Menus in Chapter Fifteen for more ideas.)

Grilled cheese and tomato
  sandwich
Fresh apple

Black Bean and Corn Salad
  with Baked Tortilla Chips
  (page 224)
Strawberry sorbet

Tostadas with Basic Black
  Beans (page 257), cheese,
  lettuce, avocado, and
  tomato
Low-fat milk
Frozen banana

Quick and Easy Lunches for Friends:

Salmon Paté (page 221) on
  crusty bread
Shrimp-stuffed avocado with
  Ranch dressing

Fresh pineapple slices
Tuna and pasta salad with
  artichoke hearts
Rye crackers
Cantaloupe quarters

Cold Sesame Beef (page 313)
  served warm over mixed
  greens
Marinated vegetables
Tropical Pudding (page 237)

Melted Boursin Cheese
  Spread (page 288) on toast
  rounds over mixed greens
  and vegetables
Wheat roll
Berry Mousse Parfait
  (page 273)

Black Bean Enchilada
  Casserole (page 294)
Carrot-apple salad
Wheat roll
Watermelon

Aspen Black Bean Soup
  (page 292)
Cornbread Toaster Biscuit
  (Entenmann's)
Grilled grapefruit

Tabouli salad with cheese
French bread
Fresh fruit salad

Pasta with Quick Alfredo
  Sauce (page 229)
Peas
Tossed salad
Wheat rolls
Frozen yogurt with
  strawberries

Light Lunch:

Thrive-on-Five Bread
(page 233) with fat-free
cream cheese
Apple Pie á la Mode Shake
(page 238)

Don't Feel Like Cooking or Eating Menu

Breakfast

Frozen melon balls
Dry toast
Fruit spread or jam
Milk or juice (later)

Snack

Pretzels or baked chips
Milk or vegetable juice

Lunch

Fresh fruit with cottage
cheese
Vanilla wafers

Snack

Lemon-lime "float" with lime
sherbet and lemon-lime
soda

Dinner

Poached or scrambled eggs
Wheat toast
Milk

Snack

Peach Popsicles (page 236)
Milk

Feel Like Staying in Bed, But Can't Menu

Before-Rising Snack

Saltine crackers or other salty
snack that appeals
Ginger-ale (later)

Snack

Jell-O with peaches
Graham crackers

Between-Meal Snack

Lemonade

Lunch

Pasta with mozzarella cheese
Sliced tomatoes

Snack

Frozen fruit juice bars

Between-Meal Snack

Pretzels
Tomato juice

Dinner

Chicken or tuna salad
Vegetables in Vinaigrette
(page 317)
Wheat crackers
Apple slices

Bedtime Snack

Raspberry Surprise Shake
(page 242)

Feel Great Menu

If you are one of the lucky ones,
you will feel close to normal and
will want to eat "as usual." You
may even feel especially hungry!
Here's an example of a good
day's diet.

Breakfast

Raisin bran
Blueberries
Pumpkin Muffin (page 235)
Milk

Snack

Dried figs or prunes

Lunch

Turkey and cheese sandwich
Fresh or canned peaches
Raw broccoli and carrots
with dip
Milk

Snack

Vegetable juice
Popcorn

Dinner

Oriental Salad (page 228)
Broiled salmon steak
Roasted New Potatoes
(page 312)
Carrots Antibes (page 226)

Snack

Tangy Salad (page 269)

Blender Breakfasts (or, Snacks-to-Go):

Banana-Orange Flip
(page 239)
Cinnamon graham crackers

Piña Colada Frappé
(page 241)
Oat-bran toast

Very Berry Shake (page 243)
½ toasted whole-wheat bagel

Peanut Butter-Chocolate
Shake (page 240)

Raspberry Surprise Shake
(page 242)
Bran muffin

Apple Pie á la Mode Shake
(page 238)
Peanut butter on crackers

Chocolate Mocha Shake
(page 240)
Biscotti

Snack Ideas

Here are snack ideas for the first, second, and third trimesters, so that you won't run out of ideas for something different!

First Trimester

Rye crisp and pimiento
cheese
Apple with peanut butter
Tangy Salad (page 269)
Cottage cheese and blue-
berries on ½ English muffin
Melba toast and reduced-fat
Laughing Cow cheese
Caramel corn cakes
and yogurt
Rice pudding with raisins
Bran flakes and granola, milk
Dried figs and farmer cheese
Apple Date Bran Muffin
(page 234)
Jell-O with peaches
Creamy Asparagus Soup
(page 220)
Health Valley Date Bake Bar
Graham crackers and milk

Stewed prunes
Favorite Snack Cake
(page 322)
Pumpkin Muffins (page 235)
Pretzels

Second and Third Trimesters

Toasted cheese and
tomato sandwich
Neufchatel cheese, raisins,
and cinnamon spread on
toasted English muffin
Deviled eggs and rye crackers
Pear and cottage cheese
Apple and colby cheese
Thin-sliced turkey breast
rolled around light
cream cheese
Oven-Fried Zucchini
(page 222) with marinara
sauce
McDonald's low-fat frozen
yogurt cone
Banana and peanut butter
Baked sweet potato
Apple slices with Caramel
Dip (page 321)
Berry Mousse Parfait
(page 273)
Popcorn cakes with
string cheese
½ pita bread stuffed with
salad, light Cheddar
cheese, and vinaigrette
dressing
Popcorn
Tuna salad with apple
and crackers
Boiled eggs and saltines

Quick and Healthier
Pancakes with fresh fruit
(page 251)
Chicken and Spinach Salad
(page 227)
Refried beans with baked
tortilla chips
Quesadilla with mushrooms,
tomato, and cheese
Tropical Pudding (page 237)
Leek and Potato Soup
(page 253), milk
Rocky Mountain Quesadillas
(page 230)
Harvest Crisp wheat crackers
with spinach cottage
cheese dip
Cheerios with peaches
and milk
Figs stuffed with light
cream cheese
Frozen yogurt with fresh
strawberries and
blueberries
Toasted wheat-berry
English muffin, yogurt
Fiber bar, milk
Leftover pizza, vegetable
juice
"Guiltless Gourmet" nachos
Raw vegetables, Ranch
dressing, crackers
Orange juice with club soda,
yogurt with Post Grape
Nuts and raisins
Strawberry Bread
(page 232), milk
Hot apple cider, Thrive-on-
Five Bread (page 233)
Ham and cheese in
wheat tortilla

Chicken salad on ½ bagel
or bagel crisps (baked)
Corn muffin with Monterey
Jack cheese, tomato juice
Orange, pimiento cheese
on celery, carrots and
cucumbers
Fruit kebob with strawberries,
kiwi, pineapple, and cheese

High-Energy Mom Snack Ideas

Peanut Butter-Chocolate
Shake (page 240)
Fig Newtons
Egg custard, ginger snaps
Oven-baked potato chips
with Parmesan cheese
and Italian seasoning
Delightful Spinach (page 223)
in a flour tortilla, milk
"Macho Nachos" (Corn
tortilla toasted and served

with melted Cheddar
cheese, refried vegetarian
beans, bell pepper strips,
lettuce, tomato, light sour
cream, and avocado)
Egg and olive salad on rye,
tomato juice
Chocolate Mocha Cake
(page 274) with strawber-
ries and vanilla yogurt
Wendy's Frosty,
graham crackers
Tortellini pasta salad
with ham
Peanut butter cookies, frozen
vanilla yogurt
English muffin with melted
part-skim mozzarella
cheese, sun-dried tomatoes,
and marinated
artichoke hearts
Fruit Pizza for a Crowd
(page 324)

Fruit Crisp (page 323) with
vanilla frozen yogurt
Fat-free chocolate frozen
yogurt with strawberry
and granola topping
Old-fashioned banana pud-
ding with vanilla wafers
Raspberry Surprise Shake
(page 242), granola bar
Refried beans with cheese,
baked tortilla chips,
vegetable juice
Low-fat cheesecake with fresh
peaches and blueberries
Pound cake with peaches and
raspberry yogurt topping,
milk
Favorite Snack Cake (page
322) with cream cheese
Avocado and shrimp salad,
hard rolls

First-Trimester Recipes

The recipes on the following pages, as well as the recipes in the following chapters, are arranged as follows: beginning with snacks and dips, following with salads, soups, main entreés, breads, muffins, and finishing with desserts.

Creamy Asparagus Soup

If you like homemade soup, but don't have much time to cook, this is the recipe for you! Precooking the asparagus in the microwave prevents destruction of its important vitamin B, folate, and other water-soluble vitamins.

Makes: 3 servings

1 10-ounce package frozen asparagus

¼ cup each onion and celery, finely chopped, or 1 tablespoon dehydrated onion flakes and a few pinches celery salt

1-2 garlic cloves, chopped, or garlic powder to taste

1 chicken bouillon cube or 1 heaping teaspoon broth mix

½ cup water, hot

1 12-ounce can skim evaporated milk

1½ tablespoons flour

½ teaspoon seasoned salt or garlic salt

⅛ teaspoon pepper, or to taste

1. Place asparagus, onion, celery, and garlic in bottom of microwave-safe dish. Add 1 tablespoon water, cover, and cook on high in microwave for 2 minutes. Rearrange spears and cook 3 minutes more, or until tender. Leave covered several minutes to cool and cut into 1-inch pieces.

2. Meanwhile, dissolve 1 bouillon cube (or enough to make 1 cup broth) in ½ cup hot water. Pour into blender pitcher. Add milk and flour. Blend on low speed; then on high, until well blended.

3. Pour mixture into large saucepan, leaving about ¾ cup in blender. Add asparagus and blend until asparagus is well puréed.

4. Add asparagus mixture to saucepan. Cook over medium-low heat stirring well until it reaches the desired thickness. Add seasoned salt and pepper.

5. Serve with Bridget's Garden Salad and bran muffins.

Variation

Use a 10-ounce package of frozen broccoli instead of asparagus for a Creamy Broccoli Soup.

Nutrient Analysis per Serving

150 calories
23 grams carbohydrates
14 grams protein
1 gram fat
2 grams fiber

Key Nutrients

Vitamin C–33%
Folate–32%
Calcium–30%
Vitamin A–26%

Diabetic Exchanges

1 Skim Milk
1 Vegetable
½ Starch

Salmon Paté

This creamy spread can be used as a dip or a sandwich filling. It tastes so good you won't believe its low fat content!

Makes: 20 servings

*1 15½-ounce can salmon with
  skin removed*

2½ tablespoons grated onion

1½ teaspoons white horseradish

2 tablespoons lemon juice

*1 teaspoon dry dill or
  1 tablespoon fresh dill*

*2 teaspoons dry parsley or
  2 tablespoons fresh parsley,
  chopped*

1 teaspoon Liquid Smoke

*8 ounces fat-free cream cheese
  or 8 ounces low-fat
  cottage cheese*

1. Place cheese in food processor and blend until smooth.

2. Add remaining ingredients and blend until smooth. When you taste it you shouldn't feel any bones.

Variations

Serve on rye crackers, toasted pita bread, or on a sandwich with thinly sliced cucumbers. For appetizers, stuff cherry tomatoes, spread on crackers, or stuff mushroom caps.

Nutrient Analysis per Serving

50 calories
1 gram carbohydrate
7 grams protein
1.5 grams fat

Key Nutrients

Vitamin B$_{12}$–48%
Selenium–22%
Calcium–4%

Diabetic Exchanges

1 Very Lean Meat

Oven-Fried Zucchini Sticks

What a great way to eat vegetables! They almost taste too good to be healthy!

Makes: 4 servings

½ cup Italian bread crumbs

2 tablespoons Parmesan cheese, freshly grated or canned

¼ teaspoon garlic powder

3 medium zucchini

Water or milk

1 cup fat-free or low-fat spaghetti sauce

Cooking spray

1. Preheat oven to 450°F. Spray cookie sheet with cooking spray.

2. Place bread crumbs, cheese, and garlic powder in a Ziploc bag and shake well to combine all ingredients. Set aside.

3. Cut each zucchini lengthwise into 8 pieces; cut each piece again in half lengthwise. Fill a pie plate with water; then dip each zucchini stick first in water, then into bag of crumb mixture. Shake until zucchini are coated on all sides. Place on cookie sheet. Repeat with rest of sticks.

4. Bake on cookie sheet for 10 to 15 minutes or until brown and tender. Serve with warm spaghetti sauce.

Variation

Use 1 medium peeled eggplant, sliced into thin rounds, instead of zucchini.

Nutrient Analysis per Serving

107 calories

17 grams carbohydrate

5 grams protein

2 grams fat

Key Nutrients

Small amounts of all nutrients.

Diabetic Exchanges

2 Vegetables

½ Starch

½ Fat

Delightful Spinach

Do you groan at the thought of eating greens? This simple recipe will tempt you to ask for seconds! The creamy sauce boosts calcium and protein content. This "delightful" dish can be used for a side dish or as a dip.

Makes: 3 servings

1 10-ounce package frozen spinach, chopped

4 ounces fat-free or low-fat cream cheese

½ teaspoon mixed herbs

Salt and pepper, to taste

2 drops Tabasco sauce (optional)

1. Cook spinach (or thaw completely) and squeeze out all its water; place in small saucepan over low heat.

2. Add cream cheese and spices and stir well until blended and warmed throughout.

Variations

You can prepare this recipe using Swiss chard, kale, mustard greens, or any greens, even cooked lettuce.

Nutrient Analysis per Serving

44 calories
4 grams carbohydrate
7 grams protein
less than 1 gram fat
1 gram fiber

Key Nutrients

Vitamin A–61%
Folate–23%
Magnesium–16%
Vitamin B$_{12}$–10%

Diabetic Exchanges

1 Very Lean Meat
1 Vegetable

Black Bean and Corn Salad with Baked Tortilla Chips and Yogurt Sauce

This easy-to-make dish is chock-full of important nutrients for you and your baby! You can prepare it for a light meal, or eat a smaller portion as a snack.

Makes: 4 servings

Salad

1 16-ounce can black beans, drained

1 cup corn, drained

½ cup fat-free Italian dressing

4 cups romaine or leaf lettuce leaves, torn

4 ounces reduced-fat Cheddar or Monterey Jack cheese

2 tomatoes

Yogurt Sauce

½ cup plain nonfat yogurt

½ teaspoon cumin

⅛ teaspoon garlic powder

Tortilla Chips

6 corn tortillas

Cooking spray

1. Mix corn, beans, and dressing. Marinate in refrigerator at least 30 minutes.

2. Spoon corn and bean mixture over lettuce. Sprinkle 1 ounce of cheese on each serving. Garnish with 2 tomato quarters.

3. Mix yogurt with cumin and garlic powder.

4. Serve with homemade tortilla chips (or Baked Tostitos or Guiltless Gourmet chips) and yogurt sauce.

Baked Tortilla Chips

1. Preheat oven to 350° F. Cut each tortilla into 6 pieces, spray with cooking spray and sprinkle with salt, and or spices.

2. Bake on cookie sheet for 20 to 30 minutes, turning once.

Nutrient Analysis per Serving

350 calories
52 grams carbohydrate
21 grams protein
8 grams fat
12 grams fiber

Key Nutrients

Vitamin C–32%
Chromium–24%
Folate–20%

Diabetic Exchanges

3 Starches
1½ Medium-Fat Meats
1 Vegetable

Bridget's Garden Salad

I often create meals from my refrigerator leftovers, or in this case, from my garden. With a little luck, many of my creations work (though my husband sometimes attests otherwise). I created this salad one week last summer when it seemed as though our garden was producing only green beans.

Makes: 4 servings

4 cups leaf or romaine lettuce, torn

2 cups green beans or a mixture of green and wax beans, cooked

½ cup purple cabbage, shredded

4 large mushrooms, sliced

2 tomatoes, coarsely chopped

4 ounces smoked turkey, cubed

½ cup kidney beans, drained

2 ounces reduced-fat cheese, grated

½ cup fat-free Italian dressing

2 tablespoons low-fat sour cream

Sesame seeds, sunflower seeds, or pine nuts (optional)

1. Toss all ingredients except cheese, dressing, and sour cream.

2. Mix sour cream and dressing in small bowl.

3. Toss salad with dressing. Sprinkle cheese on top. Garnish with toasted sesame seeds or sunflower seeds, if desired.

Variation

Substitute 4 cups of pasta (rotini or shells work well) for lettuce. Increase fiber content by using whole-wheat pasta.

Nutrient Analysis per Serving

177 calories
16 grams carbohydrate
17 grams protein
6 grams fat
5 grams fiber

Key Nutrients

Vitamin C–50%
Vitamin A–26%
Vitamin B$_6$–19%
Zinc–10%

Diabetic Exchanges

2 Lean Meats
2 Vegetables
½ Starch

Carrots Antibes

While visiting my husband's family in France, I ate this dish in a restaurant located on the Mediterranean coast. Europeans love puréed vegetables, and once you try Carrots Antibes, you'll know why! This is my version of the dish, which even kids will love!

Makes: 4 servings

**8 carrots (about 1 pound),
   peeled and sliced**

½ cup water

1 egg

½ teaspoon sugar

¼ teaspoon nutmeg

1. Place carrots and water in microwave-safe dish. Cover and cook 10 minutes in microwave on high, turning half-way once during cooking. Drain off liquid.

2. Place carrots in blender or food processor with egg and spices. Blend until well puréed.

3. Return mixture to microwave dish and cook 4 minutes, rotating once.

4. Serve as a side dish or as a snack with crackers.

Nutrient Analysis per Serving

82 calories

15 grams carbohydrate

3 grams protein

2 grams fat

5 grams fiber

Key Nutrients

Vitamin A–509%

Potassium–24%

Vitamin C–19%

Diabetic Exchanges

3 Vegetables

Chicken and Spinach Salad

This dish from the cookbook, *Quick and Healthy Recipes and Ideas,* by Brenda Ponichtera, makes a wonderful summertime lunch. Substitute other fruit if fresh strawberries are not available. Try using leftover grilled chicken and prewashed spinach for an especially quick meal.

Makes: 7 servings

Salad

6 ounces spinach, fresh

2 oranges, peeled and cut into chunks

2 cups chicken, cooked and cubed

2 cups strawberries, sliced

Dressing

3 tablespoons red wine vinegar

3 tablespoons orange juice

1½ tablespoons canola oil

¼ teaspoon dry mustard

⅓ teaspoon poppy seeds

1. Mix dressing ingredients in a bowl and refrigerate.

2. Wash spinach and tear into bite-size pieces into a large bowl.

3. Add oranges, chicken, and strawberries.

4. Serve with dressing.

Source: Reprinted with permission from *Quick and Healthy Recipes and Ideas,* by Brenda J. Ponichtera, R.D. (ScaleDown Publishing, Inc.)

Nutrient Analysis per Serving

152 calories
9 grams carbohydrate
14 grams protein
7 grams fat

Key Nutrients

Vitamin C–88%
Niacin–41%
Vitamin A–27%
Selenium–23%
Folate–19%

Diabetic Exchanges

1½ Lean Meats
1 Fruit
1 Vegetable (free)

Oriental Salad

Makes: 6 servings

Salad

4 cups romaine lettuce, shredded

1 celery stalk, finely chopped

1 or 2 green onions, sliced

½ cup sliced water chestnuts, rinsed

1 10-ounce package frozen snow peas, thawed or steamed; then cooled

1 teaspoon toasted sesame seeds

½ cup mung bean sprouts

1 11-ounce can mandarin oranges (optional)

Dressing

¾ cup white wine vinegar

¼ cup sugar

½ teaspoon sesame oil

1 teaspoon soy sauce

¼ teaspoon pepper

1. Toss salad ingredients in large salad bowl.

2. Add dressing and toss with salad.

(If you are accustomed to having more oil in your salad dressing, add a few extra teaspoons of vegetable oil.)

Nutrient Analysis per Serving

76 calories
12 grams carbohydrate
1 gram protein
3 grams fat

Key Nutrients

Vitamin C–16%
Folate–15%
Vitamin A–14%

Diabetic Exchanges

1 Vegetable
½ Fat
½ Starch

Pasta with Quick Alfredo Sauce

Do you love alfredo sauce, but hate its rich ingredients? Try this delicious, more healthful version.

Makes: 4 servings

1 cup low-fat cottage cheese

¼ cup Parmesan cheese, preferably freshly grated

¼ teaspoon garlic salt

¼ to ⅓ cup skim evaporated milk or fresh milk

2 dashes nutmeg

1 cup frozen peas, thawed or lightly cooked

4 cups cooked pasta

1. Purée all ingredients except peas and pasta in food processor or blender.

2. Pour into microwave-safe container and cook on medium-high for 2 minutes. Or place in saucepan and cook on a low flame until warm.

3. Toss pasta with peas.

4. Pour sauce over pasta. Garnish with more Parmesan cheese.

Variation

Use canned mushroom pieces instead of peas. Add several ounces of chopped lean ham.

Nutrient Analysis per Serving

313 calories
46 grams carbohydrate
20 grams protein
5 grams fat

Key Nutrients

Vitamin B$_{12}$–24%
Calcium–16%
Folate–10%

Diabetic Exchanges

3 Starches
1½ Lean Meats

Rocky Mountain Quesadillas

This can be served as a snack, an appetizer, or a light meal. The figs give this dish a real nutritional boost!

Makes: 1 serving

1 small whole-wheat flour tortilla

1 ounce farmer cheese, grated or sliced

4 figs

1. Cut figs in half. Arrange them on one half of flour tortilla.

2. Top with cheese.

3. Broil until cheese is just melting; then fold over.
OR
Fold over tortilla and cook in microwave on medium-high for 45 seconds to 1 minute.

Nutrient Analysis per Serving

268 calories
44 grams carbohydrate
10 grams protein
7 grams fat
4 grams fiber

Key Nutrients

Calcium–23%
Potassium–15%
Magnesium–11%

Diabetic Exchanges

2 Fruit
1 Lean Meat
1 Starch

Spring Vegetables in Cream Sauce

This recipe is very versatile: it can be a side dish, a light meal over angel hair pasta, or a filling for crepes. You can also add cooked chicken breast, shrimp, crab, or white beans for a complete meal.

Makes: 4 servings

Sauce

1½ cups fat-free chicken broth

1 cup skim milk

1 package Butter Buds

3 tablespoons cornstarch

½ teaspoon tarragon

¼ teaspoon each dill and basil

½ teaspoon onion powder

½ teaspoon garlic salt

1 teaspoon lemon pepper

1 teaspoon lemon juice

Vegetables

1 1-pound package Green Giant California Style Vegetables (*has cauliflower, carrots, asparagus*) *or use other frozen vegetable mixtures*

1 7- or 14-ounce can artichoke hearts, quartered

½ red bell pepper, sliced thinly

1. Put chicken broth, milk, cornstarch, and Butter Buds in blender. Blend on high until blended well.

2. Pour mixture into large saucepan and add rest of sauce ingredients.

3. Cook over medium heat, stirring often until thickened.

4. Meanwhile, steam vegetables or cook in microwave.

5. Add steamed vegetabels to thickened sauce and serve.

Nutritional Analysis per Serving

103 calories
22 grams carbohydrate
6 grams protein
0 grams fat
4 grams fiber

Key Nutrients

Vitamin A–124%
Vitamin C–56%
Folate–19%

Diabetic Exchanges

1 Starch
2 Vegetables

Strawberry Bread

My friend, Peggy Conner, made and served this bread at my baby shower. Serve with fat-free cream cheese that's been whipped with strawberry fruit spread.

Makes: 16 pieces

1½ cups sifted flour

½ cup whole-wheat flour

½ cup old-fashioned rolled oats

2 tablespoons wheat germ

½ teaspoon baking soda

2 teaspoons baking powder

½ teaspoon salt

2½ teaspoons cinnamon

¼ cup sugar

2 tablespoons vegetable oil

2 10-ounce packages of frozen, sliced, sweetened strawberries, thawed, drained to equal 1¾ cups

½ cup unsweetened applesauce

2 eggs

½ cup pecans, chopped (optional)

Cooking spray or margarine to grease the pan

1. Preheat oven to 325° F.

2. Combine first 8 ingredients. Mix well.

3. Add the rest of ingredients except nuts and mix just until moistened. Gently fold in nuts, if desired.

4. Pour into 8-by-8-inch pan that has been sprayed with cooking spray or lightly oiled and bake for 45 to 55 minutes.

Quick Tip

No applesauce in the house? Peel a medium-sized apple, place in a microwave-safe dish, cover, and cook in microwave 5 minutes. When cool, remove core and mash with fork. One cooked apple equals about ½ cup applesauce.

Nutrient Analysis per Serving

131 calories

24 grams carbohydrate

3 grams protein

3 grams fat

3 grams fiber

Key Nutrients

Manganese–17%

Vitamin C–16%

And small amounts of many nutrients.

Diabetic Exchanges

1½ Starches

½ Fat

Thrive-on-Five Bread

Experimenting with a basic zucchini bread recipe of mine, I added ingredients until I came up with a bread that contained five different fruits and vegetables!

Makes: one 15-slice loaf

½ cup each whole-wheat flour, white flour and wheat germ

2 teaspoons baking soda

1 teaspoon baking powder

½ teaspoon cinnamon

¼ teaspoon cloves

¼ teaspoon ginger

¼ cup vegetable oil

1 egg

¼ cup brown sugar

⅓ cup molasses

½ cup crushed pineapple in juice, drained well

½ cup applesauce

1 cup each carrot and zucchini, grated

½ cup raisins

Cooking spray or margarine to grease pan

1. Preheat oven to 350° F.

2. Mix together in a bowl all dry ingredients except for sugar and set aside. In a separate bowl, mix together oil, egg, brown sugar, and molasses. Add vegetables and fruits.

3. Gradually add dry ingredients to sugar mixture. Mix just until moistened.

4. Pour mixture into 9-by-5-inch loaf pan that is lightly oiled or sprayed with cooking spray. Bake 50 to 60 minutes.

Nutrient Analysis per Serving

136 calories
23 grams carbohydrate
3 grams protein
5 grams fat
2 grams fiber

Key Nutrients

Manganese–24%
Vitamin A–17%
Iron–7%

Diabetic Exchanges

1½ Starch
1 Fat
A tiny portion of Fruit and Vegetable

Apple Date Bran Muffins

This recipe was developed by Deborah Compton who loves to cook. Muffins can be baked and served fresh or kept as ready-to-bake dough in the refrigerator for up to one week!

Makes: 24 muffins

1 cup oat-flake cereal

2 cups 100% bran cereal

1 cup low-fat buttermilk, scalded, or 1 cup plain nonfat yogurt, heated

2 large eggs or ½ cup egg substitute

½ cup margarine, at room temperature

1½ cups brown sugar, packed

1 cup low-fat buttermilk or 1 cup plain nonfat yogurt

1 cup unsweetened applesauce (choose one with vitamin C)

2 cups all-purpose flour

½ cup whole-wheat flour

2½ teaspoons baking soda

¼ teaspoon salt

1 cup dates, chopped

Cooking spray, margarine, or muffin liners

1. Preheat oven to 400° F. In a large bowl, combine oat and bran cereals; pour scalding buttermilk over the cereal mixture and stir.

2. Add eggs, margarine, sugar, the second cup of buttermilk, and applesauce; mix to blend.

3. Mix flour, soda, and salt in a separate bowl and then stir into cereal mixture just until moistened.

4. Fold in dates.

5. Grease muffin tins, spray with cooking spray, or line with paper liners. Fill muffin tins ⅔ full. Bake 20 to 25 minutes.

Diabetic Variation

Reduce brown sugar to ½ cup and substitute ½ cup thawed apple juice concentrate.

Nutrient Analysis per Serving

147 calories
27 grams carbohydrate
3 grams protein
4 grams fat
2 grams fiber

Key Nutrients

Small amounts of all nutrients.

Nutrient Analysis per Serving
(Diabetic Variation)

134 calories
24 grams carbohydrate
3 grams protein
4 grams fat
2 grams fiber

Diabetic Exchanges

1½ Starches
1 Fat

Pumpkin Muffins

Makes: 12 muffins

2 egg whites or 1 egg

1 tablespoon whipped margarine

¾ cup + 2 tablespoons canned unsweetened pumpkin

⅔ cup brown sugar

¾ cup skim milk

2 cups all-purpose flour

2 teaspoons baking powder

½ teaspoon baking soda

½ teaspoon salt

¼ teaspoon ground ginger

½ teaspoon each ground cinnamon and nutmeg

½ cup raisins (optional)

Cooking spray

1. Preheat oven to 400° F. In large bowl, combine egg whites, margarine, pumpkin, sugar, and milk.

2. In small bowl, combine remaining ingredients.

3. Fold the wet ingredients into the dry ingredients just until blended. Fold in raisins, if desired.

4. Spray muffin pan with cooking spray. Pour batter into pan and bake for 20 to 25 minutes.

5. Remove from pan and cool on wire rack.

Serving Suggestion

Serve with Orange Cream Cheese Spread: Mix fat-free cream cheese, orange marmalade, and powdered sugar, to taste.

Nutritional Analysis per Serving

169 calories
36 grams carbohydrate
4 grams protein
1 gram fat

Key Nutrients

Vitamin A–50%
Thiamin–16%
Iron–12%

Diabetic Exchanges

2½ Starches

Peach Popsicles

This recipe is from *Quick and Healthy* by Brenda Ponichtera and may be just the trick for "morning sickness." This treat also makes a great warm-weather snack. If you like "chunky" popsicles, experiment with adding a few fresh blueberries, grape halves, or other small pieces of fruit to fruit purée before pouring into popsicle containers.

Makes: 8 servings

1 can (16 ounces) sliced peaches, packed in juice, not drained

2 tablespoons sugar

1. In a blender, blend all ingredients until smooth.

2. Pour into popsicle containers and freeze until firm, about 3 to 5 hours.

Diabetic Variation

Omit sugar or use an equivalent of Equal.

Source: Reprinted with permission from *Quick and Healthy, Volume II*, by Brenda J. Ponichtera, R.D. (ScaleDown Publishing, Inc.)

Nutrient Analysis per Serving

36 calories
10 grams carbohydrate
0 grams protein
0 grams fat

Key Nutrients

Contains small amounts of many nutrients.

Diabetic Exchanges

⅔ Fruit

Tropical Pudding

Women who can't tolerate milk will enjoy this dessert.

Makes: 4 servings

*1 package vanilla instant
  pudding*
½ cup orange juice
1 cup plain nonfat yogurt
*½ cup crushed pineapple,
  well drained*
½ teaspoon coconut extract

1. Mix juice into pudding mix using wire whisk.

2. Stir in yogurt and coconut extract. Follow package directions.

3. Stir in pineapple.

4. Chill at least 30 minutes.

5. Garnish with pineapple slice.

Diabetic Variation

Substitute sugar-free instant pudding for regular pudding.

**Nutrient Analysis
per Serving**

*157 calories
36 grams carbohydrate
4 grams protein
0 grams fat*

**Key Nutrients for
Regular and
Diabetic
Variations**

*Vitamin B₁₂–35%
Vitamin C–22%
Calcium–10%*

**Nutrient Analysis
per Serving**
(Diabetic Variation)

*86 calories
18 grams carbohydrate
3.5 grams protein
0 grams fat*

**Diabetic
Exchanges**

*½ Fruit
½ Starch*

Shakes

These shakes can be made with plain yogurt or milk. Yogurt adds a little tanginess and makes the shake very thick.

Apple Pie á la Mode Shake

Makes: 2 servings

½ *cup applesauce, frozen*

2 *tablespoons brown sugar*

1 *cup skim milk or plain nonfat yogurt*

½ *teaspoon cinnamon or apple pie spice*

½ *teaspoon vanilla extract*

Ice as needed

1. Blend all in blender and serve.

Diabetic Variation

Instead of brown sugar, use Equal to taste.

Nutrient Analysis per Serving

120 calories
26 grams carbohydrate
4 grams protein
0 grams fat
1 gram fiber

Key Nutrients

Vitamin B$_{12}$–21%
Potassium–15%
Calcium–13%

Nutrient Analysis per Serving
(Diabetic Variation)

86 calories
17 grams carbohydrate
4 grams protein
0 grams fat
1 gram fiber

Diabetic Exchanges

⅔ *Fruit*
½ *Skim Milk*

Banana-Orange Flip

Makes: 2 servings

½ cup skim milk or plain nonfat yogurt

½ cup orange juice

1 frozen banana

1. Blend all in a blender and serve in tall glasses. Add ice as needed.

Nutrient Analysis per Serving

100 calories
22 grams carbohydrate
3 grams protein
0 grams fat

Key Nutrients

Vitamin C–38%
Potassium–21%
Riboflavin–10%

Diabetic Exchanges

1¼ Fruit
¼ Skim Milk

Peanut Butter-Chocolate Shake

This shake is filling–drink it when you're hungry, trying to gain weight, or when you don't feel like preparing or eating an entire meal.

Makes: 1 serving

1 cup plain nonfat yogurt or skim milk

1 package chocolate instant breakfast mix

2 tablespoons smooth peanut butter

Ice as needed

1. Blend all in blender and serve in tall glasses.

Variations

Chocolate Mint: Omit peanut butter and substitute ½ teaspoon peppermint flavoring.

Vanilla Fruit: Use vanilla instant breakfast mix and substitute frozen unsweetened berries, frozen pineapple and banana, or peaches.

Chocolate Mocha: Dissolve 1 teaspoon of instant decaffeinated coffee mix to milk before blending.

Note: This recipe contains significant amounts of sugar. Use sugar-free hot cocoa mix or sugar-free instant breakfast mix instead of regular.

Nutrient Analysis per Serving

351 calories
43 grams carbohydrate
24 grams protein
9 grams fat

Key Nutrients

Vitamin A–66%
Calcium–46%
Magnesium–46%
Vitamin C–41%
Zinc–37%

The reason for this recipe's high nutrient content is the use of the instant breakfast mix, which is fortified. If you eat more than one fortified food in a day, such as instant breakfast and a fortified cereal, PLUS your prenatal vitamin, you will be getting more than your day's requirements of some vitamins and minerals.

Piña Colada Frappé

Makes: 2 servings

½ cup frozen pineapple

½ frozen banana

1 cup plain nonfat yogurt

½ teaspoon coconut extract

2 teaspoons of sugar or 1 packet of Equal (optional)

1. Blend all in a blender and serve in tall glasses.

Nutrient Analysis per Serving

127 calories
25 grams carbohydrate
7 grams protein
0 grams fat
1 gram fiber

Key Nutrients

Potassium—23%
Calcium—20%
Vitamin C—14%

Diabetic Exchanges

1 Fruit
¾ Skim Milk

Raspberry Surprise Shake

Makes: 2 servings

*1 cup plain nonfat yogurt
or 1 cup skim milk*

*2 fresh peaches or nectarines,
peeled, sliced, and frozen*

*½ of one 10-ounce package
frozen sweetened raspberries*

1. Blend all in a blender and serve in tall glasses.

Variation

Use frozen strawberries instead of raspberries.

Diabetic Variation

Use unsweetened fruit and add Equal, to taste.

Nutrient Analysis per Serving

174 calories
36 grams carbohydrate
8 grams protein
0 grams fat
3 grams fiber

Key Nutrients

Vitamin B$_{12}$–31%
Potassium–27%
Vitamin C–26%

Nutrient Analysis per Serving
(Diabetic Variation)

135 calories
26 grams carbohydrate
8 grams protein
3 grams fiber
0 grams fat

Diabetic Exchanges

1½ Fruit
½ Milk

Very Berry Shake

This is my favorite shake. If you have children at home, they will love its pretty purple color.

Makes: 2 servings

1 cup unsweetened frozen strawberries and blueberries, or any combination of berries

1 cup vanilla nonfat yogurt or skim milk plus 1 teaspoon vanilla and sugar, to taste

1. Blend all in a blender and serve in tall glasses.

Diabetic Variation

Use vanilla sugar-free nonfat yogurt.

Nutrient Analysis per Serving

112 calories
23 grams carbohydrate
6 grams protein
0 grams fat
2 grams fiber

Key Nutrients

Vitamin C–60%
Potassium–18%
Calcium–17%

Diabetic Exchanges

1 Fruit
½ Skim Milk

CHAPTER FOURTEEN

Menus and Recipes for the Second Trimester

A Month of Breakfast Ideas

Do you ever get tired of eating the same things, day-in, day-out, for breakfast? Here is a whole month's-worth of meal and recipe ideas to help relieve your boredom.

- Peanut butter on toast with banana
- Frozen Nutri-Grain waffles topped with blueberries
- Vanilla yogurt with Health Valley Granola, bran muffin
- Oat bran cereal with strawberries
- Country Brunch Casserole (page 302), oat toast, milk
- Apple Date Bran Muffins (page 234), mixed fresh fruit salad, milk
- Orange slices, wheat berry English muffin with farmer cheese
- Strawberry Bread (page 232) with light or fat-free cream cheese, mango slices, milk
- French French Toast (page 252), broiled grapefruit, milk
- Microwaved scrambled eggs with low-fat cheese, mushrooms, and tomato slices, toast, milk
- Krusteaz Oat Bran Belgium Waffles with peaches
- Cantaloupe and cottage cheese, blueberry bagel
- Bran cereal with mixed dried fruit, milk
- Oatmeal with raisins, peanut butter on graham crackers, milk
- Poached egg and ham on English muffin, tangerine, milk
- Mixed fresh fruit salad, Quick and Healthier Pancakes (page 251), yogurt
- Bran muffin, honeydew melon, milk

- Thrive-on-Five Bread (page 233) with fat-free cream cheese, hot cocoa
- Breakfast Pancakes with Raspberry Sauce (page 250), milk
- Hot wheat cereal with chopped dried figs, milk
- Berry Mousse Parfait (page 273), cinnamon toast triangles, milk
- Melted Swiss cheese on rye bread, apple pieces, milk
- Cantaloupe, wheat toast with peanut butter, milk
- Vegetable juice, boiled eggs, wheat bagel, milk
- Cheerios, banana, milk
- Corn muffins, refried beans with cheese, fresh pear, milk
- Vegetarian Breakfast Tacos (page 319), kiwi, milk
- Peanut butter and honey on whole-wheat bread, kiwi and peaches, milk
- Banana-Orange Flip (page 239), oat-bran toast
- Leftover Broccoli Quiche (page 296), watermelon cubes, milk
- Cinnamon bread with Caramel Dip (page 321)
- Raspberry Surprise Shake (page 242), poppy-seed muffin
- Very Berry Shake (page 243), bran muffin

Menus for a Hungry Appetite

Mixed green salad
Stuffed Eggplant Creole (page 268)
Wheat baguette
Frozen yogurt with berries

Vegetable juice
French French Toast (page 252)
Mixed fruit salad

Leek and Potato Soup (page 253)
Chicken Roll-Ups (page 258)
Carrots Antibes (page 226)
Wheat rolls
Fruit Crisp (page 323)

Salad with grated carrot, red cabbage, garbanzo beans, and corn
Pasta with Quick Alfredo Sauce (page 229)
Garlic bread
Tropical Pudding (page 237)

Raw veggies with Boursin Cheese Spread (page 288)
Tortellini with Creamy Pesto Sauce (page 259)
Wheat rolls
Chocolate Mocha Cake (page 274) with strawberries

Caesar salad
Spinach-Stuffed Shells (page 314)
Carrots, zucchini, and yellow squash
Hard rolls
Frozen melon balls

Coleslaw with pineapple
Vegetarian Chili (page 320)
Baked Tortilla Chips (page 224)
Frozen yogurt with blueberries
Sugar cookies

Chicken and Shrimp with Fruit Salsa (page 299)
Broccoli and carrot stir-fry
Roasted New Potatoes (page 312)
Strawberry Bread (page 232)

Piña Colada Frappé (page 241)
Breakfast Pancakes with Raspberry Sauce (page 250)
Turkey sausage slices
Milk

Creamy Broccoli Soup (page 220)
Greek Island Pita Pockets (page 263)
Banana pudding

▼

I Could Cook All Day Menus

Sesame Beef (page 313)
Oriental noodles
Stir-fried vegetables
Tangy Salad (page 269)

Vegetables in Vinaigrette
(page 317)
Turkey Pot Pie (page 271)
Chocolate Mocha Cake
(page 274)

Mushroom and Barley Soup
(page 255)
Grilled pork loin chops
Ratatouille (page 311)
over rice or bulgur
Frozen yogurt with fresh fruit

Orange-glazed Cornish hens
Thanksgiving Sweet Potatoes
(page 270)
Green beans almondine
Pumpkin Roll (page 275)

Three-bean salad
Crab Marinara over
angel hair pasta (page 303)
Herbed dinner rolls
Sunshine Sorbet (page 325)

Homemade cream of
tomato soup
Hoppin' John (page 306)
Cheese cornbread rolls
Lime sorbet with blueberries

▼

Company's Coming! Menus

Brunch Menus

Watermelon and
cantaloupe balls
Country Brunch Casserole
(page 302)
Apple Date Bran Muffins
(page 234)
Steamed milk with amaretto
flavoring

Oriental Salad (page 228)
Broccoli Quiche (page 296)
Strawberry Bread (page 232)

Very Berry Shake (page 243)
Breakfast Pancakes with
Raspberry Sauce (page 250)
Vegetarian breakfast sausage

Creamy Broccoli Soup
(page 220)
Chicken and Spinach Salad
(page 227)
French bread
Apple slices with Caramel
Dip (page 321)

Pineapple-orange juice
spritzers
Crepes with various fillings
(page 261)
(you could also turn this
into a "Bring Your Own
Filling" party)
Grilled Canadian bacon

Berry Mousse Parfait
(page 273)
Strawberry Bread (page 232)
and Pumpkin Muffins
(page 235)
Lite or fat-free cream cheese
whipped with orange
marmalade and
powdered sugar
Cinnamon-orange herb tea

Lunch or Dinner Menus

Boursin Cheese Spread
(page 288) with fresh vegetables and French bread
Cranberry juice and
sparkling water spritzers
Company Fondue (page 260)
Fruit Pizza for a Crowd
(page 324)

Spinach-Stuffed Shells
(page 314)
Garlic bread sticks
Tossed salad
Frozen blueberry yogurt
with raspberries

Mushroom and Barley Soup
(page 255)
Chicken with Dijon Sauce
(page 304)
Bulgur and Veggie Mix
(page 297)
Wheat rolls
Blueberry Cobbler (page 276)

Apricot-Glazed Chicken
(page 295)
Steamed asparagus
with lemon
Rice wheat-berry pilaf
Mixed fruit salad
Apple Date Bran Muffin
(page 234)

Mixed green salad
Corn muffins
Spanish Steak Roll with
Sautéed Vegetables
(page 267)
Potatoes Marie Louise
(page 265)
Raspberry sorbet

Salmon en Papillote with juli-
enne vegetables (page 266)
Spaghetti squash with warm
tarragon vinaigrette
Country sourdough bread
Peaches and blueberries
topped with lemon yogurt

Sliced tomatoes and cucum-
bers in vinaigrette dressing
Spring Vegetables in Cream
Sauce over linguini
(page 231)
Peach Cobbler (page 276)

Coleslaw
Quick Grilled Fish (page 310)
Carrots Antibes (page 226)
Wild rice pilaf
Chocolate Mocha Cake
(page 274) with strawber-
ries and Lite Cool Whip

Minute Minestrone
(page 254)
Crepes (page 261):
Ham and Cheese Crepes
Spinach and Cheese crepes
Fruit crepes with yogurt

Oven-Fried Zucchini
(page 222) with Ranch dip
Crab Marinara (page 303)
Sunshine Sorbet (page 325)

Vegetables in Vinaigrette
(page 317)
Veal Piccata with Roasted
Red Pepper and Cream
Sauce (page 316)
Spinach pasta with vegetables
Apple tart

Tossed salad
Cheese-Topped Orange
Roughy (page 298)
French-style green beans
and corn
Roasted New Potatoes
(page 312)
Fresh melon

Mexican Kale and Pork Soup
(page 290)
Stuffed Eggplant Creole
(page 268)
Low-fat cheesecake with
raspberries

Second-Trimester Recipes

These recipes were developed for your second-trimester eating moods. Most women feel their best during these months, so the recipes are hearty and require a bit more preparation time in the kitchen than recipes for the other trimesters. The recipes are loosely arranged in the following order: breakfast, soup, lunch/dinner, and dessert.

Breakfast Pancakes with Raspberry Sauce

With this dish, Margo Marrow won first place in the bread category of the Delicious and Nutritious Recipe Contest. Margo has a special interest in nutrition since she works for the WIC program, a nutrition program for children and pregnant women. Her recipe shows her love of good food and nutrition. The variety of grains boosts the recipe's nutrient and fiber content and the raspberry sauce is high in vitamin C.

Makes: 3 servings

Pancakes

¾ **cups soy-wheat pancake flour (or use ¼ cup soy flour and ½ cup wheat flour)**

¼ **cup each corn meal, oatmeal, and white flour**

3 **egg whites**

¾ **cup skim evaporated milk or skim milk**

½ **cup orange juice**

Margarine, canola oil, or vegetable spray to grease griddle

Raspberry Sauce

1 **10-ounce package frozen raspberries (unsweetened) or 1¼ cup fresh berries**

3 **tablespoons sugar**

1 **tablespoon cornstarch**

1 **teaspoon vanilla**

⅓ **cup any juice (orange, apple, or cranberry)**

Pancakes

1. Lightly beat egg whites. Add milk, flours, and orange juice. Using paper towel, lightly grease pan with oil or spray with cooking spray.

2. Pour 3-inch pancakes using 1 full tablespoon for each.

3. Serve on plates kept hot in the oven.

Raspberry Sauce

1. Strain thawed berries, reserving juice. Heat raspberry juice in saucepan until it simmers.

2. Dissolve cornstarch in cold juice. Add with sugar to simmering raspberry juice. Stir occasionally to prevent sticking.

3. Cook until slightly thick and clear. Add vanilla and berries.

4. Serve warm over pancakes.

Nutrient Analysis
(Diabetic Variation)

292 calories
55 grams carbohydrate
13 grams protein
2 grams fat
5 grams fiber

Key Nutrients
(Diabetic Variation)

Vitamin C–90%
Potassium–31%
Folate–20%

Nutrient Analysis per Serving

298 calories
58 grams carbohydrate
12 grams protein
2 grams fat
5 grams fiber

Key Nutrients

Vitamin C–32%
Magnesium–20%
Calcium–13%

Diabetic Variation

Omit sugar and use ⅕ cup diluted frozen juice concentrate instead of regular juice in sauce.

Diabetic Exchanges

2 Starches
1 Fruit
½ Skim Milk
½ Fat

Quick and Healthier Pancakes

I developed this recipe for those who aren't quite ready for 100 percent whole-grain pancakes, but yet want something healthier than "all white" pancakes.

Makes: 4 servings

1 reduced-fat Bisquick mix

½ cup old-fashioned oatmeal

½ cup wheat germ

4 tablespoons molasses

½ cup skim or 1% milk (or low-fat yogurt)

1 teaspoon cinnamon

1 egg or 2 egg whites

Cooking spray or oil to grease the pan

1. Mix all ingredients together just until well blended.

2. Spray pan with cooking spray or use small amount of oil. Pour about ⅛ cup of batter for each pancake.

3. Cook over medium heat until bubbles form on top and batter looks "set."

4. Turn and cook briefly until the pancake reaches desired shade of brown.

Variation

After pouring batter, add raisins and/or thinly sliced bananas on top of batter. Gently push into batter. Cook as usual. This makes the pancake sweet, so you can cut down or omit the syrup. The leftovers also make a good snack.

Nutrient Analysis per Serving

279 calories

47 grams carbohydrate

10 grams protein

5 grams fat

2 grams fiber

Key Nutrients

Selenium–38%

Zinc–19%

Iron–17%

Calcium–16%

Diabetic Exchanges

3 Starches

1 Fat

French French Toast

When you're married to someone from another country, you find out which ethnic foods are "real." Although our version of "French" toast doesn't exist in France, my mother-in-law remembers eating French French Toast as a child. This dish is great for those with a hearty appetite or for those who need to gain more weight.

Makes: 2 servings

2 large eggs or 4 egg whites

3 tablespoons skim or low-fat milk

Salt and pepper to taste

6 slices of stale French bread or 4 slices regular bread

Cooking spray

2 ounces ham

1½ ounces Swiss cheese

1. Mix eggs, milk, salt, and pepper. Soak bread pieces in egg mixture. Spray pan with cooking spray.

2. Place bread in pan and cook over medium heat for several minutes.

3. Turn bread pieces over and add ham and cheese to each piece. Cook several more minutes, and remove when cheese is melted.

Nutrient Analysis per Serving

347 calories

29 grams carbohydrate

24 grams protein

14 grams fat

1 gram fiber

Key Nutrients

Selenium—80%

Calcium—25%

Chromium—23%

Diabetic Exchanges

2½ Medium–Fat Meats

2 Starches

½ Fat

Leek and Potato Soup

When you taste this soup, you may swear it has ham in it–it doesn't! This soup is great on a fall or winter day with cheese toast and fresh fruit. Spinach, combinations of leftover green vegetables, or vegetable mixtures can also be substituted.

Makes: 16 servings

2 pounds of leeks
4 medium carrots
8 potatoes
2 cups evaporated skim milk
Salt and pepper, to taste

1. Peel potatoes and carrots. Cut leeks down the center and rinse thoroughly. Cut all vegetables into 1-to-2-inch pieces.

2. Place all vegetables into large pot of hot water. Bring to a boil and simmer, covered, for 45 minutes, or until potatoes and carrots are tender. (Since carrots take longer to cook, you may want to give them a head start in the pot.)

3. Drain 90 percent of the water. Purée in batches in blender, adding a small amount of milk to each batch.

4. Place all puréed soup in large bowl. Stir well, adding additional milk if needed. Add salt and pepper, to taste.

Nutrient Analysis per Serving

141 calories
30 grams carbohydrate
6 grams protein
0 grams fat
3 grams fiber

Key Nutrients

Vitamin A–74%
Vitamin B₆–24%
Folate and
*   Vitamin C–17%*

Diabetic Exchanges

2 Vegetables
1 Starch
½ Skim Milk

Minute Minestrone

This hearty vegetable soup can't be beat for a quick, nutritious meal on a cold night.

Makes: 4 servings

5 ounces frozen spinach, thawed, or cooked and minimal amount of water, not drained

1 8-ounce can tomato sauce

1 14½-ounce can diced tomatoes

1 cup green beans

1 cup garbanzo or kidney beans

¾ to 1 cup pasta, cooked

1 cup water

½ teaspoon onion powder

½ teaspoon garlic powder

1 teaspoon Italian spices

½ teaspoon basil, dried

Parsley, 1 teaspoon dried or 2 teaspoons fresh

1. Combine all ingredients in a 1½-quart saucepan.

2. Simmer 10 to 15 minutes, until heated. Add more water for a thinner soup.

Variation

Omit green beans and spinach and add one 10-ounce package frozen mixed vegetables to soup. Cook until vegetables are done.

Nutrient Analysis per Serving

182 calories

36 grams carbohydrate

9 grams protein

2 grams fat

Key Nutrients

Vitamin A–51%

Vitamin C–46%

Potassium–41%

Iron–15%

Diabetic Exchanges

3 Vegetables

1½ Starches

½ Fat

Mushroom and Barley Soup

This can become a main dish soup by adding 2 cups cooked chicken or white beans.

Makes: 6 servings

½ cup pearl barley, uncooked
4½ cups water
1 medium onion, chopped
2 medium cloves garlic, minced
1 pound mushrooms, sliced
1-2 tablespoons dry sherry
3 cups fat-free chicken broth
Freshly ground black pepper

1. Place the barley and 1½ cups of the water in a large saucepan. Bring to a boil, cover, and simmer until the barley is tender (20 to 30 minutes).

2. Meanwhile, heat 1 to 2 tablespoons water in a skillet. Add the onions and sauté for about 5 minutes over medium heat; add garlic and mushrooms. Cover and cook, stirring occasionally, until everything is very tender, about 10 to 12 minutes.

3. Add the sauté with all its liquid to the cooked barley, along with the remaining 2 cups water, sherry, and broth. Grind in a generous amount of black pepper and simmer, partially covered, another 20 minutes over very low heat. Season to taste and serve.

Nutritional Analysis per Serving

87 calories
17 grams carbohydrate
3 grams protein
0 grams fat
3 grams fiber

Key Nutrients

14% Niacin
14% Selenium
10% Potassium

Diabetic Exchanges

1 Starch
½ Vegetable

Basic Bean Cooking

Soaking

Quick Soak

Add 6 to 8 cups hot water to 1 pound of beans. Bring to a boil and boil for 2 minutes; set aside and cover. Let soak 1 hour.

Overnight Soak

Add 6 cups cold water to 1 pound dry beans. Let soak overnight or at least 6 hours in a cool place; do not refrigerate. After soaking, drain the soaking water and rinse the beans before adding more water for cooking.

Cooking Methods

Standard Method

Place beans in large pot with 6 cups hot water. Boil gently with lid tilted until desired tenderness is reached.

Savory Method

Place beans in large pot with 3 cups hot water. **Add:**
  2 teaspoons onion salt,
  ¼ teaspoon garlic salt,
  ¼ teaspoon white pepper,
  1 tablespoon chicken-stock base or 3 consommé cubes.
Boil gently with lid tilted until desired tenderness is reached. Add water as needed to keep beans covered.

General Tips for Cooking Beans

- Simmer beans slowly; cooking too fast and stirring frequently breaks skins.
- Add 1 to 2 tablespoons of oil to prevent foaming.
- Acid slows down cooking. Add tomatoes, vinegar, etc., last.
- At high altitudes, beans take longer to cook.
- When cooking in hard water, add ⅛ to ¼ teaspoon baking soda (no more) per pound of beans to shorten cooking time.
- When cooking large lima beans, for casseroles and stews, which require longer cooking, avoid overcooking (the beans should not be falling apart). To purée or mash, cook until soft.
- Some old-time recipes call for cooking unsoaked lima beans with meats, vegetables, etc. This is acceptable. However, soaking and discarding soaking water improves the beans' flavor and digestibility and shortens their cooking time. Nutrient loss is minimal.
- Long, slow cooking in water is essential for rehydration and digestibility of dry beans.
- Microwave ovens can be used for reheating cooked or canned beans.

Source: *Favorite Recipes of Four Generations, Featuring California's Large Lima Beans,* by the Large Lima Council of the California Dry Bean Advisory Board.

Dry Bean Arithmetic

1-pound package
    = 2 cups beans
    = 5 cups soaked beans
1 15½-ounce can
    = 1⅜ cups beans

Basic Black Beans

Black beans often fill my craving for something creamy and rich that sticks to my ribs. This recipe can easily be turned into soup or a dip. I often eat them for lunch with fresh tomatoes and cheese melted on top. Or make a soft taco or tostado. If you don't have time to cook beans from scratch, keep a stock of canned beans on hand.

Makes: 10 servings

**1 pound dry black beans
or any dry bean**

4 cloves garlic

**3 medium shallots or 1 onion,
chopped**

**1 teaspoon each cumin and
chili powder**

½ teaspoon pepper

**2-3 pieces turkey bacon or ham
(optional)**

1. Soak beans overnight or use the quick-soak method. Discard soaking water.

2. Combine all ingredients in large pot. Add enough water to cover, about 6 cups.

3. Cook 4 to 6 hours, or until beans are tender.

Variations

"Refried" Black Beans: To 2 cups cooked beans, add 1 to 2 cloves minced garlic, or garlic powder, cumin, and salt, to taste. Mash by hand or in food processor or blender.

Quick Soup: Blend cooked beans and chicken broth in blender until desired consistency is reached. Add onion and garlic powder, cumin and chili powder, to taste. (See Aspen Black Bean Soup, page 292.)

Dip: Place 1½ cups of cooked beans in food processor. Add 1 tablespoon vinegar, 1 to 2 cloves mashed garlic, and ½ teaspoon salt (or use garlic salt, to taste, in place of garlic and salt). Process until smooth. Serve with baked tortilla chips or pita crisps.

Nutrient Analysis
per ⅔-Cup Serving

201 calories
34 grams carbohydrate
14 grams protein
1 gram fat
6 grams fiber

Key Nutrients

Folate–64%
Magnesium–37%
Zinc and Iron–12%

Diabetic Exchanges

2½ Starches
1 Very Lean Meat

Chicken Roll-Ups

This can be an elegant meal for company or just a casual meal for family.

Makes: 4 servings

4 skinless, boneless chicken breast halves

3 tablespoons light or fat-free cream cheese

2 teaspoons fresh parsley, minced

2 ounces lean ham, thinly sliced

⅓ cup Italian-style bread crumbs

1 teaspoon lemon pepper

½ teaspoon garlic salt

½ teaspoon basil

1 tablespoon Parmesan cheese, grated, fresh or canned

1 egg plus 1 tablespoon milk, beaten

Fresh parsley and lemon wedges for garnish

Cooking spray

1. Preheat oven to 350°F. Place all chicken breast halves between wax paper or plastic wrap and pound flat until they're almost ¼-inch thick.

2. In a small bowl, combine cream cheese with parsley. In a shallow dish, mix bread crumbs, spices, and Parmesan cheese.

3. Lay out one chicken breast half on a clean surface (plate, board, etc.). Place 1 slice of ham (½ ounce) on top. Spread ½ tablespoon of cream cheese mixture evenly over ham.

4. Roll up chicken breast, starting with small end. Secure with tooth picks, if necessary.

5. Beat 1 egg and 1 tablespoon milk in a shallow bowl. Dip the rolled chicken breast in egg mixture and roll in bread crumb mixture. Place in a small baking dish coated with cooking spray.

6. Repeat steps 3 to 5 with remaining chicken halves.

7. Bake uncovered for 30 minutes or until tender. Increase oven heat to broil last 2 to 3 minutes of cooking. Remove toothpicks before serving.

8. Serve sprinkled with fresh chopped parsley and lemon wedges.

Nutrient Analysis per Serving

270 calories

38 grams protein

8 grams carbohydrate

8 grams fat

Key Nutrients

Niacin—84%

Selenium—60%

Vitamin B$_6$—30%

Chromium—21%

Diabetic Exchanges

4½ Very Lean Meats

½ Starch

Creamy Pesto Sauce

If you like a lot of flavor without a lot of fat, you'll love this recipe. Try the sauce over fettuccine or small shells.

Makes: 4 servings

1 cup low-fat cottage cheese

¼ cup Parmesan cheese (preferably freshly grated)

1 cup plain nonfat yogurt

¼ cup prepared pesto sauce (can usually be purchased in produce department)

2 teaspoons tarragon vinegar

Freshly ground pepper

Salt

1. Combine all ingredients except yogurt in food processor or blender.

2. Blend until smooth, adding yogurt until desired thickness is achieved.

3. Pour into microwave-safe bowl and heat 2 minutes on medium-high. Or cook slowly, stirring frequently, on the stove until hot.

Nutrient Analysis per Serving

179 calories
8 grams carbohydrate
15 grams protein
9 grams fat

Key Nutrients

Vitamin B$_{12}$–36%
Calcium–20%
Potassium–14%

Diabetic Exchanges

1½ Lean Meats
1 Fat
½ Skim Milk

Company Fondue

The first time I ate this dish was at a gathering of coworkers. It was great fun because everyone brought a small portion of the meal, so the host didn't have much to prepare! For a last-minute company meal, I can't think of a faster meal to cook and serve.

Makes: 8 servings

Fondue

6 cups chicken or beef broth

4 pounds any combination of beef, chicken, shellfish, or tofu

1 pound fresh spinach, washed and trimmed

2 pounds fresh mushrooms, washed and trimmed

Dipping Sauces

Teriyaki sauce

Dijon cream sauce:
Mix ½ cup plain nonfat yogurt with ½ cup low-fat sour cream and 1 or 2 tablespoons Dijon mustard (to taste).

Sweet and sour sauce:
Heat ½ cup fruit spread (apricot or plum) with 1 tablespoon soy sauce and 1 or 2 teaspoons vinegar (to taste).

Horseradish mayonnaise:
Mix 1 tablespoon white horseradish with ½ cup low-fat or fat-free mayonnaise.

Honey-mustard sauce

Steak sauce/barbecue sauce

1. Cut meat and chicken into 1-inch pieces.

2. Heat broth to boiling. Pour into fondue pot or crock pot.

3. Arrange meats and vegetables on separate platters.

4. Using fondue forks, guests cook meat and vegetables to desired doneness and dip in sauces.

5. When everyone is finished eating, pour a dash of sherry or sherry vinegar into the broth, divide it among the guests, and pass out soup spoons.

Variation

Serve fondue with noodles or brown rice and tossed green salad.

Nutrient Analysis per Serving
(not including broth or sauces)

259 calories
3 grams carbohydrate
41 grams protein
9 grams fat

Key Nutrients

Zinc–20%
Vitamin B₆–20%
Folate–17%
Iron–17%

Diabetic Exchanges

5½ Lean Meats
½ Vegetable

Crepe Dinner

I had to include one of our family favorites. Crepes are versatile; you can have them for breakfast, an elegant lunch, dinner, or dessert. Have the leftovers as a snack. Or host a "Make-Your-Own-Crepe Party!"

Makes: 10 to 12 servings

Batter

1 whole egg or 2 egg whites

2 teaspoons canola oil

¼ teaspoon salt

2 cups flour

2 cups skim or evaporated skim milk

1 cup plus 2 tablespoons water

Cooking spray

For dessert crepes add:
  1 teaspoon vanilla and
  2 tablespoons sugar

1. In a large bowl, beat eggs, oil, and salt. Alternate flour, milk, and water. Add vanilla and sugar for sweet crepes. Beat until smooth. Let stand several minutes.

2. Using ladle, pour 2 to 3 tablespoons of batter into heated 10-inch nonstick skillet sprayed with cooking spray. It is essential to use a pan that is in good shape that doesn't have nicks or scratches. After pouring batter into pan, quickly rotate the pan so that the batter completely covers the bottom of pan.

3. Cook over medium to medium-high heat until one side starts browning. Turn crepe over and cook briefly on other side.

4. Fill immediately with one of the fillings listed below (or use your own filling), or place between pieces of waxed paper or foil to use later or to freeze.

5. Unused batter may be kept several days in refrigerator. Before using, let the batter sit at room temperature a few minutes; then beat well.

Variations for Fillings

Breakfast

Peanut butter and banana

Berries and strawberry fruit spread or powdered sugar

Ham and cheese

Margarine and sugar or honey

Applesauce and cinnamon

Fresh fruit and yogurt *(continued on next page)*

Crepe Dinner
(continued)

Lunch or Dinner

Spinach filling from Spinach-Stuffed Shells (page 314)

Ham and Swiss cheese, topped with Dijon Sauce (page 304)

Chicken and mushrooms topped with thick cream-of-mushroom soup

Ratatouille (page 311) and mozzarella cheese

Salmon Paté (page 221) with Cucumber Yogurt Sauce (page 263)
Sautéed or steamed shrimp and scallops with white sauce

Boursin Cheese Spread (page 288)

Dessert

Peaches with Caramel Dip (page 321)

Fresh fruit with vanilla yogurt

Chocolate frozen yogurt topped with raspberries

Margarine and sugar or honey

Vanilla frozen yogurt and blueberries with heated strawberry all-fruit spread

Vanilla frozen yogurt with bananas that are cooked in orange juice
and brown sugar

Nutrient Analysis per Serving
(2 unfilled crepes)

120 calories
22 grams carbohydrate
5 grams protein
1 gram fat

Key Nutrients

Contains small amounts of all nutrients. Depending upon the fillings you choose, your crepes can be chock-full of nutrients.

Diabetic Exchanges

1 Starch
½ Fat

Greek Island Pita Pockets
with Cucumber Yogurt Sauce

This dish mimics the flavor of a gyro sandwich, but uses less fat.

Makes: 4 servings

Pita Stuffing

**1 pound boneless pork loin
or loin chops**

1 clove garlic, minced

½ cup lemon juice

1 teaspoon dry oregano

1 tablespoon Dijon mustard

**4 pieces of whole-wheat
pita bread**

1 tomato, chopped

**Leaf or romaine lettuce,
shredded**

Cucumber Yogurt Sauce

½ cup plain low-fat yogurt

**½ small clove garlic (or less if
you can't tolerate garlic well.
You may just want to put a few
dashes of garlic powder.)**

¼ teaspoon oregano

1 teaspoon lemon juice

½ cucumber, peeled and chopped

⅛ teaspoon salt

1. Cut pork into ½-inch slices.

2. Mix together garlic, lemon juice, and spices in Ziploc bag or glass container. Add pork and marinate at least 1 hour.

3. Stir-fry 3 to 5 minutes until pork is no longer pink and is thoroughly cooked. Stuff meat, lettuce, and tomato inside pita bread.

4. To make the sauce, place all sauce ingredients in food processor or blender and blend until cucumbers are finely chopped but not puréed. Or, chop cucumber finely by hand and mix with all other ingredients.

5. Top your stuffed pita with Cucumber Yogurt Sauce.

Nutrient Analysis per Serving	**Key Nutrients**	**Diabetic Exchanges**
417 calories	*Thiamin–82%*	*4½ Lean Meats*
26 grams carbohydrate	*Niacin–46%*	*1½ Starches*
38 grams protein	*Vitamin B₆–24%*	*½ Vegetable*
15 grams fat	*Zinc–19%*	
2 grams fiber		

Leg of Lamb

If not for my husband, I may never have had the joy of discovering leg of lamb. The French usually eat it with flagolet (a legume similar to a northern bean), green beans, and some type of potato. The leftovers are good served cold with Dijon mustard or eaten as a sandwich on an onion roll. Bon appetit!

1 leg of lamb, with or without bone

4-6 garlic cloves, peeled and sliced into 2 or 3 pieces

1½ teaspoons each rosemary, oregano, thyme, and marjoram

OR

3-4 teaspoons Herbes de Provence (found in gourmet shops)

1. Preheat oven to 450° F.

2. Cut small slits in leg. Insert garlic clove pieces as deep as possible into the slits.

3. Sprinkle outside of leg with spices.

4. Reduce oven heat to 325° F.

5. Bake 30 minutes per pound. If you prefer pink or rare meat, reduce cooking time to 15 or 20 minutes per pound. Internal temperature of meat should be 175° to 180° for well-done and 160° to 165° for medium-rare.

6. Serve with pan juices or mint jelly.

Nutrient Analysis per Serving
(1 serving is 4 ounces)

217 calories
0 grams carbohydrate
32 grams protein
9 grams fat

Key Nutrients

Zinc—46%
Iron—16%
Folate—14%

Diabetic Exchanges

4 Lean Meats

Potatoes Marie Louise

This is another favorite dish we serve in our home–it's a great way to include more vegetables in your diet (and to encourage picky children to gobble up their veggies!). Vary the amount of carrots used for a different flavor and color.

Makes: 18 servings

10 medium potatoes (about 7 ounces each), peeled and cubed

5 medium carrots, peeled and sliced

1 to 1½ cups evaporated skim milk

2 tablespoons soft margarine

Salt and pepper, to taste

1. Place potatoes and carrots in large pot; cover with water. Cook 45 minutes to 1 hour, or until both are tender.

2. Drain; place vegetables in large bowl. Whip with electric beater, adding milk, margarine, and seasoning. Add more milk until desired consistency is reached.

Variation

Add 3 ounces Light Velveeta cheese while beating for a richer, creamier dish.

Nutrient Analysis per Serving

127 calories
26 grams carbohydrate
3 grams protein
1 gram fat
2 grams fiber

Key Nutrients

Vitamin A–70%
Potassium–23%
Vitamin C–12%

Diabetic Exchanges

1½ Starch
1 Vegetable

Salmon en Papillote

The beauty of fish is that it cooks so quickly. This recipe is based on the "a dash of this and a dash of that" principle–so use your imagination! This dish is traditionally cooked in parchment paper; I use aluminum foil. Some people like to add a teaspoon of dry white wine or tarragon vinegar for more flavor. Salmon is a good source of omega-3 fatty acid, which is important for the development of your baby's nervous system and brain.

Makes: 4 servings

*4 pieces of salmon steak
  (about 1 pound)*

Lemon pepper

Dill, preferably fresh

Green onion and garlic, chopped

Basil, fresh

*Lemon juice (from a fresh lemon
  or in a bottle)*

Wine, soy sauce, or vinegar

Tomatoes, chopped

Garlic powder

*Zucchini and carrots,
  cut julienne-style (optional)*

Lemon slices

1. Preheat oven to 400° F. Place each piece of fish on top of a piece of foil or parchment paper big enough to wrap fish in.

2. Top each piece of fish with spices and lemon juice, dash of wine, soy sauce, or vinegar. Add or delete any spices according to your mood. Add herbs and vegetables. Top with several very thin lemon slices.

3. Bring together the ends of the paper above the fish and crimp the sides and ends of paper so that fish is enclosed in an almost air-tight package.

4. Place on cookie sheet and bake for 10 minutes per each inch of thickness of fish. Or cook on a medium-hot grill for 15 to 20 minutes.

5. Serve the fish still wrapped in its baking paper, so your guests can open their package and enjoy the aroma.

Nutrient Analysis per Serving

210 calories
0 grams carbohydrate
31 grams protein
9 grams fat

Key Nutrients

Niacin–56%
Selenium–53%
Magnesium–13%

Diabetic Exchanges

4 Lean Meats

Spanish Steak Roll with Sautéed Vegetables

Sandy Collins won first place with this recipe in a National Beef Cookoff. I'm sure you'll agree that this dish is delicious! Omit the chilies if you can't tolerate spicy foods.

Makes: 6 servings

1½ pounds boneless 1-inch-thick
beef top sirloin steak

1 teaspoon garlic powder,
divided in half

¼ teaspoon black pepper,
freshly ground

2 teaspoons vegetable oil,
divided in half

1 teaspoon butter

¾ teaspoon salt, divided in half

1 red and 1 green bell pepper,
cut lengthwise into strips

1 small white onion, thinly sliced

1 cup fresh mushrooms, sliced

⅓ cup walnuts, chopped

¼ teaspoon chili powder

1 tablespoon sour cream
or low-fat yogurt

1 4-ounce can green chilies,
chopped

Lemon slices

Cilantro sprigs

1. Pound boneless beef top sirloin steak to about ¼-inch thickness. Sprinkle with ½ teaspoon garlic powder and pepper.

2. Heat 1 teaspoon oil and butter in 12-inch heavy frying pan over medium-high heat until hot.

3. Pan-fry steak 5 to 7 minutes for medium-rare doneness, turning once.

4. Remove steak to heated platter and sprinkle with ½ teaspoon salt. Keep warm.

5. Add remaining 1 teaspoon oil to frying pan. Add red and green peppers, onion, mushrooms, and walnuts. Cook 2 minutes, stirring frequently.

6. Add remaining ½ teaspoon garlic powder, ¼ teaspoon salt, and chili powder; continue cooking 2 minutes, stirring frequently.

7. Spread steak with sour cream and top with chilies.

8. Starting at long side of steak, roll up jelly-roll fashion; secure with 6 wooden picks. Place vegetables around steak roll; garnish with lemon slices and cilantro sprigs. To serve, slice steak roll between wooden picks, then remove and discard wooden picks.

Reprinted with permission, 1991 National Beef Cookoff.

Nutrient Analysis per Serving

320 calories
7 grams carbohydrate
37 grams protein
16 grams fat
2 grams fiber

Key Nutrients

Vitamin C–58%
Zinc–52%
Magnesium–18%
Iron–15%

Diabetic Exchanges

5 Lean Meats
1 Vegetable

Stuffed Eggplant Creole

This recipe is pretty mild, so most pregnant women should be able to tolerate it!
Add more Tabasco sauce if you like it hot!

Makes: 4 servings

2 small eggplants
  (1 pound each)

1 tablespoon vegetable oil

1 pound shrimp, crawfish,
  ground beef, or tofu
  (or a combination)

1 clove garlic, crushed

¼ cup each: finely chopped
  onion, green pepper,
  and celery

1 14½-ounce can tomatoes,
  undrained

¼ teaspoon dried thyme

½ teaspoon salt

Dash of Tabasco sauce or
  cayenne pepper (optional)

1 cup seasoned or unseasoned
  dry bread crumbs

½ cup low-fat sour cream

1. Preheat oven to 375° F.

2. Wash eggplant; cut in half lengthwise. Place in large pan and cover with water. Bring to a boil, cover, and simmer 15 minutes. Drain and cool.

3. Scoop out pulp from eggplant, taking care to leave ¼ inch of the shell thickness intact.

4. In skillet, heat vegetable oil. Sauté garlic with either beef, seafood, or tofu.

5. Add raw vegetables and cook 5 minutes over low flame, stirring occasionally.

6. Stir in tomatoes, thyme, salt, and dash of Tabasco or cayenne pepper, if desired.

7. Add ½ cup of bread crumbs. Add eggplant pulp and sour cream. Stir.

8. Stuff this mixture back into 4 eggplant shells and top with remaining bread crumbs.

9. Place in baking dish and bake 30 minutes.

Nutrient Analysis per Serving

347 calories
37 grams carbohydrate
29 grams protein
9 grams fat
6 grams fiber

Key Nutrients

Vitamin C–35%
Magnesium–25%
Iron–19%
Zinc–15%

Diabetic Exchanges

3 Lean Meats
3 Vegetables
1½ Starches

Tangy Salad

Gwen Shaw often serves this to her family. Even picky children should enjoy this. It tastes like a Waldorf salad, but yummier!

Makes: 4 servings

Salad

1 green apple, peeled and chopped

1 large carrot, peeled and thinly sliced

1 celery stalk, chopped

1 medium orange, peeled, seeded, and sectioned (or use 1 11-ounce can mandarin oranges, drained)

4 tablespoons raisins

2 tablespoons walnuts, chopped

4 pieces of leaf lettuce

Dressing

¾ cup plain nonfat or low-fat yogurt

1½ tablespoons honey

1 tablespoon lemon juice

¼ teaspoon each: cinnamon and nutmeg

Fresh mint or orange twists for garnish

1. Combine ingredients for dressing in small bowl. Set aside.

2. Wash and drain lettuce. Line 4 plates with 1 whole lettuce leaf per plate.

3. Combine fruits and vegetables and toss with dressing. Divide into equal protions onto plates. Garnish each with orange slice and/or mint sprig.

Diabetic Variation

Substitute 2 packets of Equal for honey.

Nutrient Analysis per Serving

170 calories
30 grams carbohydrate
5 grams protein
3 grams fat
3 grams fiber

Key Nutrients

Vitamin A–67%
Vitamin C–37%
Potassium–19%

Nutrient Analysis
(Diabetic Variation)

145 calories
23 grams carbohydrate
5 grams protein
3 grams fat
3 grams fiber

Diabetic Exchanges

1 Fruit
1 Vegetable
½ Fat

Thanksgiving Sweet Potatoes

Have Thanksgiving anytime with this variation of a classic French dish!

Makes: 6 servings

3 medium sweet potatoes, peeled and thinly sliced

2 tablespoons margarine, melted

2 tablespoons brown sugar

1 teaspoon ginger root, minced or in a jar (prepared)

Cooking spray

1. Preheat oven to 400° F.

2. Spray a 9-inch glass pie plate with cooking spray.

3. Toss potatoes with 1 tablespoon melted margarine, sugar, and ginger.

4. Arrange potatoes in an overlapping circle around the bottom of the pie plate, adding a layer around the sides of the plate.

5. Brush the remaining melted margarine on top. Cover with foil and place another pie plate upside down on top.

6. Bake on the bottom rack for 30 minutes. Remove foil and top pie pan and bake another 30 minutes, or until potatoes are brown and caramelized.

Nutrient Analysis per Serving

126 calories
18 grams carbohydrate
1 gram protein
2 grams fiber

Key Nutrients

Vitamin A–158%
Vitamin C–20%

Diabetic Exchanges

1 Starch
1 Fat

Turkey Pot Pie

This recipe is a great way to use those holiday leftovers. Divide leftovers into individual microwave/freezer containers for your own "pot-pies-to-go."

Makes: 4 servings

Filling

4 medium carrots, peeled and sliced

1 teaspoon oil

¼ cup hot water

2 green onions, thinly sliced

1 clove garlic, minced

2 tablespoons cornstarch

¾ cup chicken broth

2 cups white turkey meat, skin removed, diced

½ cup frozen peas, thawed

½ cup evaporated skim milk

2 tablespoons parsley, chopped

¼ teaspoon each: thyme, salt, and pepper

Topping

1 can (8 biscuits) of prepared biscuit dough

1. Preheat oven to 375° F.

2. Place carrots, green onions, garlic, and oil in microwave-safe dish; add ¼ cup hot water and cover. Cook 5 to 8 minutes on high. Drain (reserving the liquid) and set aside.

3. Mix cornstarch with ¼ cup broth. Then stir in rest of broth, cooking liquid from carrots, and evaporated skim milk. Cook, stirring constantly until thickened, about 5 minutes.

4. Stir in remaining ingredients. Pour into pie pan or baking dish.

5. Arrange 8 pieces of biscuit dough over "pie." Bake 15 to 20 minutes or until biscuits are browned.

Nutrient Analysis per Serving

326 calories
39 grams carbohydrate
29 grams protein
6 grams fat

Key Nutrients

Vitamin A–247%
Vitamin B$_6$–28%
Zinc–15%
Iron–10%

Diabetic Exchanges

3 Lean Meats
2 Starches
1½ Vegetables

Turkey with Hoisin Sauce

I've discovered that turkey breast is even more versatile than chicken breast. It's larger, so you can cook it as a "roast," slice it into "fillets" or "scallopini" (as in veal), or slice it thin for stir-fry dishes. An added benefit is that turkey is often less expensive than boneless chicken breast!

Makes: 4 servings

2 teaspoons canola oil

1 clove garlic, minced

1 pound turkey cutlets,
or turkey tenderloin,
sliced in ½-inch slices

2 green onions, chopped

1 teaspoon cornstarch

½ cup water

2 tablespoons frozen orange
juice concentrate, thawed

2 tablespoons soy sauce

1 tablespoon hoisin sauce
(found in the oriental section
of your grocery)

1. Heat oil in nonstick pan over medium-high heat.

2. Add garlic. Sauté for 1 to 2 minutes.

3. Add turkey and sauté for 2 to 3 minutes on each side Remove and keep warm.

4. Add green onions to pan and sauté briefly.

5. In a small saucepan, mix cornstarch with ½ cup water. Add this mixture to pan along with orange juice, soy sauce, and hoisin sauce. Bring to a boil and cook until slightly thickened.

6. Pour sauce over turkey and serve.

Serving Suggestions

Serve with brown rice and stir-fried vegetables.

Nutrient Analysis per Serving

197 calories

3 grams carbohydrate

34 grams protein

4 grams fat

Key Nutrients

Niacin–50%

Vitamin B₆–29%

Vitamin B₁₂–20%

Diabetic Exchanges

5 Very Lean Meats

Berry Mousse Parfait

This delicious dish can be dessert or a snack. You can vary the types of yogurt and fruit.

Makes: 4 servings

2 8-ounce containers or fat-free or low-fat blueberry yogurt

1 cup Lite Cool Whip

2 cups strawberries and blueberries, sliced

1. Gently stir Cool Whip into blueberry yogurt.

2. In 4 parfait or wine glasses, layer yogurt mixture, then berries, then yogurt mixture.

3. Garnish with additional Cool Whip, a few berries and a sprig of mint.

Diabetic Variation

Use sugar-free yogurt instead of regular yogurt.

Nutrient Analysis per Serving

152 calories
31 grams carbohydrate
5 grams protein
2 grams fat
2 grams fiber

Key Nutrients

Vitamin C–52%
Potassium–19%
Calcium–15%

Nutrient Analysis per Serving
(Diabetic Variation)

106 calories
19 grams carbohydrate
5 grams protein
2 grams fat
2 grams fiber

Diabetic Exchanges

1 Fruit
½ Skim Milk

Chocolate Mocha Cake

Just because you're pregnant doesn't mean you need to give up your chocolate! (Just make it a little healthier!) This cake is so moist, it reminds me of chocolate cheesecake, and just a small piece should be enough to satisfy your craving.

Makes: 15 servings

1¾ cups flour

½ cup brown sugar, packed

¼ cup canola oil

¾ cup evaporated skim milk

¼ cup cocoa powder

½ cup applesauce

1 cup strong decaffeinated coffee

1 teaspoon baking powder

1 teaspoon baking soda

1 teaspoon vanilla

Margarine and flour for greasing pan

1. Preheat oven to 375° F.

2. Mix all ingredients until well blended, about 1 to 2 minutes with electric mixer.

3. Pour into an 8-by-8-inch or 9-inch round cake pan that has been lightly greased and floured.

4. Bake 35 to 40 minutes.

5. Sprinkle cake with powdered sugar and serve with low-fat frozen yogurt and strawberries for a special treat!

Nutrient Analysis per Serving

155 calories
26 grams carbohydrate
3 grams protein
4 grams fat

Key Nutrients

Potassium—11%
Thiamin—10%
Calcium—6%

Diabetic Exchanges

2 Starches
1 Fat

Pumpkin Roll

Although this recipe may look complicated, it is actually easy to prepare. It makes a very elegant (and healthy) dessert for company or a pot-luck.

Makes: 12 servings

Cake

3 eggs (or 2 eggs and
2 egg whites)

⅔ cup unsweetened pumpkin

¾ cup sugar

¾ cup whole-wheat or white flour

1 teaspoon baking soda

1½ teaspoons cinnamon

Powdered sugar

Filling

1 8-ounce package
any type cream cheese
(fat-free, light, or regular)

½ cup powdered sugar

1 teaspoon vanilla

1. Preheat oven to 375°F. In a bowl, beat together eggs, pumpkin, and sugar.

2. In a separate bowl, mix together flour, baking soda, and cinnamon; then add to pumpkin mixture. Spread on jelly roll pan (15-by-10-by-1-inch) that has been covered with wax paper and/or well-sprayed with cooking spray or greased. Bake 15 minutes.

3. Sift a generous amount of powdered sugar onto a clean tea towel.

4. Turn hot cake onto towel and roll up towel with cake–jelly-roll fashion. Refrigerate at least 1 hour.

5. In a bowl, beat together cream cheese, sugar, and vanilla.

6. Unroll cake. Spread filling onto cake, roll up, wrap in foil, and keep chilled until ready to serve. Freezes well.

7. When you're ready to serve, sprinkle again with powdered sugar.

Nutrient Analysis per Serving

141 calories
28 grams carbohydrate
5 grams protein
1.4 grams fat

Key Nutrients

Vitamin A–40%
Manganese–9%
Selenium–9%

Diabetic Exchanges

2 Starches

Quick and Easy Blueberry Cobbler

If you like cobbler, you'll find this one to be worth the small effort.

Makes: 6 servings

1 cup flour

⅔ cup sugar

1½ teaspoons baking powder

½ teaspoon salt

1 package dry Butter Buds

1 teaspoon almond extract

*¾ cup canned evaporated
skim milk*

*1 21-ounce can "more fruit"
blueberry pie filling*

Slivered almonds (optional)

Cooking spray

1. Preheat oven to 350°F.

2. Spray 2-quart casserole with cooking spray.

3. Mix together flour, sugar, baking powder, salt, Butter Buds, almond extract, and milk. Pour into casserole.

4. Spoon pie filling on top.

5. Bake for 35 to 40 minutes or until golden brown. If desired, sprinkle almonds on top of cobbler the last 10 minutes of baking.

Variation

Use peach pie filling instead of blueberry to make a Peach Cobbler.

Note: This recipe is high in simple sugar. Diabetic moms should eat only a small amount of this dessert or none at all.

Nutrient Analysis
per Serving

275 calories

64 grams carbohydrate

5 grams protein

0 grams fat

Key Nutrients

Riboflavin–13%

Calcium–12%

Diabetic Exchanges

3½ Starches

½ Fruit

Menus and Recipes for the Third Trimester

Menus from the Grocery Deli

Most foods in these menus are from the deli; some are from other parts of the grocery store. Some menus don't include a fruit; add your favorite.

Note: Because a small number of cases of Listeriosis, a type of food poisoning, has been associated with delicatessen foods, the Food and Drug Administration has advised that "pregnant women may choose to avoid these foods or to thoroughly reheat cold cuts before eating."

Cool Supper for a Hot Summer Night

Pasta salad with ham
Greek salad
Fresh fruit

___

Bean burrito
Guacamole
Fiesta coleslaw

___

Roasted chicken
Mashed potatoes/potato salad
Carrot raisin salad

___

Stir-fried vegetables
Chicken skewers
Chinese slaw
Frozen yogurt

Ready-to-make pizza
Marinated vegetables
Fruit salad

___

Celery, broccoli, and carrots
   with dip
Spaghetti and meatballs
Fruit sorbet

___

Tropical seafood pasta salad
Toasted whole-wheat bagels
Waldorf salad

Meatless Meals

Baked beans
Pea salad with cheese
Ambrosia salad

Cheese manicotti
Ratatouille
Jell-O with fruit

Garlic bread
Spinach quiche
Tossed salad
Fresh fruit

Carrot raisin salad
Ham and Swiss cheese on rye
Vanilla pudding with banana

Coleslaw
BBQ chicken
Potato salad

Cucumber and tomato salad
Meat loaf
Twice-baked potato
Blueberries

Shrimp fried rice
Green pepper steak
Chinese coleslaw

Boiled shrimp
Pasta with pesto sauce
Fresh fruit salad

At Your Own Risk Due to Spiciness!

Cajun chicken breast
Red cabbage
Rice pudding

Sloppy Joes
California slaw
Ambrosia salad

Beef tamales
Chile rellenos
Spanish rice

▼

Using Leftovers with Flair

Day 1

Tossed salad
Grilled chicken
Rotini pasta
Steamed zucchini and yellow
  squash

Day 2

Colorado Stuffed Peppers
  (page 301)
  (cook black beans in crock
  pot during day)
Cornbread
Fresh fruit salad

Day 3
Lunch

Grilled chicken (from Day 1)
  in pita pocket with lettuce,
  tomatoes, and vinaigrette
  dressing
OR
Chicken and spinach salad

Day 4

Bridget's Garden Salad (page
  225)(rotini pasta and leftover veggies from Day 1)
Strawberries and vanilla
  yogurt

Day 5

Black bean soup with cheese
  (beans from Day 2)
Cornbread
Tomato/avocado slices, fat-
  free Italian dressing

Day 6

Fajitas with chicken, beef, or
  shrimp
Guacamole dip (tomato and
  avocado from Day 5)
Lettuce, tomato, reduced-fat
  cheese

Day 7

Salmon en Papillote
  (page 266)
Steamed asparagus
Easy Microwave Potatoes
  (page 305)
Sorbet

Day 8
Lunch

Tossed salad with leftover
  fajita strips (from Day 6),
  canned kidney beans,
  tomatoes, carrots, and
  cheese

Black bean soup (black beans
from Day 5)
Baked tortilla chips

Day 9

Linguine with salmon,
canned artichoke hearts,
and Parmesan cheese
(fish from Day 7)
Delightful Spinach (page 223)
Crusty whole-wheat French
bread
Coleslaw
Fruit salad

Day 10

Creamy Asparagus Soup
(page 220) (asparagus from
Day 7)
Baked chicken (from grocery
deli if in a hurry)
Potatoes Marie Louise
(page 265)
Green beans
Tangerine

Day 11

Lunch

Spinach, mushroom, and
cheese quesadillas with
tomatoes (spinach from
Day 9)
OR
Curried chicken salad and
romaine lettuce (chicken
from Day 10) in pita pocket
Fresh melon

Day 12

Grilled fish with grilled
pineapple
Grilled vegetable shish-
kebabs: zucchini, mush-
rooms, eggplant, tomatoes
Bulgur or brown rice pilaf

Day 13

Fish on a Kaiser roll
Tossed salad with vinaigrette
dressing
Black Bean and Corn Salad
(page 224)
Apple slices with Caramel
Dip (page 321)

Day 14

Tangy Salad (page 269)
Vegetable tacos with zucchini,
mushrooms, eggplant,
tomatoes, and cheese
(vegetables from Day 12)
Roasted New Potatoes/Home
Fries (page 312)

Day 15

Ratatouille (page 311)
Brown rice (from Day 12)
with poached egg
Kiwi and peaches over angel
food cake

Day 16

Chicken with Dijon Sauce
(page 304)
Pasta with steamed
vegetables
Fruit Crisp (page 323)

Day 17

Ratatouille (from Day 15) and
cheese on Boboli bread
Tossed salad
Frozen melon balls

Day 18

Lunch

Crepes (page 261) with
chicken and Dijon Sauce
(from Day 16)
Black Bean and Corn Salad
(from Day 13)
Frozen vanilla yogurt with
Fruit Crisp (from Day 16)
as topping

Day 19

Vegetarian Chili (page 320)
Coleslaw
Sunshine Sorbet (page 325)

Day 20

Vegetarian tacos or taco salad
(chili from Day 19)
Tossed salad
Berry Mousse Parfait
(page 273)

▼

Meals in Minutes

Cup of wonton soup
Turkey with Hoisin Sauce
(page 272)
Instant brown rice with
snow peas
Frozen banana

Healthy Choice split pea
soup
Microwaved grilled cheese
sandwich
Tomato slices
Fresh fruit

Bean tostadas with lettuce
and tomato
Frozen yogurt with strawberries

Scallop and shrimp stir-fry
with frozen veggie mix
Angel hair pasta
Fresh peach

Salad with smoked turkey,
cherry tomatoes,
and romaine lettuce
Breadsticks
Fresh orange

Hoppin' John (page 306)
Steamed broccoli
Strawberries and banana
slices

Minute steak on wheat bun
Spinach salad (in a bag)
Banana pudding

Minute Minestrone
(page 254)
Turkey breast and cheese
quesadilla in whole-wheat
tortilla
Apple

Turkey with Hoisin Sauce
(page 272)
Kid's Carrots (page 307)
Spinach pasta twists

Tomato soup
Cheese-Topped Orange
Roughy (page 298)
Bulgur and Veggie Mix
(page 297)
Mixed fruit salad

Raw vegetables with
ranch dip
Hoppin' John (page 306)
Very Berry Shake (page 243)

Apricot-Glazed Chicken
(page 295)
Easy Microwave Potatoes
with Italian seasoning
(page 305)
Delightful Spinach (page 223)

Quick Grilled Fish (page 310)
with grilled vegetables
Angel hair pasta, fresh
Tropical Pudding (page 237)

Caesar salad (in a bag)
Shrimp cocktail
Garlic French bread with
melted low-fat cheese
Frozen grapes
Sugar cookies

European-style salad
(in a bag)
Aspen Black Bean Soup
(page 292)
Baked tortilla chips with salsa
Fresh pineapple rings

Salad with leftover grilled
chicken, romaine lettuce,
corn, and tomato
Bread sticks
Cantaloupe chunks
Strawberry ice milk

Bean tostada
Sliced tomatoes and cucumbers
Frozen fruit salad (peaches,
raspberries, grapes)

Tossed salad
Crab Marinara (page 303)
over linguini
Lemon sorbet with fresh
raspberries

Feel Full Menus

These menus give you the very most nutrition per bite when you can't eat much!

Crab Marinara (page 303)
Romaine tossed salad
Cantaloupe slices

Spanish Steak Roll (page 267)
Delightful Spinach (page 223)
Bulgur pilaf

Leg of Lamb (page 264)
Green beans and Northern
  beans
Potatoes Marie Louise
  (page 265)
Raspberries

Sesame Beef (page 313)
Stir-fried bell peppers and
  tomatoes
Brown rice or bulgur pilaf
Berry Mousse Parfait
  (page 273)

Black Bean and Corn Salad
  (page 224)
Baked Tortilla Chips
  (page 224)
Fresh orange

Oriental Salad (page 228)
Cheese-Topped Orange
  Roughy (page 298)
Steamed broccoli
Mango slices

Stuffed Eggplant Creole
  (page 268)
Brown rice or quinoa
Sunshine Sorbet (page 325)

Country Brunch Casserole
  (page 302)
Very Berry Shake (page 243)

Raw veggies with Boursin
  Cheese Spread (page 288)
Spinach-Stuffed Shells
  (page 314)
Bread sticks
Watermelon balls

Chicken and Shrimp with
  Fruit Salsa (page 299)
Carrots Antibes (page 226)
Barley pilaf

Veal Piccata with Roasted Red
  Pepper Sauce (page 316)
Whole-wheat pasta
Strawberry and banana slices

Broccoli Quiche (page 296)
Tomato slices
Wheat baguette
Fruit Crisp (page 323)

Spanish Steak Roll with
  Sautéed Vegetables
  (page 267)
Roasted New Potatoes
  (page 312)
Cantaloupe

Apricot-Glazed Chicken
  (page 295)
Romaine lettuce salad
Piña Colada Frappé
  (page 241)

Vegetables in Vinaigrette
  (page 317)
Black Bean Enchilada
  Casserole (page 294)
Tangy Salad (page 269)

Best Bite Snacks

These snacks have the most nutrients per calorie.

Boursin Cheese Spread
  (page 288)
Favorite Snack Cake
  (page 322)
Spiced refried beans with
  Baked Tortilla Chips
  (page 224)
Very Berry Shake (page 243)
Raspberry Surprise Shake
  (page 242)
Stuffed Figs (page 48)
Berry Mousse Parfait
  (page 273)
Pumpkin Muffins (page 235)
Thrive-on-Five Bread
  (page 233)
Layered Mexican Dip
  (page 210)
Tropical Pudding (page 237)
Tangy Salad (page 269)
Oven-Fried Zucchini
  or Eggplant (page 222)
Aspen Black Bean Soup
  (page 292)
Peach Popsicles (page 236)

Vegetarian Budget Menus

The following two weeks of sample menus can help if you are becoming vegetarian, or are just looking for ways to cut food costs. Meatless meals can certainly cut costs and are also very healthy! The first week menus require ingredients found in your pantry and little preparation. The second week introduces meals using some common recipes. The menus do include milk and eggs. If you are vegan, you can substitute egg replacers, soy milk, and soy cheese.

Another recommended vegetarian cookbook for busy people is *Meatless Meals for Working People–Quick and Easy Vegetarian Recipes,* available from the Vegetarian Resource Group, P.O. Box 1463, Baltimore, M.D. 21203.

These menus use 2% low-fat milk and may contain fats (such as margarine, butter, or oil) added while cooking. The menus average 2,200 calories and assume serving sizes such as one and a half cups of cereal or soup, half to one cup fruit, half to one cup of vegetables, two tablespoons peanut butter, one cup milk, and so on. Unlike other menus, the vegetarian menus include beverages because they have been included in calculating calories and nutrients.

Week 1

Monday

Breakfast

Quick and Healthier Pancakes with sliced peaches (page 251)
Low-fat milk

Lunch

Tomato soup
Grilled cheese sandwich with whole-wheat bread
Apple

Dinner

Vegetarian Chili (page 320)
Cornbread muffins
Coleslaw
Watermelon
Low-fat milk

Snacks

Crackers with peanut butter
Low-fat milk

Tortilla chips with bean dip
Tomato juice

Tuesday

Breakfast

Total Raisin Bran
Banana
Low-fat milk

Lunch

Sloppy Joes made with TVP (textured vegetable protein–found in large health food stores)
Carrot and raisin salad
Low-fat milk

Dinner

Broccoli Quiche (page 296) (a good way to use leftovers)
Wheat toast
Broiled tomato halves
Roasted New Potatoes or Home Fries (page 312)

Snacks

Graham crackers
Low-fat milk

Canned pineapple with cottage cheese
Fruit juice

Wednesday

Breakfast

Oatmeal with raisins and molasses
Banana bread
Low-fat milk

Lunch

Black Bean and Corn Salad (page 224)
Baked corn tortillas with cheese
Fruit Crisp (page 323)

Dinner

Hoppin' John (leave out ham–page 306)
Cornbread
Collard greens or spinach
Carrot sticks
Grapes

Snacks

Popcorn
Low-fat milk

Piña Colada Frappé
(page 241)
Ginger snaps

Thursday

Breakfast

Poached eggs on
wheat toast
Grapefruit
Low-fat milk

Lunch

Macaroni and cheese
Tossed salad with kidney
beans and tomato slices
Kiwi

Dinner

Vegetables in Vinaigrette
(page 317)
Colorado Stuffed Peppers
(page 301)
Fresh cantaloupe slices
Low-fat milk

Snacks

Cheese and crackers

Pumpkin Muffins (page 235)
Low-fat milk

Friday

Breakfast

Hot wheat cereal
Peanut butter and banana
on toast
Low-fat milk

Lunch

Bean and brown rice burritos
Spinach salad with orange
pieces
Apple

Dinner

Tossed salad with chick peas
Whole-wheat pasta with
marinara sauce and cheese
Wheat rolls
Cinnamon grilled peach
halves

Snacks

Oatmeal cookies
Low-fat milk

Brown-rice pudding with
raisins

Saturday

Breakfast

Cheese toast
Apple and pear salad
Low-fat milk

Lunch

Lentil Soup (page 289)
Celery/carrot sticks
Strawberries with yogurt
Low-fat milk

Dinner

Whole-wheat couscous
with mushrooms, zucchini,
tomato sauce, and
Parmesan cheese
Kid's Carrots (page 307)
Garlic bread
Fruit salad
Low-fat milk

Snacks

Hot cocoa
Fig bars

Very Berry Shake (page 243)
Favorite Snack Cake
(page 322)

Sunday

Breakfast

Vegetarian Breakfast Tacos
(page 319)
Mango slices
Low-fat milk

Lunch

Grilled vegetable and cheese
sandwich on rye toast
Banana
Low-fat milk

Dinner

Cabbage salad
Tofu Loaf (page 315)
Steamed zucchini
Strawberry Bread (page 232)
with light cream cheese
Fresh orange

Snacks

Frozen yogurt sundae

Granola bar
Low-fat milk

Week 2

Monday

Breakfast

French toast with strawberries
Low-fat milk

Lunch

Leek and Potato Soup
  (page 253)
Whole-wheat English muffins
Celery with low-fat cream
  cheese
Frozen grapes
Low-fat milk

Dinner

Ratatouille (page 311) over
  brown rice or bulgur
Macaroni, black beans,
  and corn
Kiwi slices

Snacks

Graham crackers with
  peanut butter
Low-fat milk

Thrive-on-Five Bread
  (page 233)

Tuesday

Breakfast

Oatmeal with raisins
Fresh orange
Apple Date Bran Muffin
  (page 234)
Low-fat milk

Lunch

Grilled Swiss cheese and
  sauerkraut on rye bread
Potato salad
Fresh apple

Dinner

Oat Nut Burgers (page 309)
Thanksgiving Sweet Potatoes
  (page 270)
Wheat rolls
Fruit cocktail
Low-fat milk

Snacks

Bran muffin
Low-fat milk

Fat-free cream cheese dip
Cauliflower and carrot sticks
Wheat crackers

Wednesday

Breakfast

Cheese grits
Cantaloupe
Wheat toast

Lunch

Boursin Cheese Spread
  (page 288) on wheat roll
  with lettuce, cucumber,
  tomato, and sprouts
Carrot and pineapple salad
Sugar cookies

Dinner

Tomatoes in vinaigrette
Black Bean Enchilada
  Casserole (page 294)
Wheat garlic toast
Fresh fruit salad
Low-fat milk

Snacks

Tangerine
String cheese

Leftover veggies and beans
  in wheat tortilla with cheese
Low-fat milk

Thursday

Breakfast

Whole-grain cereal
Sliced banana
Low-fat milk

Lunch

Sliced avocado, cheese,
  tomato, and lettuce on
  wheat bread
Salad
Plums
Low-fat milk

Dinner

Bean and Cornbread Bake
  (page 293)
Coleslaw
Strawberries over angel food
  cake
Low-fat milk

Snacks

Yogurt with fruit

Refried vegetarian beans
Homemade tortilla chips or
  toasted pita bread triangles

Friday

Breakfast

Poached eggs
Cinnamon raisin bagels
Apple juice
Low-fat milk

Lunch

Minute Minestrone
(page 254)
Cottage cheese with raw
vegetables
Cornbread
Grapes

Dinner

Oriental Salad (page 228)
Vegetable and Tofu Stir-Fry
(page 318)
Chinese noodles or
brown rice
Pineapple slices

Snacks

Crackers and peanut butter
Low-fat milk

Granola bar
Low-fat milk

Saturday

Breakfast

Country Brunch Casserole
(page 302)
Raisins/prunes
Toast
Low-fat milk

Lunch

Oven-Fried Eggplant Slices
(page 222) with marinara
sauce and cheese
Crusty French bread
Watermelon
Low-fat milk

Dinner

Spring Vegetables in Cream
Sauce (page 231)
Spinach salad
Garlic bread
Low-fat milk

Snacks

Berry Mousse Parfait
(page 273)

Vegetarian nachos made with
baked tortilla chips
V-8 juice

Sunday

Breakfast

Frozen waffles
Frozen strawberries
Low-fat milk

Lunch

Aspen Black Bean Soup
(page 292)
Crackers
Carrot/celery sticks
Apple slices with Caramel
Dip (page 321)
Low-fat milk

Dinner

Spinach-Stuffed Shells
(page 314)
Three-bean salad with
cherry tomatoes
Melon

Snacks

Popcorn
Tomato juice

Banana
Peanut butter
Low-fat milk

Third-Trimester Recipes

As in the previous chapters, these recipes on the following pages are arranged as follows: beginning with snacks and dips, following with salads, soups, main entrees, breads, muffins, and finishing with desserts.

Boursin Cheese Spread

This recipe is from *More Low-Fat Favorites* by Ceacy Thatcher. Try it with pita bread crisps, crackers, raw vegetables, or in crepes with veggies. Or thin it with a little skim milk to make a sauce for pasta or vegetables or to use as salad dressing.

Makes: 12 servings

8 ounces fat-free margarine

16 ounces fat-free cream cheese

*2 cloves fresh garlic, minced,
    or 1 teaspoon chopped garlic,
    in jar*

½ teaspoon leaf oregano

¼ teaspoon leaf marjoram

¼ teaspoon leaf thyme

¼ teaspoon leaf basil

¼ teaspoon dill weed

¼ teaspoon white pepper

1. Using a hand mixer or spoon, mix all ingredients until well blended.

2. Chill 1 hour before serving.

Nutrient Analysis per Serving

40 calories
2.6 grams carbohydrate
5 grams protein
0.7 gram fat
373 milligrams sodium

Key Nutrients

Contains small amounts of all nutrients.

Diabetic Exchanges

½ Very Lean Meat
¼ Milk

Lentil Soup

The beauty of lentils is that they cook quickly and they don't need to be soaked before cooking. They are also delicious!

Makes: 6 servings

2 medium onions, chopped

6 large garlic cloves, crushed

2 stalks celery, chopped

1 pound dry lentils

7 cups water

1 cup chicken broth

½ teaspoon basil

1½ teaspoons each thyme and oregano

1 bay leaf

1 to 2 teaspoons salt

2 to 3 medium carrots, sliced

Freshly ground black pepper, to taste

Cooking spray

Garnish

Red wine vinegar

Tomatoes, chopped

1. Brown onions, garlic, and celery in a pan sprayed with cooking spray, adding 1 tablespoon of water as needed.

2. Place lentils, water, chicken broth, spices, and salt in a kettle. Bring to a boil, lower heat to a very slow simmer, and cook covered for 20 to 30 minutes.

3. Add carrots and black pepper. Cover, and let simmer another 30 to 45 minutes, stirring occasionally. Remove bay leaf.

4. Serve hot, with a sprinkle of red wine vinegar and chopped tomatoes on top of each bowl.

Nutrient Analysis per Serving

182 calories

33 grams carbohydrate

13 grams protein

0.7 gram fat

9 grams fiber

Key Nutrients

Folate–62%

Vitamin A–38%

Magnesium–17%

Diabetic Exchanges

2 Starches

1 Very Lean Meat

Mexican Kale and Pork Soup

This recipe offers an interesting combination of flavors and textures.

Makes: 8 servings

1 teaspoon canola oil

1 medium onion, chopped

1 clove garlic, minced

16 ounces pork loin or
    loin chops, trimmed of all fat
    and cut into 1-inch cubes

5 cups water

1 bunch fresh kale, trimmed
    and cut into 1-inch pieces

1 16-ounce can whole peeled
    tomatoes

5 Roma tomatoes, halved and
    sliced, or 3 medium tomatoes,
    chopped

1½ teaspoons ground cumin

¾ teaspoon chili powder

1 15-ounce can hominy grits

½ can tomato paste

Salt, pepper, and hot pepper
    sauce, to taste

1. In saucepan, heat oil over medium heat. Add onion, garlic, and pork. Cook about 10 minutes, stirring occasionally.

2. Place pork in large microwave-safe dish. Add water. Cook 5 minutes on high.

3. Add kale. Cook 5 minutes on high.

4. Add canned and fresh tomatoes, spices, hominy grits, and tomato paste; cook 15 minutes on high, or until kale reaches desired tenderness. Add more tomato paste for thicker soup.

Serving Suggestion

Serve with homemade corn chips and guacamole.

Vegetarian Variation

Substitute tofu or pinto beans for the pork.

Nutrient Analysis per Serving

229 calories
19 grams carbohydrate
19 grams protein
9 grams fat
4 grams fiber

Key Nutrients

Vitamin C–49%
Thiamin–40%
Vitamin A–40%
Vitamin B₆–18%

Diabetic Exchanges

2 Medium-Fat Meats
2 Vegetables
½ Starch

Know Your Beans, and
Commit to the "Bean Routine"!

Dry beans are a nutritional gold mine for today's mom-to-be! They are high in protein, complex carbohydrate, and fiber, low in fat, and full of important nutrients. They make a great main dish when you can't tolerate meat. Beans will save you money on your food budget and you can save time by using canned beans.

One cup of cooked dried beans provides 27 percent of a pregnant woman's need for protein, 25 percent of her requirement for manganese, 18 percent of her requirement for iron, and 31 percent of her requirement for folacin. Plus, beans provide about 9 grams of fiber (20 to 35 grams per day is recommended for pregnant women).

Beating Bean Bloat

One common concern about beans is that they can cause gas. A University of California, Berkeley, study reported greater intestinal tolerance after three weeks of eating beans regularly. Here are some tips for adjusting to the bean routine!

1. Build up your body's tolerance. Eat small servings at first; then increase your intake slowly over a period of weeks.

2. Soak beans overnight, cook your beans properly, and *always* pour off the soaking water and add fresh water for cooking. Proper cooking can break down starches, making the beans more digestible.

3. Chew well and slowly. This assists in digestion and can minimize your bloating problem.

4. Drink enough fluids. Sufficient fluid intake helps your digestive system handle the increased dietary fiber.

Source: *Good Health is Habit-Forming...Commit to the Bean Routine,* by the American Dry Bean Board.

Aspen Black Bean Soup

Serve this hearty, delicious soup after your morning walk.

Makes: 6 servings

Soup

1 medium onion, chopped

3 cloves garlic or 3 teaspoons chopped garlic in jar

1 teaspoon dried whole oregano

½ teaspoon dried whole thyme

½ teaspoon cumin

¼ teaspoon cayenne pepper (optional)

2 15-ounce cans (3 cups) black beans, drained and rinsed

3 cups fat-free chicken broth

Cooking spray

Garnish

½ cup part-skim mozzarella cheese

2 tomatoes, chopped

1 onion, finely minced (optional)

1. Spray skillet with cooking spray. Cook onion and garlic until tender, about 5 minutes; add water if needed.

2. Stir in spices, cook 2 to 3 minutes.

3. Place ½ of beans in blender and purée until smooth, adding broth as needed to help make smooth.

4. Add puréed beans, remaining broth, and remaining beans to onion mixture. Bring to boil and then lower to medium heat and simmer 20 to 30 minutes.

5. Serve garnished with chopped tomatoes, onions, and cheese.

Serving suggestion

For a complete meal, add a salad, fruit and cornbread, or a grilled vegetable sandwich.

Nutritional Analysis per Serving

240 calories

37 grams carbohydrate

15 grams protein

4 grams fat

8 grams fiber

Key Nutrients

Folate–38%

Magnesium–23%

Zinc–18%

Chromium–15%

Diabetic Exchanges

2 Starches

1 Lean Meat

1 Vegetable

Bean and Cornbread Bake

This one-dish meal is easy to make and it's high in fiber, too!

Makes: 6 servings

Beans

1 16-ounce can pinto beans, drained

1 16-ounce can kidney, black beans, or black-eyed peas, drained (any combination will work!)

¼ cup each of chopped green pepper, onion, and celery

2 tablespoons ketchup

1 8-ounce can tomato sauce

1 teaspoon dry mustard

Oil or cooking spray to grease the baking dish

Cornbread Topping

1 small package (7 to 8½ ounces) cornbread mix

¼ cup reduced-fat or fat-free Cheddar cheese, grated

¼ cup green chilies (optional)

1. Preheat oven to 375° F.

2. Mix together all but last 4 ingredients on the "Beans" list. Pour into baking dish that has been lightly oiled or sprayed with cooking spray.

3. Prepare cornbread according to package directions, adding cheese and chilies if desired. Pour over beans.

4. Bake for 30 to 35 minutes or until cornbread is golden brown.

5. Serve with a spinach salad and fresh fruit.

Nutrient Analysis per Serving

360 calories
53 grams carbohydrate
16 grams protein
10 grams fat
7 grams fiber

Key Nutrients

Folate–38%
Potassium–29%
Magnesium–23%
Iron–11%

Diabetic Exchanges

3½ Starches
1½ Fats
1 Lean Meat

Black Bean Enchilada Casserole

This quick and easy casserole was modified from Janet Boyd's recipe.

Makes: 4 servings

1 15-ounce can Southwestern style black beans (with spices), undrained

1 15-ounce can Del Monte Chili Style Tomatoes

¼ cup picante sauce

3 corn tortillas

4 to 6 ounces fat-free or low-fat cheese

Cooking spray

1. Preheat oven to 350° F.

2. In bowl, mix beans, tomatoes, and sauce. Spray 2-quart, round casserole dish with cooking spray.

3. Place 1 corn tortilla in bottom of dish. Add ⅓ of bean mixture, ⅓ of cheese, another tortilla, ⅓ of bean mixture, another tortilla and rest of bean mixture.

4. Bake 20 minutes. Sprinkle remaining 2 tablespoons cheese on top during last 5 minutes of cooking.

5. To make this recipe in a 9-by-13 pan, use 3 cans of black beans, 3 cans of tomatoes, and 12 tortillas, overlapping 6 tortillas on each layer.

Low-Sodium Variation

Cook 1 sliced onion, 1 teaspoon chopped garlic, and 1 sliced bell pepper until tender. Add 15-ounce can stewed tomatoes and ¾ cup picante sauce. Use 1½ cups cooked black beans with 1½ teaspoons cumin and 1 teaspoon chili powder.

Nutritional Analysis per Serving

269 calories
35 grams carbohydrate
20 grams protein
8 grams fat
10 grams fiber

Key Nutrients

Folate—42%
Magnesium—31%
Vitamin C—26%
Copper—18%

Diabetic Exchanges

2 Starches
1½ Lean Meats
1 Vegetable
½ Fat

Apricot-Glazed Chicken

You can cook this chicken in a flash and serve it to family or friends.

Makes: 4 servings

4 chicken breast halves, skinned and boned

2 teaspoons margarine

Salt and pepper, to taste

⅓ cup apricot or peach all-fruit spread

1½ tablespoons tarragon wine vinegar or other flavored vinegar

2 teaspoons ginger, grated fresh, or in a jar

¼ cup cashews, chopped

1. Rinse chicken and pat dry with paper towels.

2. Melt margarine in nonstick pan.

3. Sauté chicken over medium heat for 8 to 10 minutes. Remove chicken and keep warm. Sprinkle with salt and pepper. Set aside pan juices.

4. Stir preserves, vinegar, and ginger into pan juices. Cook over medium heat until hot.

5. Spoon glaze over chicken breasts. Sprinkle with cashews.

Nutrient Analysis per Serving

240 calories
11 grams carbohydrates
28 grams protein
9 grams fat

Key Nutrients

Niacin—70%
Vitamin B$_6$—24%
Magnesium—14%

Diabetic Exchanges

4 Lean Meats
1 Fruit

Broccoli Quiche

This recipe, from the book, *Quick and Healthy, Volume II,* by Brenda Ponichtera, is great for a women's luncheon or brunch. Serve with a fruit cup or orange wedges.

Makes: 6 servings

3 flour tortillas
(7½-inch diameter)

2 cups broccoli, chopped into
bite-sized pieces

½ cup green onion, sliced

4 ounces reduced-fat Cheddar
cheese, grated

8 eggs or 2 cups egg substitute

¼ cup skim milk

¼ teaspoon paprika

Salt and pepper (optional)

6 tomato slices

Cooking spray

1. Preheat oven to 350° F.

2. Spray a 9-inch pie pan with cooking spray.

3. Cut 2 tortillas in half and place each half in the pan so that the rounded edge is ¼ inch above the rim. Place the remaining tortilla in the center of the pan. Add broccoli, onion, and cheese.

4. In a separate bowl, mix eggs with milk and add salt and pepper (if desired). Pour over top; sprinkle with paprika.

5. Bake 45 minutes or until knife inserted in the center comes out clean. Let sit 10 minutes before cutting into 6 wedges.

6. Top each piece with a tomato slice.

Source: Adapted with permission from *Quick and Healthy, Volume II,* by Brenda Ponichtera, R.D. (ScaleDown Publishing, Inc.)

Nutrient Analysis
per Serving

213 calories
14 grams carbohydrate
16 grams protein
11 grams fat

Key Nutrients

Vitamin A–33%
Vitamin C–28%
Riboflavin–27%
Calcium–17%

Diabetic Exchanges

2 Medium-Fat Meats
½ Starch
½ Vegetable

Bulgur and Veggie Mix

Bulgur is a quick and healthy alternative to rice. It is also very versatile.

Makes: 5 servings

**2 cups fat-free chicken broth
   or water**

¼ teaspoon salt (optional)

**2½ cups broccoli, chopped,
   or other vegetable in season**

1 cup dry bulgur

½ teaspoon thyme

1. In saucepan, bring broth or water to boil. Add salt and broccoli. Simmer 5 minutes.

2. Place bulgur in a heat-proof serving bowl. Pour water and broccoli over bulgur.

3. Cover and let sit until most of the water is absorbed.

4. Pour off excess water and fluff with a fork.

Variation

Substitute any vegetable, or vegetable combinations, fresh or frozen, for the broccoli. California-style frozen vegetable mix also works well.

Nutritional Analysis per Serving

103 calories
22 grams carbohydrate
6 grams protein
0 grams fat
6 grams fiber

Key Nutrients

Vitamin C–103%
Magnesium and
   Vitamin A–16%
Chromium–14%

Diabetic Exchanges

1 Starch
1 Vegetable

Cheese-Topped Orange Roughy

This recipe is from *Simply Colorado,* a cookbook project of the Colorado Dietetic Association. Using this recipe, you can serve dinner in 15 to 20 minutes!

Makes: 6 servings

2 pounds orange roughy
(sole, cod, or red snapper
also can be substituted)

Cooking spray

Topping
⅓ cup light mayonnaise
⅓ cup Parmesan cheese, grated
¼ cup green onion, sliced
½ teaspoon lemon juice
¼ to ½ teaspoon garlic powder
Hot sauce to taste (optional)

1. Preheat oven to 350° F.

2. Place fish in a shallow glass casserole coated with cooking spray; bake 8 minutes or until fish flakes easily when tested with a fork.

3. Meanwhile, mix topping ingredients. Spread topping evenly over cooked fish fillets. Broil 6 inches from heat for 5 minutes or until topping is lightly browned.

Source: Reprinted with permission from Simply Colorado, Inc.

Nutrient Analysis per Serving

164 calories
2 grams carbohydrate
27 grams protein
5 grams fat

Key Nutrients

Vitamin B₁₂–121%
Magnesium–19%
Potassium–18%
Niacin–13%

Diabetic Exchanges

3 Very Lean Meats
½ Fat

Chicken and Shrimp with Fruit Salsa

My friend Debbie Russell is a wizard in the kitchen. She has won several regional and national cooking contests. This recipe is one of her winners.

Makes: 6 servings

1 pound large shrimp, shelled and deveined

1 pound boneless, skinless chicken breasts, cut into pieces

Marinade

¼ cup mild picante sauce

1 tablespoon lime or lemon juice

1 tablespoon soy sauce

½ teaspoon coriander, ground

½ teaspoon fresh ginger root, grated

1 clove garlic, crushed

Fruit Salsa

½ cup peaches, diced

½ cup pineapple, diced

½ cup green apple, diced

½ cup red bell pepper, diced

2 tablespoons green onion, chopped

1 teaspoon lime or lemon juice

1 teaspoon sugar

Garnish

12 thin slices pineapple or peaches

Cilantro or parsley sprigs

1. In dish or plastic bag, combine the marinade ingredients.

2. Add shrimp and chicken, turning to coat pieces well. Cover dish or close bag and let marinate at least 30 minutes in refrigerator.

3. In small bowl, combine salsa ingredients. Cover and set aside.

4. Drain shrimp and chicken, reserving marinade for basting. Thread shrimp and chicken alternately on skewers.

5. Broil chicken and shrimp over medium-hot coals or broil at 400° F until shrimp turns pink and chicken is well cooked, 7 to 10 minutes, basting often with marinade.

6. Serve with fruit salsa on the side. Garnish with pineapple or peach slices and cilantro or parsley.

(continued on next page)

Chicken and Shrimp with Fruit Salsa
(continued)

Variations

• Stir-fry the chicken and shrimp instead of broiling.

• Serve with Peanut Butter Sauce instead of Fruit Salsa:

½ cup plain nonfat yogurt

2 teaspoons peanut butter

½ teaspoon Dijon mustard

⅛ teaspoon Worcestershire sauce

Combine yogurt, peanut butter, mustard, and Worcestershire sauce; mix well.

Nutrient Analysis per Serving
(with Fruit Salsa)

256 calories
18 grams carbohydrate
37 grams protein
4 grams fat
1 gram fiber

Key Nutrients

Selenium–90%
Niacin–68%
Vitamin C–30%
Vitamin B$_6$–26%

Diabetic Exchanges

5 Very Lean Meats
1 Fruit
½ Vegetable

Nutrient Analysis per Serving
(with Peanut Butter Sauce)

223 calories
4 grams carbohydrate
38 grams protein
5 grams fat

Key Nutrients

Selenium–92%
Niacin–68%
Vitamin B$_6$–24%
Magnesium–16%

Diabetic Exchanges

5 Very Lean Meats

Colorado Stuffed Peppers

Makes: 4 servings

*3 Roma tomatoes or 2 medium
  tomatoes, chopped coarsely*

2 green onions, chopped

*¼ medium red onion, finely
  chopped*

1 clove garlic, minced

½ sweet red pepper, chopped

2 teaspoons olive or canola oil

*1 cup cooked brown rice
  or bulgur*

1½ cups cooked black beans

*½ cup plus 2 teaspoons reduced-
  fat Cheddar cheese, grated*

4 bell peppers, cored and seeded

1. Sauté tomatoes, both onions, garlic, and red pepper in oil until cooked to desired tenderness. (The less the tomato and pepper are cooked the more vitamin C they retain.)

2. Add brown rice, black beans, and ½ cup cheese to pan and gently stir until warm and cheese is melted.

3. Meanwhile, steam whole peppers in microwave until tender crisp; then fill with bean mixture.

4. Use remaining 2 teaspoons of cheese to sprinkle on top before serving. (To increase protein content, add some lean meat, chicken, tofu, or more cheese to the filling.)

**Nutrient Analysis
per Serving**

237 calories
37 grams carbohydrate
12 grams protein
6 grams fat
5 grams fiber

Key Nutrients

Vitamin C–106%
Selenium–32%
Folate–30%
Magnesium–27%

Diabetic Exchanges

2 Starch
1½ Vegetables
1 Lean Meat
½ Fat

Country Brunch Casserole

This recipe is from *Simply Colorado,* a cookbook project of the Colorado Dietetic Association. It's perfect to serve visiting in-laws–just prepare the dish the night before, and enjoy a leisurely brunch.

Makes: 8 servings

½ cup onion, chopped

2 tablespoons water

3 cups bread stuffing cubes

⅓ pound Canadian bacon, thinly sliced and cut into bite-sized pieces (you can also use very lean ham)

1 cup (4 ounces) reduced-fat Cheddar cheese, shredded

3 eggs

2 egg whites

2 cups skim milk

½ teaspoon dry mustard

½ teaspoon onion salt

Cooking spray

1. Microwave onion and water on high for 2 minutes, stirring occasionally.

2. Place stuffing cubes in bottom of a 12-by-8-by-2-inch baking dish that has been coated with cooking spray.

3. Sprinkle pan with microwaved onion, sliced ham, and shredded cheese.

4. In a separate bowl, mix eggs, egg whites, milk, and seasonings; pour over stuffing mixture. Cover and refrigerate overnight.

5. Bake uncovered at 325° F for 1 hour. Let stand 10 minutes before serving.

Source: Reprinted with permission from Simply Colorado, Inc.

Nutrient Analysis per Serving

202 calories

13 grams carbohydrate

18 grams protein

9 grams fat

Key Nutrients

Vitamin B$_{12}$–22%

Calcium–16%

Riboflavin–15%

Vitamin A–12%

Diabetic Exchanges

1½ Medium-Fat Meats

1 Starch

Crab Marinara

This is a very quick, delicious meal. If tomato sauce usually gives you heartburn, you may be able to tolerate this dish because the sour cream cuts the acidity of the sauce. You can keep the "crab" on hand in the freezer for those times when you have no time to cook. Freeze leftovers for lunch.

Makes: 6 servings

12 ounces spaghetti, uncooked

4 cups prepared marinara sauce

¾ cup fat-free sour cream

¼ cup olives, sliced

1 7-ounce or 14-ounce can artichoke hearts (depending on how well you like artichokes)

½ teaspoon tarragon

¼ teaspoon dill

12 ounces imitation crab, or other shellfish, cooked

1. Cook spaghetti according to package directions.

2. Meanwhile, drain artichokes and chop into ½-inch pieces.

3. In a saucepan, combine marinara sauce with sour cream, olives, artichokes, and spices.

4. Break crab into bite-sized pieces, add to sauce, and stir until thoroughly combined. Heat over medium heat until warm.

5. Serve sauce over pasta with salad and whole-wheat garlic bread.

Nutrient Analysis per Serving

351 calories
64 grams carbohydrate
17 grams protein
3 grams fat

Key Nutrients

Thiamin–47%
Vitamin C–30%
Magnesium–25%

Diabetic Exchanges

3½ Starch
1½ Vegetables
1 Very Lean Meat
½ Fat

Dijon Sauce

In France, this sauce is made with Crème Fraîche and makes any meat taste divine!
This healthy version goes well with chicken breast, pork tenderloin chops, or can
be drizzled over new potatoes.

Makes: 4 servings

½ cup low-fat or fat-free
   sour cream

½ cup plain nonfat yogurt

1-2 tablespoons Dijon mustard

Salt, pepper, and garlic powder,
   to taste

1. Mix all ingredients in saucepan.

2. If you are serving with meat, blend the sauce with the
pan juices. Heat until very warm.

Nutrient Analysis per Serving

52 calories
6 grams carbohydrate
3 grams protein
1.5 grams fat

Key Nutrients

Contains a small
amount of all
nutrients.

Diabetic Exchanges

½ Skim Milk

Easy Microwave Potatoes

With the help of a microwave, the potato can be a very quick and nutritious side dish!

Potatoes, any amount, peeled or unpeeled, cut into 1-inch pieces
2-3 tablespoons water
Salt and pepper, to taste

1. Cook potatoes in water and spices in a covered microwave-safe dish on high for 5 minutes. Rotate dish. Cook 5 more minutes on high. Continue cooking until fork can easily pierce potatoes.

Variations

Italian: Add Italian spices before cooking and top potatoes with Parmesan cheese the last few minutes of cooking.

German: Add sautéed onions and bacon bits or ham to potatoes the last few minutes of cooking. Sprinkle with vinegar and toss.

Nutrient Analysis per Serving
(1 medium potato)

178 calories
41 grams carbohydrate
4 grams protein
0 grams fat
2 grams fiber

Key Nutrients

Potassium–38%
Vitamin C–36%
Vitamin B$_6$–26%

Diabetic Exchanges
(per ½-cup serving)

1 Starch

Hoppin' John

This southern classic dish can be prepared in a flash with canned beans and quick-cooking brown rice or bulgur.

Makes: 4 servings

2 16-ounce cans red kidney beans or black-eyed peas, undrained

2 cups cooked brown rice or bulgur

6 ounces lean ham, chopped

¼ teaspoon onion powder

Pepper and salt, to taste

Garnish

Fresh parsley and red onion, chopped (optional)

1. Combine undrained beans with rice, ham and spices. Cook over medium heat, stirring frequently.

2. Serve topped with parsley and chopped onion, if desired. If you can't tolerate raw onion, cook onion with the beans.

Nutrient Analysis per Serving

262 calories

39 grams carbohydrate

17 grams protein

4 grams fat

2 grams fiber

Key Nutrients

Selenium—89%

Zinc—17%

Vitamin B$_6$—16%

Diabetic Exchanges

2½ Starches

1½ Lean Meats

Kid's Carrots

You're never too young to be in the kitchen! That philosophy paid off for 12-year-old Andy Hawk, who placed third in the vegetable category of the "Delicious and Nutritious" Recipe Contest.

Makes: 5 servings

1 1-pound package frozen baby carrots

2 tablespoons honey

Mint, 1 tablespoon minced, fresh or 1½ teaspoons dried

1. Cook carrots according to package directions. Drain.

2. Stir in honey to coat carrots. Stir in mint. Serve.

Nutrient Analysis per Serving

48 calories
19 grams carbohydrate
1 grams protein
0 grams fat
3 grams fiber

Key Nutrients

Vitamin A–167%

Diabetic Exchanges

1 Vegetable
¼ Starch

Mock Egg Foo Young

This recipe provides a good way to incorporate tofu into your diet.

Makes: 4 servings

16 ounces firm, low-fat tofu

2 eggs, beaten

4 green onions, finely chopped

1 cup mung bean sprouts,
   cut into 1-inch pieces

1 garlic clove, minced,
   or ¼ teaspoon garlic powder

1 tablespoon soy sauce

1 teaspoon salt

2 tablespoons old-fashioned
   oatmeal

1 carrot, finely grated

½ teaspoon sesame oil

1. Stir all ingredients together until well blended.

2. Form into 3-inch patties and cook in small amount of oil until lightly browned.

Nutrient Analysis per Serving

119 calories

7 grams carbohydrate

13 grams protein

5 grams fat

4 grams fiber

Key Nutrients

Vitamin A–73%

Iron–42%

Magnesium–38%

Calcium–21%

Diabetic Exchanges

2 Lean Meats

1 Vegetable

Oat Nut Burgers

This recipe is modified from a recipe in *Meatless Meals for Working People*. When my "picky eater" friends ate these, they wanted seconds! If you have hamburger lovers at your house, you can put just about any type of "burger" between the bun and they'll love it!

Makes: 3 to 4 servings

⅔ *cup rolled oats*

⅔ *cup cashews (or other nuts), chopped*

1 onion, chopped

3 stalks celery, chopped

2 carrots, grated (or use 1 carrot and ½ small zucchini, grated)

¼ *cup whole-wheat flour*

¼ *cup water*

1 teaspoon soy sauce (optional)

Salt and pepper, to taste

Oil or cooking spray

1. Mix all ingredients. Season to taste with salt, pepper, or soy sauce.

2. Shape into 6 burgers.

3. Cook in lightly oiled pan (or pan sprayed with cooking spray) until brown on both sides; or broil burgers in oven.

4. Serve on toasted buns with lettuce, tomato, etc. Oven-fried potatoes go great with these burgers.

Nutrient Analysis per Serving

189 calories
25 grams carbohydrate
7 grams protein
8 grams fat
4 grams fiber

Key Nutrients

Vitamin A–49%
Magnesium–25%
Zinc–11%

Diabetic Exchanges

1½ Fats
1½ Starches
1 Vegetable

Quick Grilled Fish

I never enjoyed thick cuts of fish until I started marinating them. Marinating adds flavor and keeps fish moist. We enjoy fish cooked this way at least twice a month!

1 pound halibut, salmon, or other "steak" cut fish

½ cup vinaigrette or fat-free Italian dressing (experiment with different dressings)

1. Pour fish and dressing into Ziploc bag. Marinate at least 1 hour; the longer the better.

2. Grill approximately 10 minutes per inch of thickness at thickest part; or broil at 450° F for same amount of time. Fish is cooked when opaque and flakes easily with fork.

Nutrient Analysis per Serving
(4 ounces)

158 calories
less than 1 gram carbohydrate
23 grams protein
6 grams fat

Key Nutrients

Selenium—81%
Vitamin B$_{12}$—55%
Magnesium—29%

Diabetic Exchanges

3 Lean Meats

Ratatouille

My husband introduced me to this wonderful and versatile dish. You can serve it over rice with cheese as a main dish, as a side dish, or as a topping on your pizza or potato. In Europe, ratatouille is often served topped with a fried egg!

Makes: 8 servings

1 eggplant, peeled and cut into 1-inch cubes

1 teaspoon olive oil

4 garlic cloves, crushed

8 tomatoes, cut into quarters

3 zucchini, sliced

1 cup mushrooms, sliced

1 teaspoon oregano

1 teaspoon basil

1 teaspoon salt

¼ teaspoon pepper

1. Brown eggplant in oil in nonstick pan. When tender, add garlic and cook until tender.

2. Add remaining ingredients. Cook over medium heat until vegetables are tender, stirring frequently.

3. Reduce heat, cover, and simmer 10 to 15 minutes.

4. Remove cover and continue cooking until most of the liquid has evaporated.

Variations

Add chopped red and bell peppers and sliced black olives.

Quick Method: Use 16-ounce can of tomatoes and ¼ cup tomato paste instead of fresh tomatoes.

Nutrient Analysis per Serving

58 calories
12 grams carbohydrate
2 grams protein
1 gram fat
4 grams fiber

Key Nutrients

Vitamin C–40%
Potassium–29%
Folate–9%

Diabetic Exchanges

2 Vegetables

Roasted New Potatoes/Home Fries

Do you like fried foods, but not the fat? Try these crispy roasted potatoes. Their secret is a high oven temperature.

Makes: 4 servings

1 pound new potatoes or baking potatoes, well scrubbed

1 tablespoon olive oil

1 to 2 cloves garlic, crushed

½ teaspoon salt

Rosemary, 1 teaspoon dried or 2 teaspoons fresh, chopped

1. Preheat oven to 450° F.

2. Cut potatoes into 1-inch pieces. Toss in a bowl with oil, garlic, salt, and rosemary.

3. Spread potatoes on a cookie sheet. Roast about 30 minutes until potatoes are tender and brown, turning once halfway through cooking.

Variations

All should cook in about 20 minutes.

Oven Home Fries: Slice white potatoes, sweet potatoes, or yams into ¼-inch slices to make home fries, or slice thinner for home-made potato chips.

Sweet Chips: Thinly sliced sweet potatoes dusted with cinnamon or pumpkin spice makes a sweet snack chip.

French Fries: Cut into thin, long strips for French fries.

Nutrient Analysis per Serving

144 calories
26 grams carbohydrate
2 grams protein
4 grams fat
3 grams fiber

Key Nutrients

Vitamin C–24%
Vitamin B₆–16%
Riboflavin–10%

Diabetic Exchanges

2 Starches
1 Fat

Sesame Beef

This recipe was modified from a recipe in the 1991 National Beef Cookoff.

Makes: 6 servings

2 pounds boneless top sirloin

Marinade

¼ cup rice wine or white vinegar

¼ cup soy sauce

2 tablespoons dark sesame oil

1 tablespoon granulated sugar

1 teaspoon fresh ginger, minced

1 teaspoon baking soda

2 teaspoons cornstarch

Sauce

8 ounces beef broth

2 tablespoons cornstarch

½ cup light brown sugar, packed

¼ cup hoisin sauce

1½ tablespoons sesame seeds

1 tablespoon teriyaki sauce

½ tablespoon molasses

1 clove garlic, minced

1 tablespoon dark sesame oil

Garnish

1 large head romaine lettuce, shredded

Sesame seeds

Crushed red-pepper pods or hot chili paste (optional)

1. Slice beef into 1-inch strips; remove all fat.

2. Mix together marinade ingredients. Toss with beef and store in plastic bag, turning occasionally. Marinate at least 30 minutes, preferably overnight.

3. Drain marinade. Cook beef quickly in nonstick pan, adding small amount of oil if needed. Keep warm.

4. Mix 2 tablespoons of broth with cornstarch; set aside. Mix remaining broth with other sauce ingredients.

5. Add garlic and ½ teaspoon oil to same pan in which you cooked the beef. Sauté 1 minute.

6. Add sauce mixture; bring to a boil. Add broth-cornstarch mixture. Cook over medium heat until thickened, stirring occasionally.

7. Arrange lettuce on platter. Top with meat and drizzle with sauce or serve sauce on the side. Sprinkle with sesame seeds and optional crushed red pepper.

Diabetic Variation

Follow directions for sauce, omitting brown sugar and molasses.

Diabetic Exchanges

6 Lean Meats

1 Vegetable

Nutrient Analysis per Serving	**Key Nutrients**	**Nutrient Analysis** *(meat and lettuce)*
451 calories	*Zinc–65%*	*357 calories*
30 grams carbohydrate	*Vitamin B$_6$–31%*	*6 grams carbohydrate*
42 grams protein	*Iron–22%*	*42 grams protein*
17 grams fat	*Folate–16%*	*17 grams fat*

Spinach-Stuffed Shells

I recently discovered large pasta shells. Shells can be the busy woman's elegant meal! They freeze well, so try doubling the recipe and freezing half.

Makes: 4 servings

1 10-ounce package frozen
  spinach, cooked or thawed
  and well drained

1 cup low-fat or fat-free cottage
  cheese

⅓ cup Parmesan cheese,
  preferably freshly grated

½ cup mozzarella cheese, grated

¼ teaspoon garlic powder,
  or to taste

½ pound large pasta shells,
  cooked until still slightly firm
  or al dente and drained

2½ cups prepared low-fat
  marinara sauce

Garnish

Mozzarella and Parmesan
  cheese, grated

1. Preheat oven to 350° F.

2. Mix all ingredients except shells until well blended.

3. Stuff shells with spinach mixture. Cover with marinara sauce. Bake 30 minutes.

4. Sprinkle with a bit of extra cheese just before serving.

Variation

Double the amounts of pasta and spinach. Drain 1 pound of firm tofu and squeeze out excess water. In food processor, blend tofu, 2 cloves, fresh garlic, and a bunch of fresh basil leaves until smooth. Add cottage cheese and blend until smooth. Remove from processor and stir in spinach. Stuff and cook shells as directed above.

Nutrient Analysis per Serving

388 calories
58 grams carbohydrate
25 grams protein
7 grams fat

Key Nutrients

Vitamin A–78%
Folate–51%
Calcium–45%
Vitamin C–42%

Diabetic Exchanges

3 Starches
2 Lean Meats
2 Vegetables

Tofu Loaf

This recipe is from Norma Robinson. The pecans give it an interesting texture and flavor.

Makes: 8 servings

16 ounces low-fat tofu, firm

¼ cup pecans, chopped

½ cup canned tomatoes, chopped

2 egg whites

¼ cup skim milk

½ cup dry seasoned bread crumbs or old-fashioned oatmeal

½ teaspoon salt

½ teaspoon each onion and garlic powder

1 teaspoon thyme, cumin, oregano, or Italian seasoning

Optional seasonings: chopped parsley, green onion, finely chopped

Celery or onion

Cooking spray

1. Preheat oven to 350° F.

2. Squeeze out excess liquid from tofu and crumble. With a spoon, mix with rest of ingredients until well blended.

3. Pour into loaf pan that has been sprayed with cooking spray. Bake 50 to 60 minutes.

4. Serve like meat loaf, with ketchup, salsa, pasta sauce, or on a bun, like a burger. Leftovers are great as sandwiches.

Nutrient Analysis per Serving

86 calories
5 grams carbohydrate
8 grams protein
4.2 grams fat

Key Nutrients

Iron–26%
Magnesium–22%
Calcium–12%

Diabetic Exchanges

1 Lean Meat
1 Vegetable
1 Fat

Veal Piccata with Roasted Red Pepper Sauce

The sauce makes this dish tasty and colorful.

Makes: 4 servings

16 ounces veal loin

3 tablespoons lemon juice

½ to 1 clove garlic, crushed

Sauce

½ green onion, chopped
   (if you can't tolerate onions,
   just use the green tops)

1 heaping cup roasted
   red bell peppers
   (can be bought in a jar)

2 tablespoons white wine vinegar
   (can be flavored)

⅓ cup parsley (or use 2 fresh
   spinach or lettuce leaves)

⅓ cup nonfat yogurt or
   reduced-fat sour cream

Dash cayenne pepper (optional)

1. Marinate veal in lemon juice and garlic in dish in refrigerator for at least 1 hour.

2. Cook over medium-high heat or grill to desired doneness.

3. Purée all sauce ingredients except yogurt in food processor or blender. Place in microwave-safe dish and heat on medium-high 2 minutes.

4. Fold in yogurt or sour cream. Return to microwave for 30 seconds on high. Stir and serve over meat. (The sauce can be made ahead of time and refrigerated.)

Variation

Turkey tenderloin or chicken breast can also be used.

Nutrient Analysis per Serving

301 calories
5 grams carbohydrate
39 grams protein
12 grams fat

Key Nutrients

Vitamin C–44%
Zinc–32%
Vitamin B₆–19%

Diabetic Exchanges

5½ Lean Meats,
1 Vegetable

Vegetables in Vinaigrette

A starting course of raw vegetables in vinaigrette dressing is a French tradition.

Makes: 4 servings

Use one or more of the following vegetables:

7 carrots, finely grated

½ celery root, finely grated (now available in the U.S., also called celeriac)

2 cucumbers, thinly sliced

⅓ head red cabbage, finely grated

Add

½ cup fat-free or low-fat vinaigrette dressing (strong flavored is best)

¼ cup parsley, finely chopped

Salt and pepper, to taste

1. Combine all ingredients. Let marinate at least 30 minutes.

Variation

Add 1 to 2 tablespoons fat-free or light sour cream to vinaigrette dressing.

Nutrient Analysis per Serving

30 calories
7.3 grams carbohydrate
0.5 gram protein
0.1 gram fat

Key Nutrients
(for carrots)

Vitamin A–194%
Small amounts
of other nutrients.

Diabetic Exchanges

1 Vegetable

Vegetable and Tofu Stir-Fry

You won't even miss the meat!

Makes: 4 servings

2 tablespoons vinegar

½ teaspoon sesame oil

2 tablespoons hoisin sauce

4 tablespoons lite soy sauce

¼ cup water

1 pound low-fat, firm tofu, cubed

2 tablespoons chicken broth

1 to 2 teaspoons fresh ginger, grated or chopped (or ginger in a jar)

2 cloves garlic, minced

3 green onions, chopped

4 cups mixed vegetables (carrots, bell peppers, bean sprouts, cabbage, broccoli, snow peas, or 1 pound of frozen vegetable mixture)

1. Mix together vinegar, sesame oil, hoisin sauce, soy sauce, and water. Add tofu and let marinate 10 to 20 minutes.

2. Heat chicken broth in a nonstick pan. Add ginger, garlic, and green onions. Sauté 2 minutes.

3. Add vegetables (except for broccoli) and stir-fry until crisp-tender. Add more chicken broth or water to pan if necessary.

4. Add tofu and cook, turning until brown on all sides. Remove from pan and set aside.

5. Add broccoli to pan along with remaining marinade and stir-fry until broccoli is crisp-tender.

6. Add tofu and continue cooking until warm.

Serving Suggestion

This dish is great served over brown rice, bulgur, or noodles.

Nutrient Analysis per Serving

117 calories

11 grams carbohydrate

15 grams protein

2.5 grams fat

3 grams fiber

Key Nutrients

Vitamin C–133%

Vitamin A–29%

Potassium–19%

Diabetic Exchanges

2 Very Lean Meats

2 Vegetables

Vegetarian Breakfast Tacos

Linda Hood developed this recipe, which won first place for entrees in a local recipe contest. Although "Mexican food" often brings to mind high fat content, this recipe is lower in fat, but full of flavor. This is not a spicy recipe, but you may make it even milder by reducing garlic and onion and using mild salsa (or chopped tomatoes with lemon juice and onion powder). You can also use parsley instead of cilantro.

Makes: 4 servings

2 teaspoons olive or canola oil

1 small clove garlic

½ cup onion, chopped

½ cup green pepper, chopped

1 medium potato, chopped

1 small zucchini, chopped

*1 egg, plus 2 egg whites
   (or 3 whole eggs)*

1 medium tomato, chopped

*1 tablespoon cilantro or parsley,
   chopped*

Salt and pepper, to taste

*4 whole-wheat flour
   or corn tortillas*

1 cup Mexican salsa

*4 ounces part-skim mozzarella
   cheese, shredded*

1. In oil, sauté garlic, onion, and green pepper.

2. Add potato and zucchini. Stir until tender.

3. Push veggies aside and scramble eggs in the middle of skillet; gradually stir in vegetables.

4. Add tomato and heat thoroughly.

5. Season with cilantro, salt and pepper.

6. Steam tortillas on top of mixture in covered skillet. Fill tortillas with vegetable-egg mixture. Fold over.

7. Spoon salsa over the folded tortilla and sprinkle cheese on top.

**Nutrient Analysis
per Serving**

255 calories

27 grams carbohydrate

16 grams protein

10 grams fat

3 grams fiber

Key Nutrients

Vitamin C–51%

Calcium–20%

Vitamin B₁₂–17%

**Diabetic
Exchanges**

1½ Lean Meats

1½ Starches

1 Fat

1 Vegetable

Vegetarian Chili

This hearty chili is chock full of nutrients and tastes great as a pot-luck or a casual dinner.

Makes: 6 servings

1 medium onion, chopped

2 large clove garlic, minced

1 medium zucchini or 1 medium bell pepper, chopped

1 28-ounce can crushed tomatoes in purée

1 15-ounce can tomato sauce

2 15-ounce cans kidney beans, drained

2 to 4 teaspoons chili powder

2 teaspoons cumin

½ teaspoon oregano

¼ cup uncooked bulgur

Cayenne or black pepper, to taste

Garnish

Parsley

Tomato, fresh, chopped

Onion, finely minced

1. Heat a small amount of water in a nonstick pot. Add onion and garlic. Sauté over medium heat about 5 to 10 minutes.

2. Add zucchini or bell pepper and sauté until all the vegetables are tender.

3. Add the tomatoes, tomato sauce, beans, spices, and bulgur. Simmer over lowest heat, stirring occasionally, for 15 minutes.

4. Season to taste and serve hot, topped with parsley, chopped fresh tomato, and onion.

Variations

• Oven baked tortilla chips topped with fat-free Cheddar cheese.
• Rolled up in a flour tortilla.
• Stuffed in a bell pepper.

Nutrient Analysis per Serving

220 calories

44 grams carbohydrate

12 grams protein

1 gram fat

11 grams fiber

Key Nutrients

Vitamin B$_6$–46%

Vitamin C–28%

Iron–22%

Folate–18%

Diabetic Exchanges

2½ Starches

1½ Vegetables

1 Very Lean Meat

Caramel Dip

This is Cindy McKee's recipe and you won't believe is fat-free! Serve it with apple slices or graham crackers.

8 ounces fat-free cream cheese, softened

⅓ cup brown sugar, packed

1 teaspoon Watkin's Caramel Flavor

1 teaspoon vanilla

Note: Watkin's caramel flavor can be ordered by calling 1-800-247-5907 Director # 47233.

1. Beat all ingredients with mixer.

Variation

Caramel Dip Sauce: Over very low heat, thin mixture with small amount of milk until desired consistency is reached. Serve over crepes, fruit, or frozen yogurt.

Diabetic Variation

Instead of brown sugar, use Equal, to taste.

Nutrient Analysis per Serving

57 calories
11 grams carbohydrate
4 grams protein
0 grams fat

Key Nutrients

Contains small amounts of many nutrients.

Nutrient Analysis per Serving
(Diabetic Variation)

23 calories
2 grams carbohydrate
4 grams protein
0 fat

Diabetic Exchanges

1 Very Lean Meat

Favorite Snack Cake

This is one of my son's favorite snacks. Unfortunately, it's also our dog's favorite—the first time I made this cake, he finished it off–on the counter!

Makes: 12 servings

1¼ cups whole-wheat flour

½ cup rolled oats

¼ cup cornstarch

1 teaspoon baking soda

1 teaspoon each ground ginger and cinnamon

½ teaspoon ground cloves

½ teaspoon salt

1 large egg

2 tablespoons canola oil

½ cup blackstrap molasses

1¾ cups applesauce (use the kind that's fortified with vitamin C)

Margarine and flour to grease the pan

1. Preheat oven to 325° F.

2. Mix together all dry ingredients and spices.

3. In a separate bowl combine egg, oil, molasses and applesauce.

4. Gradually add egg mixture to dry ingredients.

5. Pour batter into a greased and floured 9-by-9 pan (in a pinch you can also use a 9-inch pie plate).

6. Bake 45 minutes, or until knife inserted in middle comes out clean. Let cool on wire rack.

Nutrient Analysis per Serving

129 calories
25 grams carbohydrate
2 grams protein
3 grams fat
2 grams fiber

Key Nutrients

Potassium–23%
Iron–9%
Calcium–8%

Diabetic Exchanges

1½ Starches
½ Fat

Fruit Crisp

This recipe from the National Heart, Lung, and Blood Institute is full of fiber and vitamins. Try the summer and winter variations, or come up with your own.

Makes: 6 servings

Winter Variation

Filling

½ cup sugar

3 tablespoons all-purpose flour

1 teaspoon lemon peel, grated

¼ teaspoon lemon juice

5 cups apples, unpeeled, sliced

1 cup fresh cranberries
or ½ cup raisins

Topping

⅔ cup rolled oats

⅓ brown sugar, packed

¼ cup whole-wheat flour

2 teaspoons ground cinnamon

1 tablespoon soft margarine, melted

1. To prepare filling, in medium bowl, combine sugar, flour, and lemon peel; mix well. Add lemon juice, apples, and cranberries and stir to mix.

2. To prepare topping, in a small bowl, combine oats, brown sugar, flour, and cinnamon. Add melted margarine and stir to mix.

3. Pour the apple mixture into a baking pan and sprinkle the oat mixture on top.

4. Bake in a 375° F oven for approximately 40 to 50 minutes. Serve warm or at room temperature. It's delicious with low-fat yogurt!

Summer Variation

Instead of apples and cranberries, substitute 4 cups fresh or unsweetened frozen (thawed) peaches and 3 cups fresh or frozen (unthawed) blueberries. If frozen, thaw peaches completely (do not drain). Do not thaw blueberries before mixing or they will be crushed.

Note: This dish contains a significant amount of carbohydrate and women with diabetes should eat it only in very small amounts.

Nutrient Analysis per Serving
(winter variation)

283 calories
62 grams carbohydrate
4 grams protein
4 grams fat
5 grams fiber

Key Nutrients

Magnesium–13%
Vitamin C–10%
Chromium–8%

Nutrient Analysis per Serving
(summer variation)

309 calories
68 grams carbohydrate
5 grams protein
4 grams fat
7 grams fiber

Key Nutrients

Manganese–37%
Vitamin C–24%
Potassium–21%
Vitamin A–11%

Diabetic Exchanges

Winter 2 Fruit
2 Starches
Summer 2½ Fruit
2 Starches

Fruit Pizza for a Crowd

This recipe is adapted from the book *Quick and Healthy Recipes and Ideas* by Brenda Ponichtera. The secret to this impressive dessert is to arrange the fruit in attractive patterns–try combinations of strawberries, raspberries, blueberries, and kiwi fruit. You can also add lite whipped topping. (See notation below for using different-size pans.) This dessert is considered a "somewhat healthy" splurge, so go easy on portion sizes!

Makes: 18 servings

1 package (20 ounces) Pillsbury Sugar Cookie Dough

1 quart strawberries, (or other fresh fruit) washed and hulled

1 large box (5.1 ounces) vanilla instant pudding

3 cups skim milk

6 ounces fat-free cream cheese product, room temperature

Cooking spray

Source: Reprinted with permission from *Quick and Healthy Recipes and Ideas* by Brenda J. Ponichtera, R.D. (ScaleDown Publishing, Inc.)

1. Preheat oven to 350° F.

2. Spray a pizza pan with cooking spray.

3. Slice cookie dough into ¼-inch slices.

4. Arrange slices on pizza pan so that they are ½ to 1 inch apart. Bake for 18 to 20 minutes or until golden and set. Cool.

5. In small mixing bowl, combine pudding mix and milk. Beat on low to mix. Add cream cheese and beat until smooth and thickened.

6. Pour over cooled cookie crust. Arrange fruit on top.

Note: This amount will also make four 8-inch pizzas or one 11-by-14-inch and an 8-inch pizza. Eight-inch cake pans work fine.

Diabetic Variation

Use sugar-free pudding instead of regular pudding. This diabetic variation still contains significant amounts of sugar. Women with diabetes should either skip this recipe or eat only in limited amounts.

Nutrient Analysis per Serving

191 calories
31 grams carbohydrate
5 grams fat
4 grams protein

Key Nutrients

Vitamin C–27%
Small amounts of many other nutrients.

Nutrient Analysis per Serving
(Diabetic Variation)

167 calories
25 grams carbohydrate
5 grams fat
4 grams protein

Diabetic Exchanges

1½ Starches
1 Fat
½ Very Lean Meat

Sunshine Sorbet

The beauty of this dessert is that it's made entirely of fruit, with no added sugar or thickener!

Makes: 5 servings

1 20-ounce can crushed pineapple, in its own juice

1 ripe banana, sliced

3 nectarines, peeled and sliced or 1 cup canned peaches, in their own juice

1 cup strawberries, fresh or frozen, unsweetened

2 teaspoons orange or lemon rind, freshly grated

Garnish

Fresh mint

1. Freeze fruit before preparing. Thaw pineapple enough to slice into chunks.

2. Place all fruit in food processor, and process until smooth. Scrape down sides occasionally.

3. Serve immediately; garnish with mint sprigs or place in 8-by-8-inch pan and freeze.

4. To serve after freezing: Thaw enough to break into chunks. Process again in food processor and store in an airtight freezer container.

Nutrient Analysis per Serving

112 calories
1.2 grams protein
less than 1 gram fat
2 grams fiber

Key Nutrients

Vitamin C–36%
Potassium–19%
Vitamin B$_6$–10%

Diabetic Exchanges

2 Fruit

References

Chapter 1

1. MRC Vitamin Study Research Group. "Prevention of Neural Tube Defects: Results of the Medical Research Council Vitamin Study." *The Lancet,* 338, July 1991: 131.

2. Center for Disease Control. "Recommendations for the Use of Folic Acid to Reduce the Number of Cases of Spina Bifida and Other Neural Tube Defects." *Morbidity and Mortality Weekly,* 11, 41 (RR-14) September 1992: 1.

3. Willett, W.C. "Folic Acid and Neural Tube Defects: Can't We Come to Closure." *American Journal of Public Health.* 82, 5, May 1992: 666.

4. Fall, C., et al. "Fetal and Infant Growth and Cardiovascular Risk Factors in Women." *British Medical Journal,* 310, 1995: 428-432.

5. Godfrey, K.M., et al. "Maternal Nutritional Status in Pregnancy and Blood Pressure in Childhood." *British Journal of Obstetrics and Gynaecology,* 101, 5, May 1994: 398.

6. Kitzmiller, J., et al. "Pre-Conception Care of Diabetes. Glycemic Control Prevents Congenital Anomalies." *Journal of the American Medical Association,* 265, 6, 1991: 731.

7. Achadi, E.L., et al. "Women's Nutritional Status, Iron Consumption and Weight Gain during Pregnancy in Relation to Neonatal Weight and Length in West Java, Indonesia." *International Journal of Gynaecology and Obstetrics,* 48, suppl., June 1995: S103.

8. Crawford, M. "The Role of Essential Fatty Acids in Neural Development: Implications for Perinatal Nutrition." *American Journal of Clinical Nutrition,* 57, suppl., 1993: S703.

9. Olds, D. "Intellectual Impairment in Children of Women Who Smoke Cigarettes during Pregnancy." *Pediatrics,* 93, 2, 1994: 221.

10. Savitz, D. "Prenatal Exposure to Parents' Smoking and Childhood Cancer." *American Journal of Epidemiology,* 133, 2, 1991: 123.

11. Pennington, J., and B.E. Young. "Total Diet Study Nutritional Elements 1980-1989." *Journal of the American Dietetic Association,* 2, 1991: 179.

12. International Food Information Council. *Food Insight; Current Topics in Food Safety and Nutrition.* March/April 1992: 1.

13. Lambert-Lagacé, L. *The Nutrition Challenge for Women.* Palo Alto, Calif.: Bull Publishing, 1990: 9.

14. Naeye, R. "Maternal Body Weight and Pregnancy Outcome." *American Journal of Clinical Nutrition.* 52, 1990: 273.

15. Werler, M., et al. "Prepregnant Weight in Relation to Risk of Neural Tube Defects." *Journal of the American Medical Association,* 275, 14, April 10, 1996: 1089.

16. Shaw, G. "Risk of Neural Tube Defect Affected Pregnancies among Obese Women." *Journal of the American Medical Association,* 275, 14, April 10, 1996: 1093.

17. Green, B., et al. "Risk of Ovulatory Infertility in Relation to Body Weight." *Fertility and Sterility,* 50, 9, 1988: 621.

18. Frisch, R. "The Right Weight, Body Fat, and Fertility." Proceedings of the Nutrition Society, 53, 1994: 113.

19. Infante-Rivard, C., et al. "Fetal Loss Associated with Caffeine Intake before and during Pregnancy." *Journal of the American Medical Association,* 270, 24, 1993: 2940.

20. Pirke, K., et al. "Dieting Influences the Menstrual Cycle: Vegetarian versus Nonvegetarian Diet." *Fertility and Sterility,* 46, 6, 1986: 1083.

21. Stewart, D. "Reproductive Functions in Eating Disorders." *Annals of Medicine,* 24, 1992: 287.

22. Ibid.

23. Rushton, D. "Ferritin and Fertility." Letter. *The Lancet,* 337, 1991: 1554.

24. Anderson, R., et al. "Ethanol-Induced Male Infertility: Impairment of Spermatoza." *Journal of Pharmacology and Experimental Therapeutics,* 225, 2, 1983: 47, 9-86.

25. Dawson, E., et al. "Effect of Vitamin C Supplementation on Sperm Quality of Heavy Smokers." *Federation of the American Societies for Experimental Biology Journal,* 5, 4, 1991: A915.

26. Dawson, E. "Effect of Ascorbic Acid on Male Fertility." *Annals of the New York Academy of Science,* 498, 1987: 312.

27. Werbach, M. *Nutritional Influences on Illness.* 2nd edition. Tarzana, Calif.: Third Line Press, 1993: 376-381.

28. Kemmann, E., et al. "Amenorrhea Associated with Carotenemia." *Journal of the American Medical Association,* 249, 7, 1983: 926.

29. Shortbridge, L. "Advances in the Assessment of the Effect of Environmental and Occupational Toxins on Reproduction." *Journal of Perinatal and Neonatal Nursing,* 3, 4, 1990: 1.

30. Fraga, C. "Ascorbic Acid Protects against Endogenous Oxidative DNA Damage in Human Sperm." Proceedings of the National Academy of Sciences, 88, December 1991: 11003.

31. *Better Homes and Gardens Magazine.* "Our Environment." *Better Homes and Gardens Magazine.* May 1992: 128.

32. Wilson, J. *The Pre-Pregnancy Planner.* Garden City, N.Y.: Doubleday & Co. Inc., 1986: 70.

33. Lindbohm, M.L., et al. "Effects of Paternal Occupational Exposure on Spontaneous Abortions." *American Journal of Public Health,* 81, 1991: 1029.

34. Shortbridge, L. "Advances in the Assessment of the Effect of Environmental and Occupational Toxins on Reproduction." *Journal of Perinatal and Neonatal Nursing,* 3, 4, 1990: 1.

35. Cochrane, C. "Women's Concerns." *The Practitioner,* 236, 1992: 300.

36. Center for Disease Control. "Recommendations for the Use of Folic Acid to Reduce the Number of Cases of Spina Bifida and Other Neural Tube Defects." *Morbidity and Mortality Weekly,* 11, 41 (RR-14), September 1992: 1, 3.

37. Ries, C., et al. "Impact of Commercial Eating on Nutrient Adequacy." *Journal of the American Dietetic Association,* 87, 1987: 463.

38. American College of Obstetricians and Gynecologists. *Planning for Pregnancy, Birth, and Beyond.* Washington, D.C.: ACOG, 1990: 10.

Chapter 2

1. International Food Information Council and the American Dietetic Association. "How Are Kids Making Food Choices?" July 1991.

2. Cong, K., et al. "Calcium Supplementation during Pregnancy for Reducing Pregnancy-Induced Hypertension." *Chinese Medical Journal,* 108, 1, January 1995: 57.

3. Committee on Diet and Health, National Research Council. *Diet and Health: Implications for Reducing Chronic Disease Risk.* Washington, D.C.: National Academy Press, 1989: 514-515.

4. Ibid: 514.

5. Slavin, J. "Whole Grains and Health: Separating the Wheat from the Chaff." *Nutrition Today,* 29, 4, 1994: 6.

6. Committee on Diet and Health, National Research Council. *Diet and Health: Implications for Reducing Chronic Disease Risk.* Washington, D.C.: National Academy Press, 1989: 678.

7. Abrams, B., et al. "Maternal Weight Gain and Preterm Delivery." *Obstetrics and Gynecology,* 74 (4), 1989: 577.

8. Office of Public Information, University of California, Berkeley. News Release. May 1992.

9. Committee to Study the Prevention of Low Birth Weight, Division of Disease Prevention and Health Promotion, Institute of Medicine. *Preventing Low Birth Weight.* Washington, D.C.: National Academy Press, 1985: 1.

10. Hickey, C., et al. "Relationship of Psychosocial Satus to Low Prenatal Weight Gain among Nonobese Black and White Women Delivering at Term." *Obstetrics and Gynecology,* 86, 2, August 1995: 177.

11. Williams, M., et al. "Cigarette Smoking during Pregnancy in Relation to Placenta Previa." *American Journal of Obstetrics and Gynecology,* 165, 1, July 28, 1991: 28.

12. Committee on Diet and Health, National Research Council. *Diet and Health: Implications for Reducing Chronic Disease Risk.* Washington, D.C.: National Academy Press, 1989: 205.

13. Stender, S., et al. "The Influence of Trans-Fatty Acids on Health: A Report from the Danish Nutrition Council." *Clinical Science* (Colch) 88, 4, April 1995: 375.

14. American Heart Association. *The American Heart Association Diet—An Eating Plan for Healthy Americans.* 1991.

15. NIH Consensus Conference. "NIH Consensus-Development Panel on Optimal Calcium Intake." *Journal of the American Medical Association,* 272, 24, December 28, 1994: 1942.

16. Committee on Diet and Health, National Research Council. *Diet and Health: Implications for Reducing Chronic Disease Risk.* Washington, D.C.: National Academy Press, 1989: 515.

17. Rothman, K. "Teratogenicity of High Vitamin A Intake." *New England Journal of Medicine*, 333, 21, November 1995: 1369.

18. Specker, B. "Do North American Women Need Supplemental Vitamin D during Pregnancy?" *American Journal of Clinical Nutrition*, 59, 2, suppl., February 1994: 484S.

19. Studzinski, G., and D. Moore. "Sunlight–Can It Prevent as well as Cause Cancer?" *Cancer Research*, 55, 18, September 1995: 4014.

20. Bailey, L. "The Role of Folate in Human Nutrition." *Nutrition Today*, September/October 1990: 12.

21. Center for Disease Control. "Recommendations for the Use of Folic Acid to Reduce the Number of Cases of Spina Bifida and Other Neural Tube Defects." *Morbidity and Mortality Weekly*, 11, 41 (RR-14), September 1992: 1.

22. Committee on Diet and Health, National Research Council. *Diet and Health: Implications for Reducing Chronic Disease Risk.* Washington, D.C.: National Academy Press, 1989: 71

23. Jameson, S. "Zinc Status in Pregnancy: The Effect of Zinc Therapy on Perinatal Mortality, Prematurity, and Placental Ablation." *Annals of the New York Academy of Science*, 15, 678, March 1993: 178.

24. Committee on Diet and Health, National Research Council. *Diet and Health: Implications for Reducing Chronic Disease Risk.* Washington, D.C.: National Academy Press, 1989: 422.

25. Ibid: 73.

26. National Academy of Sciences Report: *Nutrition during Pregnancy*: 15.

27. Ibid: 16, 254.

28. Rothman, K. "Teratogenicity of High Vitamin A Intake." *New England Journal of Medicine*, 333, 21, November 1995: 1369.

29. Belizan, J., et al. "Calcium Supplementation to Prevent Hypertensive Disorders of Pregnancy." *New England Journal of Medicine*, 325, November 14, 1991: 1399.

30. Villar, J., and J. Repke. "Calcium Supplementation during Pregnancy May Reduce Preterm Delivery and Preterm Labor." *American Journal of Obstetrics and Gynecology*, 163, 4 Pt 1, October 1990: 1124.

31. Marcoux, S., et al. "Calcium Intake from Dairy Products and Supplements and the Risks of Preeclampsia and Gestational Hypertension." *American Journal of Epidemiology*, 133, 12, June 15, 1991: 1266.

32. Greeley, A. *FDA Consumer*, July/August 1991: 27-28.

33. Hallberg, L., et al. "Calcium Effect of Different Amounts on Nonheme and Heme Iron Absorption in Humans." *American Journal of Clinical Nutrition*, 53, 1991: 112.

34. Kahn, A. "Prenatal Exposure to Cigarettes in Infants with Obstructive Sleep Apnea." *Pediatrics*, 93, 5, May 1994: 778.

35. Olds, D."Intellectual Impairment in Children of Women Who Smoke Cigarettes during Pregnancy." *Pediatrics*, 93, 2, February 1994: 221.

36. Savitz, D. "Prenatal Exposure to Parents' Smoking and Childhood Cancer." *American Journal of Epidemiology*, 133, 2, 1991: 123.

37. Federick, J., and A. Anderson. "Factors Associated with Spontaneous Preterm Birth." *British Journal of Obstetrics and Gynaecology*, 83, 1976: 342.

38. Department of Health, Education, and Welfare. *Smoking and Health: Report of the Surgeon General,* 1979. Washington, D.C.: U.S. Department of Health and Welfare; DHHS (PHS) DHEW publication 79-50066.

39. Meyer, M.B., and J.A.Tonascia. "Maternal Smoking, Pregnancy Complications, and Perinatal Mortality." *American Journal of Obstetrics and Gynecology*, 128, 1977: 494.

40. Subcommittee on Nutritional Status and Weight Gain during Pregnancy. *Nutrition during Pregnancy.* Washington, D.C.: National Academy Press, 1990: 394.

41. Greeley, A. *FDA Consumer,* July/August 1991: 27-28.

42. *Consumer Reports Magazine.* "Lead in Water, Pipe Nightmares." *Consumer Reports Magazine,* July 1995: 463.

43. Franklin, D. "Lead: Still Poison after All These Years." *Hippocrates,* September 1991: 33.

44. Kling, M. March of Dimes. Personal communication. May 1996.

45. Eliason, M., and J. Williams. "Fetal Alcohol Syndrome and the Neonate." *Journal of Perinatal and Neonatal Nursing,* 3, 4, 1990: 65.

46. *Diet and Health*: 450.

47. Rosenthal, R. "When a Pregnant Woman Drinks." *The New York Times Magazine,* February 4, 1990: 30.

48. Ibid.

49. Fenster, L., et al. "Caffeine Consumption during Pregnancy and Fetal Growth." *American Journal of Public Health*, 81, April 1991: 458.

50. Infante-Rivard, C., et al. "Fetal Loss Associated with Caffeine Intake before and after Pregnancy." *Journal of the American Medical Association*, 270, 24, December 1993: 24.

51. Wilcox, A., et al. "Caffeinated Beverages and Decreased Fertility." *The Lancet*, 2, 8626/8627, December 24, 1988.

52. Jacobson, M., et al. *Safe Food; Eating Wisely in a Risky World*. Los Angeles, Calif.: Living Planet Press, 1991: 45.

53. *The Boston Globe*. December 13, 1989: 1.

54. Sullivan, K. "Maternal Implications of Cocaine Use during Pregnancy." *The Journal of Perinatal and Neonatal Nursing*, 3, 4, 1990: 12.

55. Ibid.

56. Haines, P., et al. "Eating Patterns and Energy and Nutrient Intakes of U.S. Women." *Journal of the American Dietetic Association*, 92, 6, June 1992: 698.

Chapter 3

1. Erick, M. *No More Morning Sickness: A Survival Guide for Pregnant Women*. New York, N.Y.: Plume, 1993.

2. Subcommittee on Nutritional Status and Weight Gain during Pregnancy. *Nutrition during Pregnancy*. Washington, D.C.: National Academy Press, 1990: 430.

3. Food and Nutrition Board. *Recommended Dietary Allowances*. 10th edition. Washington, D.C.: National Academy Press, 1989.

4. National Academy of Sciences. *Nutrition during Pregnancy*. Washington, D.C.: National Academy Press, 1990: 386.

5. Scholl, T. "Low Zinc Intake during Pregnancy: Its Association with Preterm and Very Preterm Delivery." *American Journal of Epidemiology*, 137, 10, May 15, 1993: 1115.

6. Slavin, J. "Whole Grains and Health: Separating the Wheat from the Chaff." *Nutrition Today*, 29, 4, July/August 1994: 6.

7. American Diabetes Association. "Position Statement of the American Diabetes Association: Diabetes Care," 15, suppl. 2, April 1992: 23.

8. National Center for Nutrition and Dietetics, The American Dietetic Association. "Whole Grain Goodness—Three Are Key." Nutrition Fact Sheet.

9. Committee on Diet and Health, National Research Council. *Diet and Health: Implications for Reducing Chronic Disease Risk*. Washington, D.C.: National Academy Press, 1989: 678.

Chapter 4

1. Subcommittee on Nutritional Status and Weight Gain during Pregnancy. *Nutrition during Pregnancy*. Washington, D.C.: National Academy Press, 1990: 12.

2. American Dietetic Association. "Position of the American Dietetic Association: Vegetarian Diets." *Journal of the American Dietetic Association*, 93, 11, November 1993: 1317.

3. Food and Nutrition Board. *Recommended Dietary Allowances*. 10th edition. Washington, D.C.: National Academy Press, 1989.

4. Anderson, J., et al. "Meta-Analysis of the Effects of Soy Protein Intake on Serum Cholesterol." *New England Journal of Medicine*, 333, 5, August 3, 1995: 276.

5. Widhalm, K. "Effect of Soy Protein Diet versus Standard Low-Fat, Low-Cholesterol Diet on Lipid and Lipoprotein Levels in Children with Familial or Polygenic Hypercholesteroloemia." *Journal of Pediatrics*, 123, 1, July 1993: 30.

6. Bresslau, N. "Relationship of Animal Protein-Rich Diet to Kidney Stone Formation and Calcium Metabolism." *Journal of Clinical Endocrinology and Metabolism*, 66, 1988: 140.

7. Food and Nutrition Board. *Recommended Dietary Allowances*. 10th edition. Washington, D.C.: National Academy Press, 1989.

8. Villar, J., et al. "Improved Lactose Digestion during Pregnancy: A Case of Physiological Adaptation." *Obstetrics and Gynecology*, 71, 5, 1988: 697.

9. Solomons, N., et al. "Dietary Manipulation of Postprandial Colonic Lactose Fermentation: Effect of Solid Foods in a Meal." *American Journal of Clinical Nutrition*, 41, 1985: 199.

10. Lee, C., and C. Hardy. "Cocoa Feeding and Human Lactose Intolerance." *American Journal of Clinical Nutrition*, 49, 5, 1989: 840.

11. Recker, R., et al. "Calcium Absorbability from Milk Products, an Imitation Milk-and-Calcium Carbonate." *American Journal of Clinical Nutrition*, 47, 1988: 93.

12. Whitney, E., and F. Sizer. *Nutrition: Concepts and Controversies*. Saint Paul, Minn.: West Publishing Company, 1988: 248.

13. CSPI Staff. *Nutrition Action Healthletter*, May 1992: 11.

Chapter 5

1. Food and Nutrition Board. *Recommended Dietary Allowances*. 10th edition. Washington, D.C.: National Academy Press, 1989: 163.

2. Subcommittee on Nutritional Status and Weight Gain during Pregnancy. *Nutrition during Pregnancy*. Washington, D.C.: National Academy Press, 1990: 265.

3. Roshon, M.S., and R.L. Hagen. "Sugar Consumption, Locomotion, Task Orientation and Learning in Preschool Children." *Journal of Abnormal Child Psychology*, 17, 1989: 349.

4. Behar, D., et al. "Sugar Challenge Testing with Children Considered Behaviorly Sugar Reactive." *Nutrition and Behavior*, 74, 1984: 876.

5. American Dietetic Association. "Position of the American Dietetic Association: Appropriate Use of Nutritive and Non-Nutritive Sweeteners." *Journal of the American Dietetic Association*, 87, 1987: 1869.

Chapter 6

1. Burr, M., et al. "Vegetarianism, Dietary Fiber, and Mortality." *American Journal of Clinical Nutrition*, 36, 1982: 873.

2. Phillips, R., et al. "Influence of Selection versus Lifestyle on Risk of Fatal Cancer and Cardiovascular Disease among Seventh-Day Adventists." *American Journal of Epidemiology*, 112, 2, 1980: 296.

3. Sacks, F., et al. "Plasma Protein Levels in Vegetarians." *Journal of the American Medical Association*, 254, 1985: 1337.

4. Cooper, R., et al. "The Selected Lipid Lowering Effects on Low-Density Lipoproteins in a Crossover Experiment." *Atherosclerosis*, 43, 1982: 71.

5. Dwyer, J. "Health Aspects of Vegetarian Diets." *American Journal of Clinical Nutrition*, 48, 3, suppl., 1988: 712.

6. Ornish, D., et al. "Can Lifestyle Changes Reverse Coronary Heart Disease?" *The Lancet*, 336, 1990: 129.

7. Marsh, A., et al. "Cortical Bone Density of Adult Lacto-Ovo Vegetarian and Omnivorous Women." *Journal of the American Dietetic Association*, 76, 1980: 148.

8. Pixley, F., et al. "Effects of Vegetarianism on Development of Gallstones." *British Medical Journal*, 1, 291, 1985: 11.

9. Gear, J., et al. "Symptomless Diverticular Disease and Intake of Dietary Fiber." *The Lancet*, 1, 1979: 511.

10. Thorogood, M., et al. "Risk of Death from Cancer and Ischaemic Heart Disease." *British Medical Journal*, 308, 6945, 1994: 1667.

11. American Dietetic Association. "Position of the American Dietetic Association: Vegetarian Diets." *Journal of the American Dietetic Association*, 93, 11, November 1993: 1317.

12. Janelle, K., and S. Barr. "Nutrient Intakes and Eating Behavior Scores of Vegetarian and Nonvegetarian Women." *Journal of the American Dietetic Association*, 95, 2, February 1995: 180.

13. Pike, R., and M. Brown. *Nutrition, an Integrated Approach*. New York, N.Y.: John Wiley and Sons, 1975: 792.

14. Food and Nutrition Board. *Recommended Dietary Allowances*. 10th edition. Washington, D.C.: National Academy Press, 1989: 176.

15. Haddad, J. "Vitamin D Solar Rays, the Milky Way, or Both." Letter. *New England Journal of Medicine*, 326, 18, April 30, 1992: 1213.

16. Freeland-Graves, J., et al. "Zinc Status of Vegetarians." *Journal of the American Dietetic Association*, 80, 12, December 1980: 655.

17. American Dietetic Association. "Position of the American Dietetic Association: Vegetarian Diets." *Journal of the American Dietetic Association*, 88, 3, March 1988: 351.

Chapter 7

1. Kitzmiller, J., et al. "Preconception Care of Diabetes. Glycemic Control Prevents Congenital Anomalies." *Journal of the American Medical Association*, 265, 6, 1991: 731.

2. American Diabetes Association. "American Diabetes Association Position Paper: Pre-Conception Care of Women with Diabetes." *Diabetes Care*, 19, suppl. 1, January 96, S25.

3. American Diabetes Association. *Diabetes and Pregnancy: What to Expect*. American Diabetes Association, 1989: 15.

4. American College of Obstetricians and Gynecologists. *Planning for Pregnancy, Birth, and Beyond*. Washington, D.C.: ACOG, 1990: 133.

5. Ibid.

6. Krall, L., and R.S. Beaser. *Joslin Diabetes Manual*. 12th edition. Philadelphia, Pa.: Lea and Febiger, 1989: 236.

7. Ruggiero, L., et al. "Impact of Social Support and Stress on Compliance in Women with Gestational Diabetes Mellitus." *Diabetes Care*, 13, 1990: 441.

8. American Diabetes Association. *Gestational Diabetes and Pregnancy: What to Expect*. Alexandria, Va.: American Diabetes Association Inc, 1989: 12.

9. Ibid:16.

10. Ibid:14-15.

11. Langer, O., et al. "Intensified versus Conventional Management of Gestational Diabetes." *American Journal of Obstetrics and Gynecology*, 170, 4, April 1994: 1036.

12. American Diabetes Association. *Gestational Diabetes and Pregnancy: What to Expect*. Alexandria, Va.: American Diabetes Association Inc, 1989: 14.

13. Ibid: 13

14. *Sweet Success Diabetes and Pregnancy Program Guidelines for Care*. Sacramento, Calif.: State of California Department of Health Services, Maternal and Child Health, 1992.

15. Spears, B. Telephone interview. April 1992.

16. Jovanovic-Peterson, L., and C. Peterson. "Is Exercise Safe or Useful for Gestational Diabetic Women?" *Diabetes*, 40, Suppl 2: 179.

17. Jovanovic-Peterson, L. *Managing Your Gestational Diabetes*. Minneapolis, Minn.: Chronimed Publishing Inc., 1994: 55-56.

18. American Dietetic Association. "Position of the American Dietetic Association: Use of Nutritive and Non-Nutritive Sweeteners." *Journal of the American Dietetic Association*, 93, 7, July 1993.

19. American Diabetes Association. "Position Statement of the American Diabetes Association; Use of Noncaloric Sweeteners." *Diabetes Care*, 14, Suppl 2, March 1991: 28.

20. London, R. "Saccharin and Aspartame: Are They Safe to Consume during Pregnancy?" *The Journal of Reproductive Medicine*, 33, 1, 1988: 17.

21. American Academy of Pediatrics, Committee on Nutrition. "Final Report: Task Force on the Dietary Management of Metabolic Disorders." *Pediatrics*, December 1985: 35.

22. Jacobson, M., et al. *Safe Food; Eating Wisely in a Risky World*. Los Angeles, Calif.: Living Planet Press, 1991: 151-165.

23. Black, R. Personal communication. March 1992.

24. DiGiacomo, J.E., and W.W. Hay, Jr. "Fetal Glucose Metabolism and Oxygen Consumption during Sustained Hypoglycemia." *Metabolism*, 39, 2, February 1990: 193.

25. American Diabetes Association. *Gestational Diabetes and Pregnancy: What to Expect*. Alexandria, Va.: American Diabetes Association Inc, 1989: 12.

26. U.S. Department of Health and Human Services. *Working Group Report on High Blood Pressure in Pregnancy, High Blood Pressure Education Program*. Washington, D.C.: NIH Publication 91-3029, 1991.

27. Ibid: 6

28. Eskenazl, B., et al. "A Multivariate Analysis of Risk Factors for Preeclampsia." *Journal of the American Medical Association*, 266, 2, July 10, 1991: 237.

29. Villar, J., and J. Repke. "Calcium Supplementation May Reduce Preterm Delivery in High Risk Populations." *American Journal of Obstetrics and Gynecology*, 1124, 1990: 103.

30. Cong, K., et al. "Calcium Supplementation during Pregnancy for Reducing Pregnancy-Induced Hypertension." *Chinese Medical Journal*, 108, 1, January 1995: 57.

31. U.S. Department of Health and Human Services. *Working Group Report on High Blood Pressure in Pregnancy*. Washington, D.C.: NIH Publication: 14.
32. Ibid: 2-3.

33. Ibid: 29.

34. Ibid: 6.

35. Subcommittee on Nutritional Status and Weight Gain during Pregnancy. *Nutrition during Pregnancy*. Washington, D.C.: National Academy Press, 1990: 12.

36. Pederson, A.L. "Weight Gain Patterns during Twin Gestation." *Journal of the American Dietetic Association*, 89, 5, May 1989: 642.

37. Luke, B., et al. "The Ideal Twin Pregnancy: Patterns of Weight Gain, Discordancy, and Length of Gestation." *American Journal of Obstetrics and Gynecology*, 169, 3, September 1993: 588.

38. Dimperio, D. Personal communication. University of Florida, December 19, 1995.

39. Ibid.

40. Subcommittee on Nutritional Status and Weight Gain during Pregnancy. *Nutrition during Pregnancy*. Washington, D.C.: National Academy Press, 1990: 212.

41. Olds, S., et al. *Maternal Newborn Nursing; A Family-Centered Approach.* 2nd edition. Menlo Park, Calif.: Addison-Wesley Publishing, 1984: 182.

42. Dubois, S., et al. "Twin pregnancy: The Impact of the Higgins Nutrition Intervention Program on Maternal and Neonatal Outcomes." *American Journal of Clinical Nutrition,* 53, 1991: 1397.

43. Cambell, D., et al. "Maternal Nutrition in Twin Pregnancy." *Acta Genetica Gemellologica,* 32, 1982: 221.

44. Dimperio, D. Personal communication. University of Florida, December 19, 1995.

45. Sassoon, D., et al. "Perinatal Outcome in Triplet versus Twin Gestations." *Obstetrics and Gynecology,* 75, 5, May 1990: 817.

46. Collins, M.S., and J.A. Bleyl. "Seventy-One Quadruplet Pregnancies; Management and Outcome." *American Journal of Obstetrics and Gynecology,* 162, 6, June 1990: 1384.

47. Ales, K.L., et al. "Impact of Advanced Maternal Age on the Outcome of Pregnancy." *Surgery, Gynecology and Obstetrics,* 17, 3, September 1990: 209.

48. Berkowitz, G. "Delayed Childbearing and the Outcome of Pregnancy." *New England Journal of Medicine,* 322, 10, March 8, 1990: 659.

49. Ales, K.L., et al. "Impact of Advanced Maternal Age on the Outcome of Pregnancy." *Surgery, Gynecology and Obstetrics,* 17, 3, September 1990: 209.

50. Berkowitz, G. "Delayed Childbearing and the Outcome of Pregnancy." *New England Journal of Medicine,* 322, 10, March 8, 1990: 659.

51. Hales, D., and T. Johnston. *Intensive Caring.* New York, N.Y.: Crown, 1990: 36.

52. Scholl, T., et al. "Maternal Growth during Pregnancy and the Competition for Nutrients." *American Journal of Clinical Nutrition,* 60, August 1994: 183.

53. The Rand Youth Poll. "The Marketing Charecteristics of American Teenagers." New York, N.Y., 1990.

54. U.S. Department of Health and Human Services. National Adolescent Student Health Survey. *A Report on the Health of America's Youth,* 1989. Public Health Service.

55. Schneck, M., et al. "Low-Income Pregnant Adolescents and Their Infants: Dietary Findings and Outcomes." *Journal of the American Dietetic Association,* 90, 4, April 1990: 555.

56. Subcommittee on Nutritional Status and Weight Gain during Pregnancy. *Nutrition during Pregnancy.* Washington, D.C.: National Academy Press, 1990: 10.

57. Hediger, M., et al. "Patterns of Weight Gain in Adolescent Pregnancy: Effects on Birth Weight and Preterm Delivery." *Obstetrics and Gynecology,* 74 1, July 1989: 6.

Chapter 8

1. Lanting, C., et al. "Neurological Differenes between Nine-Year-Old Children Fed Breast Milk or Formula Milk as Babies." *The Lancet,* 344, 1994: 1319.

2. Ford, R., et al. "Breastfeeding and the Risk of Sudden Infant Death Syndrome." *International Journal of Epidemiology,* 22, 1993: 885.

3. Subcommittee on Nutritional Status during Lactation. *Nutrition during Lactation.* Washington, D.C.: National Academy Press, 1990: 169.

4. Freudenheim, J., et al. "Exposure to Breast Milk in Infancy and the Risk of Breast Cancer." *Epidemiology,* 5, 1994: 324.

5. Newcomb, P., et al. "Lactation and a Reduced Risk of Premenopausal Breast Cancer." *New England Journal of Medicine,* 330, 2, January 13, 1994: 81.

6. La Leche League International Staff. *The Womanly Art of Breastfeeding.* 4th revised edition. Franklin Park, Ill.: La Leche League International, 1987: 8.

7. U.S. Department of Health and Human Services. *Healthy People 2000.* Washington, D.C.: U.S. Department of Health and Human Services, 1991. DHHS (PHS) Publication 91-50212: 379.

8. Committee on Nutrition. "Iron-Fortified Infant Formulas." *Pediatrics,* 84, 6, December 1989: 114.

9. American Academy of Pediatrics. "Infant Feeding Practices and Their Possible Relationship to the Etiology of Diabetes Mellitus." *Pediatrics,* 94, 5, November 1994: 752.

10. Shannon, M., and J. Graef. "Hazards of Lead in Infant Formula." Letter. *New England Journal of Medicine,* 326, 2, January 9, 1992: 137.

11. Crase, B. Personal communication. May 1996, 1992.

12. Ibid.

13. Ibid.

14. Krebs, N., M.D. Presentation; Colorado Dietetic Association Annual Meeting. May 14, 1992.

15. Nafziger, S., M.D. Reprinted with permission of author from *Community Network Newsletter,* 1st quarter, 1992; Pueblo, Colo.

16. Krebs, N. Personal communication. June 1992.

17. Subcommittee on Nutritional Status during Lactation, et al. *Nutrition during Lactation.* Washington, D.C.: National Academy Press, 1990: 74

18. Strode, M.A., et al. "Effects of Short-Term Caloric Restriction on Lactational Performance in Well-Nourished Women." *Acta Paediatrica Scandinavica,* 75, 1986: 222.

19. Butte, N., et al. "Effect of Maternal Diet and Body Composition on Lactational Performance." *American Journal of Clinical Nutrition,* 39, February 1984: 296.

20. Food and Nutrition Board. *Recommended Dietary Allowances.* 10th edition. Washington, D.C.: National Academy Press, 1989.

21. Subcommittee on Nutritional Status during Lactation, et al. *Nutrition during Lactation.* Washington, D.C.: National Academy Press, 1990: 219.

22. Food and Nutrition Board. *Recommended Dietary Allowances.* 10th edition. Washington, D.C.: National Academy Press, 1989.

23. Chandra, R.K., and A. Hamed. "Cumulative Incidence of Atopic Disorders in High-Risk Infants Fed Whey Hydrosylate, Soy, and Conventional Cow Milk Formulas." *Annals of Allergy,* 67, 1991: 129.

24. Subcommittee on Nutritional Status during Lactation, et al. *Nutrition during Lactation.* Washington, D.C.: National Academy Press, 1990: 168.

25. Ibid: 14

26. Mathur, N.B. "Anti-Infective Factors in Preterm Human Colostrum." *Acta Paediatrica Scandinavica,* 79, 1990: 1039.

27. Lucas, A., et al. "Breast Milk and Subsequent Intelligence Quotient." *The Lancet,* 339, 1992: 261.

28. Little, R., et al. "Maternal Alcohol Use during Breastfeeding and Infant Mental and Motor Development at One Year." *New England Journal of Medicine,* 321, 7, August 1989: 425.

29. Mennella, J. "The Transfer of Alcohol to Human Milk." *New England Journal of Medicine,* 325, 14, October 1991: 981.

30. Subcommittee on Nutritional Status during Lactation, et al. *Nutrition during Lactation.* Washington, D.C.: National Academy Press, 1990: 177.

31. Ibid: 171

32. *Environmental Nutrition,* 15, 6, June 1992: 1.

33. Subcommittee on Nutritional Status during Lactation, et al. *Nutrition during Lactation.* Washington, D.C.: National Academy Press, 1990: 171.

34. Dewey, K. "Nutrient Needs during Lactation." *Nutrition and the MD,* 18, 3, March 1992: 3.

35. Dusdieker, L.B., et al. "Is Milk Production Impaired by Dieting during Lactation?" *American Journal of Clinical Nutrition,* 59, 1994: 833.

36. Merchant, K., et al. "Maternal and Fetal Responses to the Stresses of Lactation Concurrent with Pregnancy and Short Recuperative Intervals." *American Journal of Clinical Nutrition,* 52, 1990: 280.

37. Nommsen, L., et al. "Determinants of Energy, Protein, Lipid, and Lactose Concentrations in Human Milk during the First Twelve Months of Lactation: the DARLING Study." *American Journal of Clinical Nutrition,* 53, 1990: 457.

38. Hayslip, C., et al. "The Effects of Lactation on Bone Mineral Content in Healthy Postpartum Women." *Obstetrics and Gynecology,* 73, 4, April 1989: 588.

39. Koetting, C., and G. Wardlaw. "Wrist, Spine, and Hip-Bone Density in Women with Variable Histories of Lactation." *American Journal of Clinical Nutrition,* 48, 1988: 1479.

40. Hreshchyshyn, M., et al. "Associations of Parity, Breastfeeding, and Birth Control Pills with Lumbar Spine and Femoral Neck Bone Densities." *American Journal of Obstetrics and Gynecology,* 159, 1988: 318.

41. Chan, G., et al. "Effects of Increasing Dietary Calcium Intake upon the Calcium and Bone Mineral Status of Lactating Adolescent and Adult Women." *American Journal of Clinical Nutrition,* 46, 1987: 319.

42. Rogan, W., et al. "Polychlorianted Biphenyls (PCBs) and Dichlorodipheynyl Dichloroethene (DDE) in Human Milk: Effects of Maternal Factors and Previous Lactation." *American Journal of Public Health,* 76, 2, 1986: 172.

43. Crase, B. Personal communication. May 1992.

44. La Leche League International Staff. *The Womanly Art of Breastfeeding.* 4th revised edition. Franklin Park, Ill.: La Leche League International, 1987: 348.

45. Nafziger, S., M.D. Personal communication. June 1992.

46. Food and Nutrition Board. *Recommended Dietary Allowances.* 10th edition. Washington, D.C.: National Academy Press, 1989: 163

47. Lovelady, C., et al. "Lactation Performance of Exercising Women." *American Journal of Clinical Nutrition*, 52, 1990: 103.

48. Siskind, V., et al. "Breast Cancer and Breastfeeding: Results of an Australian Case Control Study." *American Journal of Epidemiology*, 130, 2, August 1989: 229.

49. Newcomb, P., et al. "Lactation and a Reduced Risk of Premenopausal Breast Cancer." *New England Journal of Medicine*, 330, 2, January 13, 1994: 81.

50. Freudenheim, J., et al. "Exposure to Breast Milk in Infancy and the Risk of Breast Cancer." *Epidemiology*, 5, 1994: 324.

Chapter 9

1. Gerlin, A. "Workplace Nursing Becoming a Benefit." *The Wall Street Journal*, December 29, 1994.

2. Dishman, R., ed. *Exercise Adherence*. Champaign, Ill.: Human Kinetics, 1988.

3. Fischman-Havstad, L., and A. Marston. *British Journal of Clinical Psychology*, 23, 1984: 265.

4. Edell, B., et al. "Self-Efficacy and Self-Motivation as Predictors of Weight Loss." *Addictive Behavior*, 12, 1, 1987: 63.

5. Sternberg, B. "Relapse in Weight Control: Definitions, Processes, and Prevention Strategies." Edited by G.A. Marlatt and J.R. Gordon. *Relapse Prevention*. New York, N.Y.: Guilford Press, 1985: 52.

6. International Food and Information Council, *Food Insight; Current Topics in Food Safety and Nutrition*, March/April 1992.

7. Greene, G., et al. "Postpartum Weight Change; How Much of the Weight Gained in Pregnancy Will Be Lost after Delivery." *Obstetrics and Gynecology*, 71, 5, May 1988: 701.

Chapter 10

1. American College of Obstetricians and Gynecologists. *Planning for Pregnancy, Birth, and Beyond.* Washington, D.C.: ACOG, 1990: 77, 82.

2. Jovanovic-Peterson, L., and C. Peterson. "Is Exercise Safe or Useful for Gestational Diabetic Women?" *Diabetes*, 40, suppl. 2, December 1991: 179.

3. Grediagin, A., et al. "Exercise Treatment Does Not Effect Body Composition Change in Untrained Moderately Overfat Women." *Journal of the American Dietetic Association*, 95, 6, June 1995: 661.

Chapter 11

1. The Food and Drug Administration. "The New Food Label." *FDA Backgrounder*, April 1994.

2. Ibid.

3. *Consumer Reports on Health*, March 1992: 18.

4. *Nutrition Action Healthletter*, January/February 1992: 11.

5. Whitmire, D. Telephone interview. June 1992.

6. Stone, M. Presentation; Colorado Dietetic Association Annual Meeting. May 17, 1992.

7. *National Council against Health Fraud Newsletter*. January/February 1990: 5.

8. Davis, H. Personal communication, May 1992.

9. Jacobson, M., et al. *Safe Food; Eating Wisely in a Risky World*. Los Angeles, Calif.: Living Planet Press, 1991: 72.

10. Wilson, L. *Producing Leaner Beef More Efficiently*. Pennsylvania State University, 1989.

11. Dairy Industry Coalition. "Facts about BST and Milk Safety."

12. Daughaday, W.H., and D.M. Barbano. "Bovine Somatotropin Supplementation of Dairy Cows; Is the Milk Safe?" *Journal of the American Medical Association*, 264, 8, 1990: 1003.

13. Kendall, P. Telephone interview. June 1992.

14. National Pork Producers Council. *Today's Pork in Foodservice*, 1988: 6.

15. Wilson, L. "Producing Leaner Beef More Efficiently." Presentation at Pennsylvania State University, 1989.

16. Texas A & M University. *Growth Promoting Hormones, a Scientific Review*, January 1989.

17. *Consumer Reports Magazine*, 57, 2, February 1992: 106.

18. Bolger, M. Telephone interview. May 1992.

19. The Food and Drug Administration. *FDA Consumer*, April 1992: 5.

20. Harsila, J. Telephone interview. May 1992.

21. Nettleton, J. *Eat Fish and Seafood Twice a Week: It Can Make a Difference*. Arlington, Va.: National Fisheries Institute.

22. Vanderbeek, C. Telephone interview. May 1996.

23. Jacobson, M., et al. *Safe Food; Eating Wisely in a Risky World*. Los Angeles, Calif.: Living Planet Press, 1991: 13.

Recommended Resources

As you may know there are many, many good books about health and nutrition. I had trouble picking out just a few.

Prepregnancy Planning
Laversen, Niels H., M.D., and Colette Bouchez. *Getting Pregnant—What Couples Need to Know Right Now.* Fawcett-Columbine.

Sussman, John R., M.D., and Blake B. Levitt. *Before You Conceive.* Bantam.

Tannenhaus, Nora. *Pre-Conceptions; What You Can Do before Pregnancy to Help You Have a Healthy Baby.* Contemporary Books.

Pregnancy
Bard, Maureen. *Getting Organized for Your New Baby.* Meadowbrook Press.

Curtis, Glade B., M.D. *Your Pregnancy Month by Month.* Fischer Books.

Erick, Miriam. *No More Morning Sickness.* Plume.

Erick, Miriam. *Take Two Crackers and Call Me In the Morning: A Real Life Guide to Surviving Morning Sickness.* Grinnen Barrett Publishing Company. (1-617-232-1993)

Graham, Janis. *Your Pregnancy Companion.* Pocket Books.

Hotchner, Tracy. *Pregnancy Pure and Simple.* Avon.

Nilsson, Lennart. *A Child Is Born.* Dell.

Noble, Elizabeth. *Essential Exercises for the Childbearing Year.* Houghton Mifflin Company.

Sears, William, M.D., and Martha Sears. *The Birth Book.* Little, Brown.

Shapiro, Howard, M.D. *The Pregnancy Book for Today's Woman.* Harper Perennial.

Simkin, Penny, Janet Whalley, and Ann Keppler. *Pregnancy, Childbirth, and the Newborn.* Meadowbrook Press. (1-800-338-2232)

Stoppard, Miriam, M.D. *Conception, Pregnancy, and Birth.* Dorling Kindersley.

Baby Names
Lansky, Bruce. *The Very Best Baby Name Book.* Meadowbrook Press. (1-800-338-2232)

High-Risk Pregnancy
The American Diabetes Association. *Diabetes: What to Expect,* and *Gestational Diabetes: What to Expect.* The American Diabetes Association. (1-800-ADA-DISC)

Hales, Diane, and Timothy Johnson, M.D. *Intensive Caring.* Crown.

Johnston, Susan, and Deborah Kraut. *Pregnancy Bedrest.* Henry Holt and Co.

Jovanovic-Peterson, Lois, M.D., with Morton Stone. *Managing Your Gestational Diabetes: A Guide for You and Your Baby's Good Health.* Chronimed Publishing.

Noble, Elizabeth. *Having Twins; A Parent's Guide to Pregnancy, Birth, and Early Childhood.* Houghton Mifflin Co.

Rich, Laurie. *When Pregnancy Isn't Perfect.* Penguin Books.

Infertility
Levitt, B. Blake. *50 Essential Things You Can Do When the Doctor Says It's Infertility.* Plume.

Raab, Diana. *Getting Pregnant and Staying Pregnant, Overcoming Infertility and Managing Your High Risk Pregnancy.* Hunter House.

Rosenberg, Helane S., and Yakov M. Epstein. *Getting Pregnant When You Thought You Couldn't.* Warner Books.

Rosenthal, M. Sara. *The Fertility Sourcebook.* Lowell House.

Teen Pregnancy and Parenthood
Arthur, Shirley. *Surviving Teen Pregnancy: Your Choices, Dreams, and Decisions.* Morning Glory Press. (1-714-828-1998)

Lindsay, Jeanne Warren, and Jean Brunelli. *Teens Parenting Series: Your Pregnancy and Newborn Journey.* Morning Glory Press.

Lindsay, Jeanne Warren. *Your Baby's First Year.* Morning Glory Press.

Lindsay, Jeanne Warren. *The Challenge of Three-Generation Living.* Morning Glory Press.

Parenthood
Black Fatherhood: The Guide to Male Parenting. Impact! Publications. (1-310-677-6311)

Brazelton, T. Berry, M.D. *Touchpoints: Your Child's Emotional and Behavioral Development.* Addison Wesley.

Cline, Foster W., and Jim Fay. *Parenting with Love and Logic.* Pinon Press.

Crary, Elizabeth. *Without Spanking or Spoiling: A Practical Approach to Toddler and Preschool Guidance.* Parenting Press (1-800-992-6657).

Einzig, Mitchell J., M.D., ed. *Baby and Child Emergency First Aid Handbook.* Meadowbrook Press. (1-800-338-2232)

Eisenberg, Arlene, et al. *What to Expect the First Year.* Workman Publishing.

Hart, Terril H., M.D., ed. *The Parent's Guide to Baby and Child Medical Care.* Meadowbrook Press. (1-800-338-2232)

Hunter, Brenda. *Home by Choice.* Multnomah Books.

Huntley, Becky. *The Sleep Book for Tired Parents.* Parenting Press. (1-800-992-6657)

Johnson, Spencer, M.D. *The One Minute Mother.* William Morrow Inc.

Kelly, Paula, M.D., ed. *First-Year Baby Care.* Meadowbrook Press. (1-800-338-2232)

Lague, Louise. *The Working Mom's Book of Hints, Tips, and Everyday Wisdom.*

Lansky, Vicki. *Getting Your Child to Sleep...and Back to Sleep, Tips for Parents of Infants, Toddlers, and Preschoolers.* (1-800-255-3379).

Lansky, Vicki. *Practical Parenting Tips.* Meadowbrook Press. (1-800-338-2232)

Saavedra, Beth Wilson. *Meditations for New Mothers.* Workman Publishing.

Any books by parenting experts Penelope Leach, T. Berry Brazelton, or William Sears.

Baby Products
Fields, Denise and Alan. *Baby Bargains.* Windsor Peak Press. (1-800-888-0385)

Jones, Sandy, with Werner Freitag and the Editors of Consumer Reports. *Guide to Baby Products, 4h edition.* Consumer Reports Books.

Pregnancy and Parenting Books with a Touch of Humor
Atalla, Bill. *The Thirteen Months of Pregnancy; A Guide for the Pregnant Father.* Oddly Enough. (1-707-833-1222)

Bernard, Susan. *The Mommy Guide: Real Life Adventures and Tips from Over 250 Moms and Other Experts.* Contemporary Books.

Glick, Eunice, Mindee Glick Garcia, and Bonnie Glick MacGinnis. *Expect the Unexpected When You're Expecting: A Hilarious Look at the Trials and Tribulations of Pregnancy.* Harper Perennial.

Gookin, Sandra Hardin. *Parenting for Dummies.* IDG Books.
Hill, Thomas. *What to Expect When Your Wife Is Expanding.* Cader Company Inc.

Justice, Jeff. *The Pregnant Husband's Handbook.* Strawberry Patch (1-800-875-7242).

Justice, Jeff, and Diane Pfeifer. *You Know You're a New Parent When...* Strawberry Patch. (1-800-875-7242)

Lovine, Vicki. *The Girlfriend's Guide to Pregnancy or Everything Your Doctor Won't Tell You.* Pocket Books.

Feeding Your Infant and Child
Huggins, Kathleen. *The Nursing Mother's Companion.* Harvard Common Press.

La Leche League International. *The Womanly Art of Breastfeeding.* La Leche League International (1-800-LA LECHE).

Lambert-Lagacé, Louise. *Feeding Your Baby from Conception to Age Two.* Surrey Books.

Lansky, Vicki. *Feed Me! I'm Yours.* Meadowbrook Press. (1-800-338-2232)

Nissenberg, Sandra, et al. *How Should I Feed My Child? From Pregnancy to Preschool.* Chronimed Publishing.

Satter, Ellyn. *Child of Mine; Feeding with Love and Good Sense.* Bull Publishing.

Satter, Ellyn. *How to Feed Your Kid–But Not Too Much.* Bull Publishing.

General Nutrition
Donkersloot, Mary. *The Fast-Food Diet: Quick and Healthy Eating on the Run.* Simon & Schuster.

Evers, Connie Liakos. *How to Teach Nutrition to Kids.* 24 Carrot Press. (1-503-524-9318)

Finn, Susan, and Linda Stern Kass. *The Real Life Nutrition Book; Making the Right Choices without Changing Your Life-Style.* Penguin Books.

Lambert-Lagacé, Louise. *The Nutrition Challenge for Women.* Surrey Books.

Tribole, Evelyn. *Eating on the Run*. Leisure Press.

Warshaw, Hope. *The Restaurant Companion*. Surrey Books.

Cookbooks
General-Healthy
The American Diabetic Association and the American Dietetic Association Family Cookbook (4 volumes). Simon & Schuster.

Cull, Julie Metcalf. *The Quality Time Family Cookbook*. Chronimed Publishing.

Mycoskie, Pam. *Butter Busters: The Cookbook*. Warner Books.

Oxmoor House. *Cooking Light Cookbook Series*. Oxmoor House.

Ponichtera, Brenda. *Quick & Healthy Recipes and Ideas and Quick & Healthy, Volume II*. ScaleDown Publishing Inc. (1-541-296-5859)

Simply Colorado Inc. *Simply Colorado: Nutritious Recipes for Busy People*. Simply Colorado Inc. (1-303-477-6314)

Smith, M.J. *365 Low-Fat Brand-Name Recipes in Minutes!* Chronimed Publishing.

Thatcher, Ceacy. *More Lowfat Favorites*. The 20% Solution. (1-719-687-3744)

Tribole, Evelyn. *Healthy Homestyle Cooking*. Rodale.

Seafood
Harsila, Janis, and Evie Hansen, National Seafood Educators. *Seafood, A Collection of Heart Healthy Recipes and Light Hearted Seafood*. P.O. Box 60006, Richmond Beach, WA 98160. (1-206-546-6410)

Vegetarian
Elliott, Rose. *The Vegetarian Mother and Baby Book*. Pantheon.
Havala, Suzanne, with Mary Clifford Simple. *Lowfat and Vegetarian*. Vegetarian Resource Group. (1-410-366-VEGE)

Hinman, Bobbie, and Millie Snyder. *Lean and Luscious and Meatless*. Prima Publishing.

Katzen, Molly. *Moosewood Cookbook, The Enchanted Broccoli Forest*, and *Still Life with Menu Cookbook*. Ten Speed Press.

Kirchner, Bharti. *Vegetarian Burgers, The Healthy Delicious Way to Eat America's Favorite Food*. Harper Perennial.

Lakhani, Mrs. *Indian Recipes for a Healthy Heart from the Kitchen of Mrs. Lakhani*. Fahil Publishing Co. (1-310-541-8099)

Mangum, Karen. *Life's Simple Pleasures; Fine Vegetarian Cooking for Sharing and Celebration*. Harvest Press. (1-800-879-4214)

Robertson, Laurel, Carol Flinders, and Brian Ruppenthal. *Laurel's Kitchen*. Ten Speed Press.

Wasserman, Debra, and Charles Stahler. *Mealtless Meals for Working People*. Vegetarian Resource Group. (1-410-366-VEGE)

Wasserman, Debra, and Charles Stahler. *Simply Vegan*. Vegetarian Resource Group.

Diabetic
Better Homes and Gardens Diabetic Cookbook. Better Homes and Gardens Books.

Franz, Marion. *Exchanges for All Occasions—Meeting the Challenge of Diabetes*. Chronimed Publishing.

Hess, Mary Abbott. *The Fine Art of Cooking for the Diabetic, 3rd edition*. Contemporary Books.

Marks, Betty. *The Microwave Diabetes Cookbook*. Surrey Books.

Palumbo, P.J., M.D., and Joyce Daly Margie. *The All in One Diabetic Cookbook*. NAL-Dutton.

Polin, Bonnie Sanders, and Frances Towner Giedt. *The Joslin Diabetes Gourmet Cookbook*. Bantam Books.

Weight Control/Weight Maintenance/Low-Fat Eating
Bailey, Covert. *The Fit or Fat Woman*. Houghton-Mifflin Co.

Berry, Frank, and Bridget Swinney. *Make the Change for a Healthy Heart*. Fall River Press. (1-800-284-6667)

Connor, Sonja, and William Connor, M.D. *The New American Diet*. Simon & Schuster.

Goor, Ron and Nancy, and Katherine Boyd. *The Choose to Lose Diet; A Food Lovers Guide to Permanent Weight Loss*. Houghton-Mifflin Co.

Lund, JoAnne. *Healthy Exchanges Cookbook*. Putnam's Sons.

McDougal, John, M.D., and Mary McDougal. *The McDougal Program for Maximum Weight Loss*. Plume/Penguine.

Moquette-Magee, Elaine. *Fight Fat and Win: How to Eat a Low-Fat Diet without Changing Your Lifestyle*. Chronimed Publishing.

Pope, Jamie. *The Last Five Pounds: A Liberating Guide to Living Thin*. Pocket Books.

Stevens, Tree. *Living and Loving Lowfat.* Northwest Publishing Inc.

Tribole, Evelyn, and Elyse Resch. *Intuitive Eating.* St. Martin's Press.

Ulene, Art, M.D. *Lose Weight with Dr. Art Ulene.* Ulysses Press.

Waterhouse, Debra. *Outsmarting the Female Fat Cell.* Warner Books.

Other Resources
Phone Numbers
The Confinement Line (offers a support network for women on bed rest) 1-703-941-7183

Consumer Product Safety Commission 1-800-638-2772
National Center for Nutrition and Dietetics–Consumer Hotline 1-800-366-1655

National Organization of Mothers of Twins Clubs Inc. 1-505-275-0955

Sidelines (support for those experiencing a high-risk pregnancy) 1-714-497-2265

Triplet Connection 1-209-474-3073/0885

Twin Services (counseling and referrals) 1-510-524-0863

Vegetarian Resource Group 1-410-366-VEGE

Newsletters and Magazines
American Health Magazine

Cooking Light Magazine

Eating Well Magazine

Environmental Nutrition, The Professional Newsletter of Diet, Nutrition, and Health

Health Magazine

Nutrition Action Health Letter, Center for Science in the Public Interest, Washington, D.C.

Pinapple Press, *A Food and Nutrition Newsletter for Parents* (1-415-381-7774)

Tufts University *Diet and Nutrition Letter*

University of California, Berkeley, *Wellness Letter*

Vegetarian Journal, Vegetarian Resource Group

Index

Recipe Index

Computerized Nutrition Analysis Form

Fill out this form to receive a computer analysis of how your diet compares to the Recommended Dietary Allowances for pregnancy. Your printout will include analysis of your diet for overy thirty nutrients, including calories, protein, fat, carbohydrate, cholesterol, and fiber. If you are doing a one-day analysis, write down what you eat during a "typical" day. If you are doing a three-day analysis, which gives you a better picture of your average eating habits, write down the food you have eaten on one weekend day and two weekdays.

Directions for filling out form:

Write down everything you eat and drink (except water) in a twenty-four hour period. Please be as specific as possible when listing the foods–include serving size and how the food was prepared (fried, baked, etc.). Also, don't forget to include such extras as margarine, oil, and salad dressing. Please include descriptions such as fat percentage (for milk), low-fat, fat-free, and so on.

Reproduce this form for each day analyzed, as needed. Send to Bridget Swinney; P.O. Box 62578; Colorado Springs, Colorado 80962-2578. Include $8.00 for each day analyzed.

Food	Amount	How Prepared

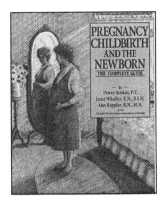

Pregnancy, Childbirth, and the Newborn
Revised and Expanded Edition
by Simkin, Whalley, and Keppler

More complete and up-to-date than any other pregnancy guide, this remarkable book is "the bible" for childbirth educators from coast to coast. Called "excellent" by the *American Journal of Nursing*.

675,500 copies in print.

ISBN: 0-671-74182-9 **$12.00**

Getting Organized for Your New Baby
Revised and Expanded Edition

by Maureen bard

This revised and expanded favorite will ensure that when baby is ready to come–the parents are ready to go! Here is an essential planning tool to help prepare parents for pregnancy, birth, and baby's first few months. It provides checklists, how-to hints, forms, charts, and bibliographies to make it easy for parents to get scheduled, budgeted, and prioritized.

57,500 copies in print.

ISBN: 0-671-53477-7 **$9.00**

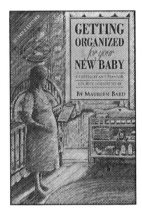

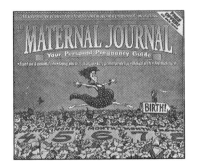

The Maternal Journal

by Matthew Bennett
illustrated by Breck Wilson

This colorful pregnancy planner/calendar is a quick and delightful way for expectant mothers to learn what to expect and do during the nine months of pregnancy and first three months of parenthood.

67,500 copies in print.

ISBN: 0-671-76031-9 **$10.00**

The Very Best Baby Name Book in the Whole Wide World

by Bruce Lansky

Introducing: the very best way to name a baby. This book has more than 30,000 popular and unusual names from around the world, complete with origins, famous namesakes, and variations.

ISBN: 0-671-56113-8 **$8.00**

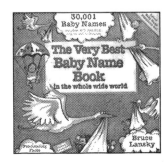

Order Form

Quantity	Title	Author	Order No.	Unit Cost	Total
	35,000+ Baby Names	Lansky, B.	1225	$5.95	
	Baby & Child Emergency First-Aid Handbook	Einzig, M.	1381	$8.00	
	Baby & Child Medical Care	Hart, T.	1159	$9.00	
	Baby Name Personality Survey	Lansky/Sinrod	1270	$8.00	
	Best Baby Name Book	Lansky, B.	1029	$5.00	
	Best Baby Shower Book	Cooke, C.	1239	$7.00	
	Dads Say the Dumbest Things!	Lansky/Jones	4220	$6.00	
	David, We're Pregnant!	Johnston, L.	1049	$6.00	
	Discipline without Shouting or Spanking	Wyckoff/Unell	1079	$6.00	
	Familiarity Breeds Children	Lansky, B.	4015	$7.00	
	Feed Me! I'm Yours	Lansky, V.	1109	$9.00	
	First-Year Baby Care	Kelly, P.	1119	$9.00	
	Gentle Discipline	Lighter, D.	1085	$6.00	
	Getting Organized for Your New Baby	Bard, M.	1229	$9.00	
	Grandma Knows Best	McBride, M.	4009	$6.00	
	Happy Helpful Grandma Guide	Spirson, L.	1290	$8.00	
	Hi, Mom! Hi, Dad!	Johnston, L.	1139	$6.00	
	Joy of Grandparenting	Lansky, B.	3502	$7.00	
	Joy of Parenthood	Blaustone, J.	3500	$6.00	
	Moms Say the Funniest Things!	Lansky, B.	4280	$6.00	
	Maternal Journal	Bennett, M.	3171	$10.00	
	Pregnancy, Childbirth, and the Newborn	Simkin/Whalley/Keppler	1169	$12.00	
	Very Best Baby Name Book	Lansky, B.	1030	$8.00	
	Working Woman's Guide to Breastfeeding	Dana/Price	1259	$7.00	
				Subtotal	
				Shipping and Handling	
				MN residents add 6.5% sales tax	
				Total	

YES! Please send me the books indicated above. Add $2.00 shipping and handling for the first book and 50¢ for each additional book. Add $2.50 to total for books shipped to Canada. Overseas postage will be billed. Allow up to four weeks for delivery. Send check or money order payable to Meadowbrook Press. No cash or C.O.D.s please. Prices subject to change without notice. **Quantity discounts available upon request.**

Send book(s) to:

Name _____

Address _____

City _____ State _____ Zip _____

Telephone (_____) _____

Purchase order number (if necessary) _____

Payment via:

☐ Check or money order payable to Meadowbrook Press (No cash or C.O.D.s please.)

   Amount enclosed $ _____

☐ Visa (for orders over $10.00 only)   ☐ MasterCard (for orders over $10.00 only)

Account # _____

Signature _____ Exp. Date _____

A *FREE* Meadowbrook catalog is available upon request.

You can also phone us for orders of $10.00 or more at 1-800-338-2232.

Mail to: Meadowbrook, Inc.
18318 Minnetonka Boulevard, Deephaven, Minnesota 55391
(612) 473-5400   Toll-Free 1-800-338-2232   Fax (612) 475-0736